Solveig Lena Hansen, Silke Schicktanz (eds.)
Ethical Challenges of Organ Transplantation

Solveig Lena Hansen, born in 1984, is a lecturer for ethics at the University of Bremen, Faculty 11 (Human and Health Sciences). Previously, she was a research associate at the University Medical Center Göttingen. After an MA in Comparative Literature, she did her PhD in Bioethics at the University of Göttingen in 2016. Her ethical research focuses on organ transplantation, health communication, and obesity. She also specializes in the field of narrative bioethics, analyzing the negotiation of bioethical issues in literature and film.

Silke Schicktanz, born in 1970, is full-professor at the Department of Medical Ethics and History of Medicine at the University Medical Center Göttingen, Germany. Her research focuses on the cultural and ethical study of biomedicine. She has lead many international cooperations and was visiting researcher at UC Berkeley, San Francisco State University, Tel Aviv University, JNU Delhi, Montreal Université and University of Lancaster.

Solveig Lena Hansen, Silke Schicktanz (eds.)

Ethical Challenges of Organ Transplantation

Current Debates and International Perspectives

[transcript]

This research was supported by the German Research Foundation (Deutsche Forschungsgemeinschaft, DFG), Grant No. SCHI 631/7-3.

Bibliographic information published by the Deutsche Nationalbibliothek
The Deutsche Nationalbibliothek lists this publication in the Deutsche Nationalbibliografie; detailed bibliographic data are available in the Internet at http://dnb.d-nb.de

© 2021 transcript Verlag, Bielefeld

Cover layout: Maria Arndt, Bielefeld
Cover illustration: Kristina Schneider, Göttingen
Proofread by Jovan Maud, Halle
Typeset by Mark-Sebastian Schneider, Bielefeld
Printed by Majuskel Medienproduktion GmbH, Wetzlar
Print-ISBN 978-3-8376-4643-6
PDF-ISBN 978-3-8394-4643-0
https://doi.org/10.14361/9783839446430
ISSN of series: 2702-8267
eISSN of series: 2702-8275

Inhalt

III. ORGAN ALLOCATION AND TRANSPLANTATION SYSTEMS

IV. ORGAN RECIPIENTS

V. ALTERNATIVES

List of Abbreviations

6MWT: Six Minute Walk Distance
ART: Assisted Reproductive Technology
ASRM: American Society for Reproductive Medicine
ATMP: Advanced Therapy Medicinal Products
AUIF: Absolute Uterine Infertility
BR: Biobank Research
CIT: Cold Ischemic Time
CKD: Chronic Kidney Diseases
CPR: Cardiopulmonary Resuscitation
DBD: Organ Donation after Brain Death
DBCDD: Organ Donation after Brain Circulation Determination of Death
DCDD: Donation after Circulatory Determination of Death
DSO: Deutsche Stiftung Organtransplantation [German Organ Transplantation Foundation]
ECD: Expanded Citeria Donors
ECMO: Extracorporeal Membrane Oxygenation
EKTAS: Eurotransplant Kidney Allocation System
ELPAT: Research Group: Ethical, Legal and Psychosocial Aspects of Transplantation
EMA: European Medicines Agency
ESKD: End Stage Kidney Disease
ESP: Eurotransplant Senior Programme
ESRD: End Stage Renal Disease
fMRI: Functional Magnetic Resonance Imaging
GKE: Global Kidney Exchange
GP: General Practitioner
HFEA: Human Fertilisation and Embryology Authority
hiPSC: Heterologous Induced Pluripotent Stem Cells
HIV: Human Immunodeficiency Virus
HLA: Human Leukocyte Antigens
HTA: Human Tissue Authority
HU: High Urgent Call
IPSC: Induced Pluripotent Stem Cells
IQWiG: Institut für Qualität und Wirtschaftlichkeit im Gesundheitswesen [Institute for Quality and Efficiency in Health Care]

IVF: In-vitro-Fertilisation
KAS: Kidney Allocation System
KDPI: Kidney Donor Profile Index
KE: Kidney Exchange
LAS: Lung Allocation Score
LD: Living Donation
LDT: Living Donor Transplants
LKTD: Living Donor Kidney Transplant
LYFT: Life Years from Transplant
MAC: Mandated Active Choice
MHRA: Medicines and Healthcare Regulatory Agency
MRKH: Mayer-Rokitansky-Keuster Hauser Syndrom
MRC: Medical Research Council
NEAD: Never Ending Altruistic Donor Chain
NHS: National Health Service
NHSBT: NHS Blood and Transplant
NICE: National Institute for Health and Care Excellence
NOTA: National Transplantation Act
OD: Organ Donation
ODNZ: Organ Donation New Zealand
OP: Organ Procurement
OPTN: Organ Procurement and Transplantation Network
PGD: Preimplantation Genetic Diagnosis
QALY: Quality Adjusted Life Years
RCT: Randomized Controlled Trial
SCD: Standard Criteria Donors
STS: Science and Technology Studies
UNOS: United Network for Organ Sharing
UT: Uterus Transplantation
VAC: Voluntary active choice
VCA: Vascularized Composite Allograft Organ
WHA: World Health Assembly
WHO: World Health Organization

Exploring the Ethical Issues in Organ Transplantation
Ongoing Debates and Emerging Topics

Solveig Lena Hansen & Silke Schicktanz

If you have not made up your mind yet about organ donation, a brief scan of the literature, internet, and media inundates you with messages. A huge variety of books, journal articles, social media campaigns, and TV shows convey information on transplantation medicine. Across this broad array of media, facts about transplantation medicine as well as individual cases of donors, donor families, health professionals, and recipients are presented to a wider audience. All this information is in one way or another linked to implicit, or sometimes explicit, moral statements: why donate, or why not. Some scholars and policies universally refer to organ donation as an act of altruistic gift giving. However, transplant rates vary widely across the globe, and so do ethical discussions. Additionally, regulations demand fair allocation of a scarce resource to those in need. Many countries invest an enormous amount into public education in this field (Hansen et al. 2018; Hansen et al. 2021).

This volume provides a systematic orientation to the main ethical questions concerning organ transplantation: Where to source the organs? How to allocate a precious resource? How do people experience their life with an organ transplant? What are the alternatives to current practices? The first two questions have been intensively discussed in research, policy, and the media in last three decades, but the latter two have not yet received the attention they deserve. Therefore, our aim in this volume is to reevaluate old debates, and consider new ones, to provide guidance to readers from moral philosophy, bioethics, health care science, social science, law, and the humanities.

Our volume has a clear international focus. Rather than confine themselves to ethical debates in specific national contexts, all contributions seek to address the main ethical issues discussed globally, but they sometimes also point out cultural specificities or discuss local solutions to delicate ethical questions. For instance, while, the English recently adopted a so-called 'opt-out' policy (without explicit objection one automatically becomes an organ donor) in May 2020 (Iacobucci 2020), some countries such as the US and Germany remain firmly in the 'opt-in' (requiring explicit consent) camp despite many attempts to change their policies (Glazier/Mone 2019). In most countries such policy changes are subject to intensive public, media, or academic debate. To be considered acceptable, they must prove both their practicability and legitimacy, which requires solid empirical exploration of the medical and social effects as well as normative reflection regarding the implications for both citizens' rights and duties as well as patients' needs or exposure to harm.

Beginning as an experimental practice, organ transplantation already provoked debates in the 1960s (Woodruff 1964; Murray 1964); and the many technical advances and legal standardizations of this practice have led to increasingly complex ethical dilemmas and debates (Diethelm 1990). Since the 1980s, organ transplantation has evolved worldwide to become a broadly established medical practice, offering a cure for chronic illness, often extending lives for many years and improving patients and their families' quality of life (Blumstein/Sloan 1989; Caplan 1989). However, despite these benefits, the clinical consequences, policy implications, and ethical relevance of organ donation have been debated right from the beginning. And although it is already subject to numerous regulations, organ donation still stimulates lively discussions in these fields of inquiry (Miller/Truog 2012; Veatch/Ross 2015).

In contrast to most other medical treatments, transplantation ethics must consider and balance not only the interests and rights of patients and physicians, but also those of donors and their relatives. Representing high-tech medicine, organ transplantation also serves as a paradigmatic case for medical progress and for controversies in bioethics (Bailey 1990). First, essential topics of discussion include brain death, organ allocation, and organ sale. Additionally, the intervention into healthy bodies for the sake of others, as in the case of living organ donation, continuous to be controversial (Garwood-Gowers 1999). Second, alternative approaches such as the use of animal organs for humans (xenotransplantation) triggered both high hopes and concerns in the 1990s and 2000s (Daar 1997) – and they are now being revived again in the context of new technological possibilities, such as genome editing (Ekser et al. 2017). Third, new topics such as face or uterus transplantation and organ printing elicit totally new debates that have yet to be sufficiently addressed. There are even more future options, such as organ allocation through artificial intelligence (Briceno 2020) or the treatment of organ failure with organoids that will require more scrutiny by ethicists (Hyun et al. 2020). However, such possibilities are not included in this volume because we felt it was too early to speculate about their ethical dimensions when their application is still very vague. But we should all keep an eye on these developments. A fourth cluster of themes we consider includes still rather marginalized topics that are, however, highly relevant to understanding the whole picture. These includes prevention, the role of old age in allocation, and the role of the family for consent.

Whereas the importance of normative theoretical problems remains unquestioned, we are convinced that the ethical challenges of transplantation medicine cannot be addressed without taking into account concrete lifeworlds with their practices, solutions, and contradictions. All these topics must therefore be examined with reference to socio-empirical, cultural, and anthropological considerations. Consequently, many invited contributions of this anthology provide an overview of the ethical debate while also considering specific socio-empirical lifeworlds through anthropological and empirical analysis. We have thus selected authors who have long-standing expertise in combining empirical methods and ethical analysis. In fields such as transplantation medicine, this is particularly important because such empirical work helps to correct false claims and assumptions about affected groups (Schweda/Schicktanz 2014; Schweda/Schicktanz 2009). Moreover, insights from medical anthropology, the social sciences, and empirical bioethics help to sensitize us to the many layers of judgements and often hidden anthropological assumptions regarding the body, the meaning of death, the social meaning of donation and the self-conception of living with a transplanted organ (Joralemon 1995; Schicktanz et al. 2017).

Various medical and scholarly insights demonstrate how the consequences, or even the idea of organ transplantation itself, challenge concepts of personal identity, the family, and the body (Lock/Crowley-Makota 2008). Such diverse attitudes seem to relate to stable sociocultural and anthropological concepts, but also to normative ideas of reciprocity and gift-giving, which influence medical and non-medical actors alike. Consequently, and often intertwined with the ethical debate, medical sociology and anthropology have accompanied developments in this field with critical observation of cases and systematic overviews (Scheper-Hughes 2008; Fox/Swazey 1992). Empirical-ethical work has scrutinized the influence of cultural concepts like identity, the family, and embodiment at the intersection of morality, anthropology and medicine, often through comparative analysis (Schicktanz/Wöhlke 2017). Thereby, we also take into account that organ donation is a field of extensive discussion, because it involves many profound challenges of our anthropological conditions. What we consider to be 'self' and 'other', 'alive' and 'dead', or 'human' and 'non-human' are contested through this medical procedures. Thereby, organ transplantation challenges many presumptions regarding what we consider as 'natural' or 'artificial'.

Such a contextualization allows us to locate such different arguments in 'grey zones' between universalism and relativism, and to examine further ethical concepts such as relational autonomy, responsibility, and trust. These ethical concepts add an important dimension to the more prominent ethical principles of autonomy, well-being, or fairness in allocation, and they therefore also feature prominently in many of our contributions.

While transplantation is now a global phenomenon, it evokes questions (and might require answers) that are very specific to certain regions and local contexts. Bringing together international perspectives allows us to make intercultural comparisons, and to learn from successes and pitfalls from around the world. Informed by empirical data, we consider the relevance of particular cultural differences and universal norms, which intersect in the field of transplantation medicine in various ways.

For instance, various models of consent exist in different countries. Still, the core ethical problem is the same everywhere: how to respect the morally autonomous decision of the potential donor. Internationally, the global exchange of organs continues to be debated, which is important due to ongoing mobility of patients as well as of organs and tissue. Other topics, such as non-heart-beating donation and models of unspecified donation, or old age, are managed and addressed in culturally different ways.

The fact that this volume revisits a long-standing discussion within bioethics and beyond is also grounded in our own research on the different forms of uneasiness and critique directed towards organ donation (Pfaller et al. 2018). Such forms of discomfort and criticism, however, are not only based on a lack of information or expertise (Hansen et al. 2021), but result from critical reflection and hidden anthropological meanings. Therefore, we see them as considered judgments and discuss them as legitimate forms of critique which ethicists, practitioners, and policy makers should consider while attempting to find and establish ameliorative strategies. In order to continue these lively debates, the book is divided into five sections, each comprising several chapters, which mirror the sequence of transplantation decisions: (i) donation of organs and tissue, (ii) human organ sources, (iii) organ allocation and transplantation systems, (iv) organ recipients, and (v) alternatives.

(i) Donation of Organs and Tissue

Anja MB Jensen and Klaus Hoeyer (Denmark) begin our anthology with a major question centered on the constant global need for organs: What motivates donor families and potential organ donors to decide for donation? Based on both an analysis of the debates on altruism, duty to donate, and incentives for organ donation as well as a decade of anthropological research in Denmark among donor families, hospital staffs, and registered organ donors, their chapter argues that deciding to donate organs is a meaning-making practice centered on consoling family members. They show that organ donation is therefore a way to make sense of death that can reflect a wish to create a legacy for the deceased. It can also be a comfort in the usability of the organs, and expose wider relations to the body, the family, and society in general.

Alberto Molina-Pérez, Janet Delgado, and David Rodríguez-Arias (Spain) systematically analyze how models of consent, autonomy, and the role of the family are intertwined in various policies. The ethics of deceased organ procurement is supposedly based on individual consent to donate, either explicit (opt-in) or presumed (opt-out). The authors propose a novel and comprehensive taxonomy of the models of consent. Depending on the country, the family may be allowed to take different kinds of actions in different situations, which may be grounded in law or simply by traditions of clinical practice. By comparing different models of consent, they show that these models rely on different concepts of autonomy, and they discuss the ethical debates surrounding two policy approaches: presumed consent and family veto.

Douglas MacKay and Katherine Saylor (USA) provide an overview of the ethical considerations relevant to nudging in organ donation policy. They first outline the different ways in which jurisdictions use nudging to facilitate the donation of organs before exploring and evaluating the ethical objections to nudging, including the claim that nudging is a form of manipulation and thus disrespectful of people's autonomy. Finally, they consider the benefits that governments may realize through the use of nudges to promote organ donation and consider whether these benefits can be great enough to outweigh any moral objections.

Solveig Lena Hansen and Katharina Beier (Germany) analyze normative implications of trust in transplantation discourses and debates on tissue donation for research. Comparing the practice of organ and tissue donation, they critically analyze how both public and academic discourses evoke a certain paradigm of trust. This paradigm follows a logic in which the application of adequate practices and regulative frameworks results in a well-informed public, thus leading to trusting donors who ultimately support donations in practice. The emergence of trust, however, is more complex than this paradigm suggests. In addition, the willingness to donate organs for transplantation and tissue for research depends not only on trust but also on other factors, such as concepts of the body, understandings of death, acceptance of research in general, as well as notions of altruism and solidarity.

(ii) Human Organ Sources

Dieter Birnbacher (Germany) observes that there is a lingering uneasiness about whether brain death is a satisfactory criterion of death. Though all legislatures identify, explicitly or implicitly, brain death with human death, sections of the public as well as a number of academic anthropologists continue to hold reservations about whether it is morally acceptable. The chapter examines the arguments for and against the identification of death and brain death, both from theoretical and ethical perspectives. Taking a pragmatic position, he argues that abandoning the brain death definition of death would seriously limit the highly beneficial practice of organ transplantation, which, in the absence of alternative methods of treatment, would be ethically undesirable.

Anne L Dalle Ave (Switzerland), *David Shaw* (Switzerland), and *James L. Bernat* (USA) analyze protocols for donation after the circulatory determination of death (DCDD). According to their analysis, this system forces physicians to decide exactly how death should be determined following the cessation of respiratory and circulatory functions. In DCDD, death is determined by the permanent cessation of circulation and respiration but before those cessations become irreversible. During this time, vital organs could regain function if circulation were restored by resuscitation. Because the cessation of brain functions is essential for the determination of death, and because the brain may regain functions with reperfusion, death cannot be determined unless brain circulation has permanently ceased. The authors conclude that organ procurement should be initiated only after the possibility of auto-resuscitation has elapsed, and after ensuring that the functions of the brain have permanently ceased.

Dominique E. Martin (Australia) examines the ethics of directed living organ donation. By permitting a healthy person to undergo an invasive surgical procedure that is both medically unnecessary and nonbeneficial to the physical health of the donor, and that further poses immediate and potentially longer term risks to their health and wellbeing, living organ donation challenges fundamental norms of health ethics. Nevertheless, living donation of kidneys and partial livers is now widely accepted, and in some countries it has become the primary source of organs for transplantation. Evaluating the proportionality of risks and benefits of donation to living donors and justifying the acceptance or non-acceptance of prospective donors remains clinically and ethically complex. The author argues that ethical concerns about living donation should be recognized as reflecting routine ethical considerations in health care, but they also require exploration in the broader context of prospective donors' lives and relationships.

Greg Moorlock and *Heather Draper* (UK) focus on ethical aspects of unspecified living donation. They first provide a brief overview of the practice, the international context, and regulation before discussing the principle of 'first do no harm'. They explore how this potential obstacle has been overcome by adding the principle of autonomy as addition to established accounts of benefits and harms. Finally, they analyze whether the medical profession should promote this practice.

(iii) Organ Allocation and Transplantation Systems

Søren Holm (UK/Norway) analyzes how postmortal organs, a rare non-fungible resource, should be allocated among potential recipients and investigates the ethical and pragmatic criteria used. The weightings of criteria used in existing organ allocation schemes are to some extent arbitrary. In addition, the chapter discusses the use of organ allocation schemes as mechanisms for incentivizing organ retrieval, and whether geographical restrictions within a country or transplant organization can be justified. Finally, while organ shortage might be hypothetically solved by replacing material scarcity with financial scarcity, the quest for fair allocation would remain.

Peter Sykora (Slovakia) analyzes the underlying moral assumptions of the current system of organ procurement, which is based on the notion altruistic organ donation but is considered by many to be 'a qualified failure'. Based on a discussion of kidney exchange programs, he argues that instead of seeing the solution in an organ market, a new approach based on indirect reciprocity holds promise.

Zümrüt Alpınar Şencan (Germany) scrutinizes how the scarcity of organs and the growing ease of internet communications have led to the rise of commercial organ transactions. The chapter presents an overview of the moral arguments in favour of and against this trend. In particular, critics to organ sale relate to various approaches, ranging from of harm and benefit, exploitation and justice, autonomy and coercion as well as social values. These arguments are either (a) guided by generally adopted principles of biomedical ethics or moral concerns without further inquiry, or (b) mostly founded on contingent factors, which are adjustable. The chapter addresses a further concern regarding the practice: a dignity-based objection to organ selling. It argues that according to a social account of dignity, the practice of organ selling, independent of whether the subject chooses to act autonomously and regardless of the external conditions, threatens human dignity by implying that some people have less value than others.

Mark Schweda and *Sabine Wöhlke* (Germany) analyze how questions of old age and generational relations are increasingly receiving attention in the field of transplantation medicine. Demographic ageing contributes to a growing demand for transplantable organs, thus intensifying the problem of 'organ scarcity' and fueling concerns about the efficient use and fair distribution of donor organs. At the same time, older people are being discovered as potential organ donors in postmortem and living organ allocation. In all these contexts, positions and arguments regarding organ donation are interwoven with morally loaded ideas of (old) age, the life course, and intergenerational relations. Against the backdrop of current research in transplantation medicine, the authors provide an overview of the social role and ethical implications of age and generational relations in organ donation, indicating open questions and the need for further empirical research and ethical debate.

(iv) Organ Recipients

Paweł Łuków (Poland) analyzes the role of embodied personal identity and conceptions of good life and how this is relevant for assessing organ transplantation. He argues that embodied identity has a central place in every conception of a good life. Instabilities in a patient's present identity, and in their conception of a good life, can prevent them from developing a sufficiently stable and instructive future identity, and therefore from having a good post-transplant life. An adequate response to such challenges may involve not only reciprocal adaptation of the patient's post-transplant identity but also a reframing of the very concept of the good life when applied to life after transplant surgery.

Rhonda M. Shaw (New Zealand) discusses insights from a large set of qualitative studies to critically examine the gift-discourse. Her analysis is based on 127 face-to-face, in-depth interviews and fieldwork undertaken in New Zealand between 2007 and 2013 with medical professionals, living organ donors, donor families, and transplant recipients. The study findings indicate that while the gift-of-life discourse is the dominant cultural script available for people to articulate their experiences of organ donation and transplantation, it is not always aligned with people's testimonies of organ transfer. To address this gap in understanding, the author draws on the philosophical concept of epistemic injustice to show why the inclusion of perspectives from organ donors, donor families, and transplant recipients is ethically needed and justified. The chapter emphasize the importance of qualitative social science research in bringing these views to bear on our collective understanding of organ donation and transplantation processes.

Sayani Mitra (UK) offers an ethical analysis of uterus transplantation (UT) using a normative critique of the existing ethical and legal debate from a feminist standpoint. By referring to a reproductive justice approach, the chapter identifies and analyses three ethical issues that require a gender-sensitive explanation. The first ethical issue revolves around the designation of UT as a 'non-vital' transplant procedure that simply improves the quality of life and the impact of this categorization on uterus retrieval procedures. The second issue concerns the strategy of uterus allocation and listing and the gendered position of the donor in the process. The third issue revolves around the questions as to whether UT needs to be regulated as another transplant procedure, like the other vascularized composite allograft organs (VCAs), or needs to be recognized as an assisted reproductive technology (ART).

(v) Alternatives

Tatjana Višak (Germany) analyzes the ethical debate on xenotransplantation, the transplantation of animal organs to humans. Her analysis features two main lines of argumentation: anthropocentric and sentientist. Anthropocentric arguments focus on harms and benefits for humans: the potential improvements to the welfare of organ recipients and their loved ones. However, the extent of this benefit is still unclear, since it depends on the quality of the organs and on the required public safety measures. The main costs for humans are the opportunity costs: the lost benefits that would have occurred if scarce health care resources had been invested in other, more cost-effective, projects. Other costs include the risk of zoonoses, namely the transfer of animal viruses to humans, a topic that due to the Coronavirus-crisis in 2020 has received new attention. By contrast, sentientist arguments consider the interests of all sentient beings on an equal basis. These arguments allow for animal rights, which are meant to protect animal interests and function as constraints against killing and injuring animals for research purposes or as organ sources. From a sentientist perspective xeno-transplantation may be unacceptable.

Charlotte Burnham-Stevens and *Niki Vermeulen* (UK) discuss case studies from the field of 3D bioprinting, a future prospect for transplantation medicine. The potential of 3D bioprinting in transplantation medicine tends to focus on its promissory power; its ability to 'solve' a number of key problems associated with traditional organ transplantation and revolutionize modern medicine. Whilst the nascent technology could indeed have some future benefits, it also raises social and ethical issues around its embedding in health care systems, including regulation, ownership, and access. For instance, organ bioprinting may risk further commodification of our bodies, or sustain or increase existing health inequalities, while its promises may heighten expectations and desires for 'ideal health'. In the context of emerging ethical debates, this chapter combines bioethical and legal scholarship with insights from Science and Technology Studies (STS), using hypothetical narratives for further exploration of ethical issues.

In the final chapter, *Hagai Boas* (Israel), *Nadav Davidovitch* (Israel), and *Michael Yudell* (USA) provide broad reflections on the public health ethics of organ transplantation. The gap between organ demand and available supply is large, and patients across the globe die every day awaiting a needed organ. The authors argue that transplant bioethics alone cannot solve many of the problems facing transplant medicine, and turn instead to public health for answers. Hereby, they discuss the critical paradox of prevention as well as how a global perspective can challenge some assumptions regarding brain death and donation policies.

Acknowledgements

This volume is also the productive outcome of a four-year project funded by the German Research Foundation (DFG) (SCHI 631/7-3). We would like to thank our reviewers, who helped to improve all texts through their critical comments and suggestions: Frank Adloff, Kristof van Assche, Dieter Birnbacher, Hagai Boas, Claudia Bozzaro, Markus Christen, Frederic Gilbert, Daniel Kersting, Nadia Primc, Ralf Stoecker, Mark Schweda, Manuel Schaper, Alfred Simon, and Claudia Wiesemann. Furthermore, we thank Jovan Maud for his copy editing and language support on most of the articles in this collection. Finally, we are particularly grateful to Kristina Schneider for allowing us to use her artwork for the book's cover image, which in our view symbolizes a cultural interpretation of living cells, production, and connectivity.

References

Bailey, Leonard L. (1990): "Organ Transplantation: A Paradigm of Medical Progress." In: The Hastings Center Report 20/1, pp. 24–28.

Blumstein, James F./Sloan, Frank A. (1989): Organ Transplantation Policy. Issues and Prospects, Durham/London: Duke.

Briceno, Javier (2020): "Artificial Intelligence and Organ Transplantation – Challenges and Expectations." In: Current Opinion in Organ Transplantation. DOI: 10.1097/MOT.0000000000000775

Caplan, Arthur (1989): "The Gift of Life: Dilemmas in Organ Transplantation." In: The Mount Sinai Journal of Medicine 56/5, pp. 395–405.

Daar, Abdallah S. (1997): "Ethics of Xenotransplantation: Animal Issues, Consent, and Likely Transformation of Transplant Ethics." In: World Journal of Surgery 21, pp. 975–982.

Diethelm, Arnold (1990): "Ethical Decisions in the History of Organ Transplantation." In: Annals of Surgery 211/5, pp. 505–520.

Ekser, Burcin/Li, Ping/Cooper, David K. C. (2017): "Xenotransplantation: Past, Present, and Future." In: Current Opinion in Organ Transplantation 22/6, pp. 513–521.

Fox, Renée C./Swazey, Judith P. (1992) (eds): Spare Parts. Organ Replacement in American Society, New York: Oxford University Press.

Garwood-Gowers, Austen (1999): Living Organ Transplantation. Key Legal and Ethical Questions, London/New York: Routledge.

Glazier, Alexandra/Mone, Thomas (2019): "Success of Opt-In Organ Donation Policy in the United States." In: Journal of the Americal Medical Association 322/8, pp. 719–720.

Hansen, Solveig L./Eisner, Marthe I./Pfaller, Larissa/Schicktanz, Silke (2018): "'Are you in or are you out?!' Moral Appeals to the Public in Organ Donation Poster Campaigns – a Multimodal and Ethical Analysis." In: Health Communication 33/8, 1020–1034.

Hansen, Solveig L./Pfaller, Larissa/Schicktanz, Silke (2021): "Critical Analysis of Communication Strategies in Public Health Promotion. An Empirical-Ethical Study on Organ Donation in Germany." In: Bioethics 35/2, pp. 161-172.

Hyun, Insoo/Scharf-Deering, J. C./Lunshof, Jeantine E. (2020): "Ethical Issues Related to Brain Organoid Research." In: Brain Research 1723. DOI: 10.1016/j.brainres.2020.146653

Iacobucci, Gareth (2020): "Organ Donation: England will have 'opt-out' System from May 2020." In: British Medical Journal 368. DOI: 10.1136/bmj.m752

Joralemon, Donald (1995): "Organ Wars: The Battle for Body Parts." In: Medical Anthropology Quarterly 9/3, pp. 335–356.

Lock, Margaret/Crowley-Makota, Megan (2008): "Situating the Practice of Organ Donation in Familial, Cultural, and Political Context." In: Transplantation Reviews 22/3, pp. 154–157.

Miller, Franklin G./Truog, Robert D. (2012) (eds): Death, Dying, and Organ Transplantation. Reconstructing Medical Ethics at the End of Life, Oxford: University Press.

Murray, Joseph E. (1964): "Moral and Ethical Reflections on Human Organ Transplantation." In: The Linacre Quarterly 31/2, pp. 54–56.

Pfaller, Larissa/Hansen, Solveig L./Adloff, Frank/Schicktanz, Silke (2018): "'Saying No to Organ Donation': an Empirical Typology of Reluctance and Rejection." In: Sociology of Health and Illness 40/8, pp. 1327–1346.

Scheper-Hughes, Nancy (2008): The Last Commodity. Post-Human Ethics, Global (In)Justice, and the Traffic in Organs, Penang: Multiversity & Citizens International.

Schicktanz, Silke/Pfaller, Larissa/Hansen, Solveig L./Boos, Moritz (2017): "A Comparison of Attitudes towards Brain Death and Body Concepts in Relation to Willingness or Reluctance to Donate: Results of a Students' Survey before and after the German Transplantation Scandals." In: Journal of Public Health 25, pp. 249–256.

Schicktanz, Silke/Wöhlke, Sabine (2017): "The Utterable and Unutterable Anthropological Meaning of the Body in the Context of Organ Transplantation." In: Dilemata 27, 107–127.

Schweda, Mark/Schicktanz, Silke (2014): "Why Public Moralities Matter – The Relevance of Socioempirical Premises for the Ethical Debate on Organ Markets." In: Journal of Medicine and Philosophy 39/3, pp. 217–222.

Schweda, Mark/Schicktanz, Silke (2009): "The 'Spare Parts Person'? Conceptions of the Human Body and their Implications for Public Attitudes towards Organ Donation and Organ Sale." In: Philosophy, Ethics, and Humanities in Medicine 4/4, pp. 1–10.

Veatch, Robert M./Ross, Lainie F. (2015) (eds): Transplantation Ethics. 2nd edition, Washington: Georgetown University Press.

Woodruff, M. F. A. (1964): "Ethical Problems in Organ Transplantation." In: British Medical Journal 1, pp. 1457–1460

I. DONATION OF ORGANS AND TISSUE

1. Making Sense of Donation
Altruism, Duty, and Incentives

Anja M.B. Jensen & Klaus Hoeyer

1. Introduction

One of the major questions in the field of postmortem organ donation revolves around reasons for donation: What motivates potential organ donors and donor families to donate organs? If it were possible first to identify a set of factors associated with willingness to donate, and then to influence these factors, answering this question might help promote donation frequency and alleviate the global lack of organs often highlighted in public debates and academic literature. In this chapter, we take another route. Instead of identifying factors, we explore how people make sense of death and donation – how they reason when confronted with the option to donate. We believe that if we understand these meaning-making practices, we might better ensure the long-term sustainability of postmortem donation as well as create positive donation experiences. This, we believe, is a fundamental precondition for the practice of organ donation, and more feasible than controlling factors that lead to donation.

Based on ethnographic studies in Denmark, we provide examples of how donor families and registered donors make sense of the act of donation. We suggest that reasons for donation reflect the way organ donation facilitates new ways for future donors to deal with the prospect of death, as well as new ways for donor families to make sense of a tragic loss. Reasons for donation are embedded in meaning-making practices that build upon wider sets of ideas and life values, hopes and ideals. This means that policymakers must stay attentive to the meanings of organ donation if they wish to align political frameworks and practical organizational arrangements with the expectations and wishes of potential donor families.

As many studies debating donor motivation have argued, donation reasoning can be explored through conceptual frameworks and principles that have their roots in philosophy and various branches of the social sciences. While acknowledging these important contributions, our chapter emphasizes the importance of understanding the social practices of donation decisions. Organ donation produces meaning for people in different ways and engage them in relationships with ambiguous effects. These meanings vary over time and across cultural contexts. Sociologist Kieran Healy has argued that donation policies have worked to establish values such as altruism as a particular form of social force. From his perspective, altruism should be seen more as a product of organ donation practices than as a pre-existing motivational cause (Healy 2006). Inspired by his work, we see reasons to donate as not necessarily the cause of donations, but rather as decisions that gradually emerge as people make sense of organ donation practices and death. As we will show, reasons for postmortem donations emerge as families attempt to align the donation decision with the values and personality of the deceased, and with their perception of 'the good death'. By constructing a post-donation narrative that transform a tragic sudden death into something meaningful because of organ donation, families orchestrate death (Jensen 2011a) and gradually articulate reasons for donation.

When discussing reasons to donate, it is important to recognize the difference between reasons based on actual donation experience (the families of potential donors) and donation wishes (registered donors). Registered donors articulate the reasons behind their donation wishes in their daily life settings and are detached from the actual turmoil of a sudden donation decision. Many are not aware that in reality, only one in 1.000 deaths occur in a manner that makes postmortem donation an option (Hoeyer/Olejaz 2020). Donor families, conversely, make decisions in the hospital in the immediate aftermath of a sudden tragedy, while they are still deeply emotionally affected. The death they encounter is no longer a potential death, but a very real one. For such families, sudden death raises many questions other than those relating to organ donation. A donation request comes in a stream of other emotionally charged questions that families have to tackle. Studies have underlined that families base donation decisions on what they consider meaningful in light of their individual situation (Berntzen/Bjørk 2014; Forsberg et al. 2014; Jensen 2011a, 2016; Sque/Payne 1996). Our point is that although altruism, duty, or incentives might all factor into 'reasons for organ donation', in practice, the concrete experiences and meanings attached to those reasons can be very different.

The chapter begins by outlining how reasons for donating interconnect with how meaning-making reflects the cultural and political context. Then we describe how three reasons for donating have featured prominently in the international literature (and in policymaking): altruism, duty, and financial incentives. Thereafter, we use more detailed examples from studies we have conducted in Denmark to discuss how Danish donor families and registered donors experience their donation decisions, and how these practices relate to attempts to make sense of death. Finally, based on these findings, we suggest that policymaking must take into account empirical insights into donors' and donor families' reasons and interests in order to balance the wish for increased donor rates with family care and public legitimacy.

2.   Donation Decisions Reflect Cultural and Political Contexts

Many studies highlight the influence of national, ethnic, social, political and religious contexts on reasons for donating and donation policies across the world (Bruzzone 2008; Joralemon 1995; Sharp/Randhawa 2016; Shaw 2015; Schicktanz et al. 2010; Schweda/Schicktanz 2009; Wakefield et al. 2011). Some studies, for example, suggest that African-Americans, based on particular experiences and historical injustices, are more suspicious towards brain death and express less trust in American organ donation agencies than the white majority population (Sharp 2006; Siminoff et al. 2006).

Many countries and big cities with diverse populations have launched campaigns targeted at specific ethnic groups and developed partnerships with religious leaders and cultural groups in order to foster cultural acceptance of donation practices (Jensen 2007; Randhawa/Neuberger 2016). Conversely, recent studies suggest that even if ethnicity plays a significant role in donation processes in clinical practice, donation reluctance cannot be directly associated with culture, religion or heritage (Cooper/Kierans 2016; Kierans/Cooper 2013). The point is not to see, for example, ethnicity as having a particular impact on donation willingness, but instead to explore the experiences that make particular positions meaningful to people in given situations – and thereby to avoid prejudice.

When people reflect on why they donate, their reasons are typically related to how death becomes meaningful, and how they envision a 'good death'. What constitutes a good death differs among individuals as well as across contexts, not only because of cultural values and traditions, but also because of the different affordances of medical organizational systems for donation and follow-up care. The use of dead bodies in medicine is and has been practiced with significant variation over time and in different locales. Anthropologist Margaret Lock (2002) has illustrated how postmortem donation was received differently in the USA and in Japan, and how policies and practices took particular forms that reflected differing ideas about dead bodies and kinship rights and obligations. Important work has illustrated similar variations in other parts of the world (Hamdy 2012; Hogle 1999; Sanal 2011), pointing to the need to engage local perceptions, values and institutions when working to ensure the acceptability and social sustainability of new initiatives.

Donations reflect the values and beliefs of the individuals of a given country; people are affected by the norms and values of the society in which they live. In Israel, some people believe that a 'heroic death' involves giving one's life for one's country, and that when soldiers die in battle, their individual bodies become symbolically a part of the collective body of the nation. Suicides or traffic accidents do not have the same social significance. Still, if the family consents to organ donation, these 'ordinary' ways of dying can be transformed into heroic deaths worthy of national attention and recognition (Ben-David 2005). Families adopting this view might find comfort in the donation and deal with the tragedy of sudden death. Likewise, in the US, organ donors are honored in a manner not dissimilar to the celebration of war heroes, and especially in the New York region, donors are compared to the heroic firefighters of 9/11. It is quite common to hold public recognition ceremonies for organ donors where their images and life stories are on display. In some instances, families are presented with 'gift of life' medals, and donor family stories are publicly celebrated (Sharp 2000, 2001, 2006; Jensen 2007, 2010, 2011a, 2011b). Such practices of recognition cannot be uncritically adapted to other cultural contexts because social dynamics differ (Hogle 1999). The importance of context for the reasoning through which support for donation emerges points to the need to study the social values of local settings before adopting policy tools developed elsewhere.

3.   Known Reasons for Donating Organs:
Altruism, Duty and Financial Incentives

People can have many different reasons for deciding to donate or for declining to become an organ donor. Providing an overview of the entire philosophical and social science literature on the full spectrum of articulated reasons is thus beyond the scope of this chapter. We have chosen instead to focus on three of the most common and most debated reasons: altruism, duty, and financial incentives. In practice, different reasons – including these three – often intersect. As argued above, they are articulated in different ways depending on political, social and cultural context – and they do not necessarily precede and cause a decision; they are sometimes retrospectively constructed as people try to make sense of an overwhelming donation situation. The three reasons chosen here have been discussed in the literature as being both descriptive (explaining why people donate) and prescriptive (as a normative guidance to how organ donation should work and why people ought to donate). We do not want to assume that one can move from 'is' to 'ought' – and thereby commit what Moore defined as a naturalistic fallacy (Moore 1903). Nor do we take sides in the debates about whether a descriptive argument can overrule a normative or vice versa. Our point is simply to introduce key elements of the literature and provide a sense of the existing scholarship on reasons for supporting post-mortem organ donation. In relation to policymaking, however, we take a clear stance. We believe that an empirical understanding of donation reasoning in local settings is imperative if policymakers are to achieve the effects they desire.

3.1   Altruism

Altruism has been defined as "behaviour intended to benefit another, even when this action risks possible sacrifice to the welfare of the actor" (Monroe 1996: 6). Concern for others has been an enduring topic in philosophy, but the modern notion of altruism is typically attributed the French philosopher August Comte, who in the beginning of the 19th Century identified an unselfish desire to "live for others". Comte wrote at a time when he feared egoism or individualism would ruin solidarity in modern urban society (Piliavin 2001). Altruism in this sense need not be directed towards specific individuals (see also chapter 10 in this book). Recently, the complexities of the concept of altruism have been central to studies of both deceased and living organ donation that discuss how altruism intersects with public policies and information, and with solidarity and self-interest in donor reasoning (cf. Hansen et al. 2018; Healy 2006; Moorlock et al. 2014; Saunders 2012; Thornton 2019).

This ideal of an unselfish act devoid of expectations of something in return has been challenged empirically by mostly anthropological scholarship drawing on gift exchange theory. Marcel Mauss (1990) famously argued that all gifting is engrained in a threefold obligation to give, receive and reciprocate. He thereby claimed that there is no such thing as pure altruism. This position has shaped a great deal of anthropological work on organ donation, which has unfolded the relational character of obligations between giver and recipient (Alnæs 2001; Fox/Swazey 1992; Jensen 2007; Sharp 1995, 2000, 2001; Sque/Payne 1994). The anthropological claim has been that gifting helps to maintain social order exactly by exerting demands for reciprocity (Mauss 1990, see also chapter 10 in this book). The articulation of the altruistic ideal might nevertheless provide the act of gifting with a particular social texture that sustains relationships between people, institutions, and the communities in which they live. The social articulation of ideals can influence practices, even if ideals do not determine practice.

The notion of altruism has shaped a rhetoric of 'gifts' often used in campaigns for organ donation (Hansen et al. 2018; Siminoff/Chillag 1999). Here, gifting relates to the idealized and normative sense of donation, not the anthropological theory. Normative discourses can thereby influence the meanings that are attributed to donation. In public campaigns, popular media and in many scientific studies, post-mortem exchange of organs is often framed through the concept 'the gift of life' (Alnæs 2001; Lock 2002). Lesley Sharp (1995: 365) suggests that a rhetoric of altruism is designed to encourage the involved parties to regard organ transplants as an unselfish and generous action that does not require any kind of reciprocal action: it is prescriptive rather than descriptive. Ideas about altruism also influence policies that aim to promote organ donation based on an assumption that provision of information about the needs of recipient will make people donate (Hoeyer et al. 2015, Nuffield 2011; Tontus 2019; Sharp/Randhawa 2014). However, other studies have shown how donor families, transplant patients, and organ procurement organizations continue to reflect on obligations of reciprocity (Jensen 2007, 2011, 2017; Sharp 2006; Siminoff/Chillag 1999).

Many donor families and members of the public embrace (or are deliberately encouraged to adopt) the organizational language of organ donation as a 'gift' (Jensen 2010; Sharp 2006). However, the social relations that are closely associated with the gift can also cause problems. Sociologists Fox and Swazey have argued that in transplantation, the psychological and moral burden is especially onerous because the gift is so extraordinary that it is inherently un-reciprocal: "It has no physical or symbolic equivalent" (1992: 40). People usually give gifts in return. Hence, the giver and the receiver are "locked in a creditor-debtor vice that binds them one to another in a mutually fettering way" (ibid). This is what they call the 'tyranny of the gift'. Their work primarily focuses on living donation between family members, but the idea that reciprocity is more or less impossible or problematic has also had tremendous impact on the field of post-mortem donation (Alnæs 2001; Lock 2002; Sharp 1995, 2006; Siminoff/Chillag 1999). While this work seeks to empirically challenge the notion of altruism as the primary reason for donation, it does not address the normative argument as such. Furthermore, the normative reasoning can be seen to have empirical effects as it is used in campaigns and shapes organizational logics, which makes altruistic reasoning an empirical phenomenon.

3.2 Duty

Another and related reason commonly discussed in the literature is *duty* (Altman 2011; Brecher 1994, Gerrand 1999; Merle 2000). In modern ethics, the normative concept of duty is mainly associated with the deontological ethics of Immanuel Kant. Kant's famous categorical imperative suggests that one should 'act only according to the maxim whereby you can at the same time will that it should become a universal law'. It can be discussed whether a universal duty to donate (or to help others) in any way follows from the imperative. However, in a narrow sense, many assume that helping those in existential need is a duty of humanity. When people articulate a duty to donate, they typically refer to this type of inclination. It is thereby not derived from a particular (Kantian) philosophical position: the word is used in ways resembling some more akin to a *social obligation*. It is an obligation that can be argued in various ways and be based on multiple values. The word 'duty' nevertheless permeates donation debates, perhaps because of (rather than despite) its ambiguous meanings.

Today, *duty* is mobilized in its more general sense to encourage donations, and often by relating it to altruism, which thereby loses its meaning as unconditioned gifting (see also chapter 14 in this book). As with altruism, the donation literature often refers to duty in a prescriptive manner. In turn, this use has empirical effects as it enters campaigns and organizational policies. When related to altruism in political campaigns, the duty principle of organ donation becomes regarded and articulated as a social obligation towards society: in public debates, statements such as 'if you want to receive, you have to be willing to give,' aim to classify organ donation as an ideally fair and socially acceptable exchange, and thus the social obligation to donate as something natural (Jensen/Larsen 2020). The work of John Rawls (1999) on 'free riders' that seek to benefit without contribution has substantiated this further. The social obligation to donate is aligned with fairness (it is not fair to benefit without contributing). Sometimes reluctance to accept this logic is even considered irrational (Almassi 2014; Eaton 1998; Hester 2004; Jarvis 1995; Steinberg 2004). Social obligation also features in some arguments favoring presumed consent legislation. In presumed consent systems, citizens are automatically regarded as organ donors unless they opt out (see also chapter 2 in this book). Such systems have been legitimized with reference to a social obligation (termed duty) to donate. Other policies articulate instead an obligation to make up one's mind about donation (Gill 2004; Hoeyer/Olejaz 2020). Recent studies have debated whether presumed consent actually promotes donation rates as intended, how it may challenge clinical end of life care, and how its inherent sense of obligation creates ethical dilemmas and high public ambivalence across Europe (Jensen/Larsen 2020; Molina-Perez et al. 2019; Prabhu 2019; Sheperd et al. 2014).

3.3   Incentives

As a third reason, we will mention how some studies discuss whether *incentives*, such as financial remuneration, can or should influence the propensity to donate. Scholarship supporting incentives adopts a view of human agency that emphasizes self-interest rather than duty or altruism, and offers a number of suggestions in terms of practical policy. Literature in this vein can be both prescriptive and descriptive. Discussions about incentivized action tend to stimulate reflections on body ownership and rest on a view of human organs as spare parts in strong demand (Brecher 1994; Burrows 2004; DeCastro 2003; Murray 1996). Some scholars even suggest financial compensation in the form of a so-called 'market model', where monetary exchange delivers the mechanism for allocation of organs (Satel 2008). Incentives are typically defended on the grounds that donation policies based on altruism and duty have failed, but incentives have also evoked ethical dilemmas and public debates (Becker 2009; Cherry 2005; Goodwin 2006; Hippen et al. 2009; Schweda and Schicktanz 2008; Taylor 2005). Some support 'softer' models of financial compensation, which can include remuneration of health care costs, or special health benefits to the family of the donor. An example of this is the priority rule allocation (Li et al. 2013). While only few states use incentive strategies to promote organ donation, priority rule allocation has been implemented in Israel since 2010 (Levy 2018; Stoler et al. 2016). It entails moving registered donors, or relatives of deceased donors, to the front of organ waiting lists. To the extent that it builds on the idea that 'if you have been willing to give, you should be allowed to receive,' it can be said to link the reasoning involved in social obligations (as discussed above) with that of incentives.

A critique of the use of financial incentives can be found in studies on the organ trade (see also chapter 11 in this book). American anthropologist Nancy Scheper-Hughes (1996, 2004), for example, has argued that the organ trade symbolizes global power structures, and the divide between rich people in high-income countries on the waiting list and poor people in low-income countries, who may, for example, sell their kidney for a minor sum, risking their health in the process. This critique is directed at a globally free market solution where organs are bought and sold, not regulated incentives via state policies. Based on studies from the US, anthropologist Lesley Sharp has argued that financial incentives involve a 'commodification' of the body, which can harm public attitudes towards organ donation because it indicates that a person only consists of valuable parts, and it "dehumanize[s] individuals in the name of profit" (2000: 293). In interesting ways, this is similar to a Kantian position. Even if organ transplantation was not a medical possibility at his time, Kant also spoke against commercializing bodily donations, fearing they would reduce bodies to means for other people and thereby undermine their inherent dignity. Commenting on the selling of teeth for transplants (a common practice during his time), Kant argued:

> Man cannot dispose over himself, because he is not a thing. He is not his own property – that would be a contradiction; for so far as he is a person, he is a subject, who can have ownership of other things... for it is impossible, of course, to be at once a thing and a person, a proprietor and a property at the same time. [...] He is not entitled to sell a tooth, or any of his members. (Kant 1997: 157)

How do contemporary citizens view incentives in this area? A review from 2013 on public attitudes towards financial incentives for organ donation identified a considerable preference for non-commercial forms of organ procurement, but also a need to consider alternative perceptions of financial means. These incentives could include remuneration of expenses in ways that could be experienced as signs of respect and reciprocity, such as payment of funeral expenses (Hoeyer et al. 2013). It is, however, important to keep in mind that what might seem like similar policies on financial incentives can have different implications in different contexts depending on, for example, available options for social security and health care and cultural perceptions of the body (Schweda/Schicktanz 2009).

4.   Denmark as Case Study: Methods and Context

In the following, we will substantiate our central claim that reasons for donations relate to how people make sense of death, dying and donation, and that this process of sense-making reflects the social context in which people contemplate these issues. We base our argument on anthropological studies of Danish donor family experiences and the attitudes of registered donors in Denmark (Hoeyer et al. 2015; Jensen 2011a, 2011b, 2016; Olejaz/Hoeyer 2016). We draw on data from twelve years of anthropological studies across several research projects, and some quotes have been published in the publications we reference. Anja Jensen has conducted field studies at neuro-intensive care units, including participant observation during organ donation cases, and she has conducted interviews with donor and non-donor families (N=102). Together and independently, we have interviewed hospital staff (N=78) and registered donors (N=48). Along with colleagues, we have also administered a national survey of public attitudes to donation in Denmark with questions based on our qualitative work (Nordfalk et al. 2016), from which we will include data on reasons for donation.

Denmark, it is worth pointing out, is a rather special context for organ donation. Denmark has low donation rates compared to other European countries, and also struggles to encourage individuals to sign up to the donor registry. In 2018, three out of four organ donors in intensive care units had not registered a prior decision in the register. Donations therefore had to be decided by their families (Jensen/Larsen 2020). Denmark was once known among the medical community internationally for its skepticism towards brain death and organ donation (Lock 2002; Rix 1999). Brain death did not become a criterion of death until 1990, after an intense public debate. More recently, in contrast to most other European countries, Denmark has rejected adopting presumed consent legislation in organ donation (Jensen/Larsen 2020). There is evidence, however, that the Danes' stance towards organ donation has changed. In 1995, just 30 per cent of the population stated that they were 'positive towards organ donation'. In 2016, that number had risen to 92 per cent (Nordfalk et al. 2016). In 2021, Denmark will follow the majority of European countries and implement donation after circulatory death.

In the following, we make three claims about the reasons for donations. We substantiate these claims with material from our fieldwork in each section. Our hope is that the three general claims might be valid in contexts other than Denmark, though we believe the particular values enacted in practice will remain local.

4.1   Organ Donation Helps Relatives Making Sense of Tragedy and Creates a Legacy for the Deceased

Danish families often articulate their donation decision as a way to ascribe some meaning to a tragic death. For them, the most important issue is not primarily saving other patients; it is about making a decision that is in accordance with the legacy of the deceased and thereby creating a meaningful aftermath (Jensen 2010, 2011a, 2011b, 2016a). Often this kind of reasoning reflects stories about the kind of person the donor used to be. Leo, a man in his thirties who lost his father, Erling, had always been in favor of organ donation and had had no doubts when deciding whether his father should become a post-mortem donor. His sister and his mother, however, found the decision very difficult and were not sure they could allow Erling's body to be submitted to surgery. Leo explained that he and his brother then talked to their sister and mother about it, using these words:

> I thought we should see it in relation to how my father lived his life and my father's
> values. And that can be very hard to apply to such a situation, and it is not something

you can redo. But my father was always helping others. He supported us no matter what and always thought of others first. He was the kind of man who helped all of us adult children renovate our bathrooms. He always worked hard so we had the freedom to educate ourselves. So in relation to how he lived his life, we had no doubts that he should donate his organs. (Jensen 2011a: 110)

After he shared his thoughts with them, Leo explained, his sister and mother agreed. They could also see that helping others to survive was in accordance with the way Erling had lived his life. In this way, by looking at the social history, the values and the previous actions of the individual, the family members could construct organ donation as a respectful and sense-making way of ending life. Here, we also see the connection between the normative arguments about altruism and the social practice of deciding: Erling's family relied on values associated with altruism to make sense of his life and death. For Leo, and also many other families in Jensen's studies, acknowledging the deceased and his life values, which included helping others, becoming a donor is a meaningful way of orchestrating death during and after a tragic loss (Jensen 2011a).

One time, Jensen sat at the kitchen table of Betty, a woman in her late 40s who had lost her brother John. John and his ex-wife had divorced ten years before his death, and after this his already serious drinking habit turned into alcohol abuse, isolating him physically and socially from his family and friends. After several attempts to treat his alcohol abuse, he ended up in a treatment center, but his drinking nevertheless persisted. Betty gave several examples of her efforts to support her brother. She blamed herself: "Why was I not able to help my brother?" she said. "I felt like a failure." Some months after entering the center, John was rushed to hospital with a brain hemorrhage. Betty and her father were told that John was brain-dead and asked if they would consider donating his organs. "We said yes right away," Betty told me. "John was that kind of person, and it made perfect sense if somebody could benefit from this." Just like Leo's relatives, she characterized her deceased brother as an altruistic person, and it helped her remember him in a positive manner, despite his difficulties with fulfilling these ideals in the course of his lived life.

Betty revealed that despite the tragic situation, she thought the time following the decision to donate was exciting. Doctors were running in and out for tests and blood samples. She was intrigued about which organs could be used, who was going to receive them, and how the transplants would turn out in the end. She told Jensen that she had even considered sneaking into the hallways of the hospital in Copenhagen to see the recipients of her brother's kidneys. "I can only imagine the newspaper headlines," Betty said, laughing: "Mysterious woman caught sneaking around in the kidney department at the Copenhagen University Hospital." Betty was not able to help John, but by donating his organs, she was able both to help others and to find meaningful closure to his life. Associating organ donation with John's personality was so much better than remembering the severe alcohol abuse, the loneliness and the many failures that characterized his last decade. "It is a good aftermath," she said (Jensen 2011a: 228–229). When discussing the fact that families in other parts of Denmark receive a 'thank you'-letter, Betty said: "I would have liked such a letter. I could have put such a letter in the folder I have with all his papers with pride. I would have placed it in the front of the folder as a way to wrap up the life of my younger brother." (Ibid: 229)

While the story of organ donation cannot change John's issues with alcohol abuse – his *life history* – it can somehow change the *story* of his life. By way of organ donation, John's death becomes a 'good death,' and, ironically, a contrast to his tragic life. Betty likes the idea of recognition of reciprocity, almost as if it can mend the failure to connect reciprocally during the period of alcohol abuse. In these ways, themes of altruism, duty and the social obligations of reciprocity become resources for sense-making when people are confronted with death and organ donation.

4.2   The Thought of Usability can be Comforting

A persistent theme in the literature on post-mortem organ donation has been the proposition that technology manipulates death in order to align it with what Lock has coined "the utilitarian interests of the transplant world" (Lock 1996: 596). The critique of utilitarian reasoning has suggested that it promotes the type of 'spare parts' view of the human body discussed above (Fox/Swazey 1992). Many studies suggest a potential conflict between dignity and utility – a conflict that resonates with famous divides in philosophy. While we do not dismiss the relevance of the normative debate about this conflict, our empirical studies among Danish donors and donor families suggest that, for some, utility can support the sense of dignity. Furthermore, it is not only the 'transplant world' (i.e. the medical staff) who objectify body parts; donors and donor families can experience objectification and utilitarian discourses as meaningful and dignified. We have encountered families and registered donors who use objectification and the image of utility when coping with despair and when trying to make sense of death and donation. Bente and Carsten, for instance, are the parents of a teenage boy, Adam, who was shot in the head. Thinking about the donation process, Carsten explained:

> Before we got the message that the left part of the brain was ruined, the hope we had that he would survive had turned around to a hope that the doctors would give us that message. As I was quoted in one of the newspapers, it was a question of vegetable or funeral. So it turned into a hope that it went fast – and a hope that his heart would last the pressure. If his heart stopped, he could not be used for organ transplantation and that would be bad! I was very cynical and said of course we are going to do that; we cannot use him for anything else. So we hoped that he would last. (Jensen 2016: 386)

For this family, hope for survival changed into a hope that death would finally come and that his body could be used for something. For Bente and Carsten, organ donation was a better alternative than a life 'as a vegetable'. Of the scenarios they could imagine, organ donation became the best outcome they could hope for. Such narratives often figured in the stories of donor families, sometimes with strong metaphors to underline their appreciation of the functionality of the dead body. Ole, who lost his adult son Tobias, explained his distinction between 'person and part' like this:

> I think I have the distinction that as soon as Tobias was declared brain-dead, the person Tobias was gone. The rest is a maintenance box, a spare parts box. And I have never had any problems or scruples about that. To repeat myself, it is with joy and pride I think

about Tobias being so conscious of wanting to help others. All we did was live up to his expectations. That's it. (Ibid: 387)

By conceptualizing Tobias' body as a 'spare parts box', Ole makes it meaningful to pass on the organs. This distinction in turn influences the way he memorializes Tobias. It gives him joy and pride to think about the determination of Tobias to become a donor. As such, organ donation shapes the legacy of the dead and accentuates a new kind of hope at a point in time where hope for survival is gone. This occurs not *despite* but *because of* and *through* the usability of the body. Though the debate about incentives emphasizes the risk of 'commodification' as a consequence of objectification, we see here that objectification can form part also of social dynamics through which families find hope and construe narratives of dignity. The transformation of a person into an object for transplantation allows families to orchestrate a good death. In many cases, utility and dignity are closely connected in donor family practices of hope (ibid).

In our interviews with registered organ donors, most highlighted a sincere wish to have their bodies used as much as possible (Hoeyer/Olejaz 2020). Benazir, for example, was a young academic woman with an immigrant background who was ambitious and socially engaged. She said: "Well, of course, if I – let's say that I die at the age of 24 – then, of course, I'd really, really hope that I would die in a manner making it possible to help others [brain death]. Compared to … dying just ordinarily and then lying there in the grave putrefying bit by bit." (ibid: 4). A part of our methodology was in every inter- view to search for limits to legitimate use as a way of understanding people's moral reasoning. When asking a young father, Jonas, about limits, he explained that he had none. Any kind of use would be better than 'being eaten by worms':

Jonas: 'You may do anything! Feed me to the cats, I'm dead [his emphasis, laughing]. Really, I'd rather not be buried in a coffin; I'd like to be used, for whatever. Bury me under an apple tree then I can be used as fertilizer.'
Klaus: 'What is the difference between fertilizing the graveyard and an apple tree?'
Jonas: 'You eat the apples off the apple tree. A churchyard is not very productive; it's not fertilization, it's waste.' (Hoeyer/Olejaz 2020: 421-422)

In a similar vein, Karen – also a registered donor – said that they could use all of her if they wanted, "…if you want to boil the meat off and make me into a skeleton, that is okay too" (Olejaz/Hoeyer 2016: 23).

Another registered donor, Ingrid, detached her person (or soul) from her dead body. Being a member of an interdenominational Christian movement, Ingrid imag- ined that the soul leaves the body upon death, living on in Heaven, and that Jesus does not need bodies in Heaven. She said: "You know, when I am dead, then I am in Heaven with the Lord and what happens with my body? If anyone can use it then I think it's wonderful" (ibid: 22). For her, imagining the body being used was not about losing bodily integrity, as some studies have suggested (Sanner 1994, Stephenson et al. 2008); rather, it informed the reasoning that made registering as a donor meaningful (Olejaz/ Hoeyer 2016, Hoeyer/Olejaz 2020).

4.3   Donation Decisions Reflect Relations to Body, Family and Society

When families contemplate donation decisions, their reasoning reflects a wider set of relations between the family and the deceased, relations within the family, as well as broader social relationships to the health care institutions and the welfare state. What might formally be an autonomous decision is embedded in social relations. We now give an example illustrating how donation is not always an easy decision, and how different relations between families and society, each with different temporalities, interact when donor families try to make up their minds.

Alice and Jim lost their 15-year-old son Morten in an accident. They came to Jensen's apartment one winter night and sat across from her with tears in their eyes, holding their coffee cups tight. Alice began explaining the course of events, and when telling Jensen about the question of organ donation, Alice emphasized her considerations about the body of her son:

> My first reaction was no. They shall not touch him. It is my child. They shall not start cutting him open. They shall let him be as intact as he is. They cannot cut into my child. I must look after him. I must protect him. It was really, really difficult for me in the time after we said yes to donation. I felt guilty towards my son [...] I really felt I let him down because I left him while his heart was beating. And then again, rationally, I knew that the heart would stop beating as soon as they removed him from the respirator. But at that time, it did not matter. I let him down. (Jensen 2011a: 168)

As his mother, it was almost impossible for Alice to leave Morten and thereby stop protecting the body of her child. Many of the parents Jensen interviewed felt that it was intrinsic to the role of a parent to protect the body of a child. Alice nevertheless explained that she had since come to the realization that organ donation was good because it was what Morten had wanted. A new relation – between Morten and the anonymous recipients – worked with a different temporality, and the mother's short-term urge to protect her child was replaced with a willingness to allow him to do good for others. Donation created a new future for Morten.

Historian Ruth Richardson (1996, 2007) provides a historical and contextual background for understanding such challenges of leaving the dead and transplanting body parts. She describes that in the UK in the early 18th and 19th centuries, it was considered a duty not to leave a dead body alone. This was based on the assumption that the dead body still had needs, the soul might still be present, and the "hopeful fear that the dead might return to life and require assistance" (Richardson 2007: 6). In addition, people believed that cutting the body could damage the soul, cause haunting, and prevent the possibility of resurrection (Richardson 1996: 71). Centuries later, in our age of modern medical technology and an information paradigm where public campaigns are carefully designed to convince the public to become organ donors (Hansen et al. 2018), it still matters how the body of a family member is handled. Trusting that death has occurred, accepting the need to say goodbye while the heart is beating, and balancing the wish to donate with the urge to keep your family member intact all influence the family's donation decisions and grieving (Jensen 2011a; Sque/Galasinski 2013).

In many instances, the sense of belonging to a particular community features in family reasoning on organ donation. After losing his ex-wife Kate, sixty-eight-year-old

Jens told the story of choosing to donate her kidneys. Jens differed from other donor families in that he did not draw heavily on his emotions when sharing his story, instead focusing on the background of his family's decision and the more general social obligations of donating organs:

> I don't see it as a gift; I see it as an attitude. As a natural thing living in the society we do. I mean, we do expect that somebody will come and pick us up if we fall, and take care of us. And if somebody is hurt and needs a kidney, then I find it reasonable if somebody that is passing away can deliver a useable kidney. I find it natural. And based on my own opinion, I have a hard time understanding the debate. [...] I consider it the same as helping an old lady who falls in the street. I would stop my car and help her to her feet. My fundamental attitude is that as a Danish citizen I can use the facilities in this country. And then it is natural for me that I also have an obligation, when I am not here anymore, that they can use whatever parts and bits they like. And I think that should be a part of Danish citizenship or whatever. (Jensen 2011b: 143)

Jens's narrative opens a window to investigate how ideas about social obligations and the perception of duties of citizenship shape his reasoning on organ donation. 'Obligation' is here part of his sense-making, and he associates it with belonging to a place and a community. His recollection connects the personal narrative with the national orchestration of a good death (Jensen 2011b). What we wish to underline here is that reasons for organ donation are deeply intertwined with the ideals and values surrounding the 'good death' in the particular time and society where the decision needs to be reached. They acquire their particular emotional flavor based on the relationships through which people negotiate and make sense of organ donation; and similar reasons might therefore be experienced very differently for different groups of people.

5.   Conclusion: Lessons for Policymaking

Important prescriptive work in philosophy and other disciplines has established a pool of reasons in favor of organ donation. In particular, reasoning based on notions of altruism, duty and incentives has been influential and shaped scholarly as well as public debates. The various lines of reasoning have supported as well as worked against the idea that donation is the right choice. Conversely, descriptive work exploring how reasoning operates in practice has illustrated the ways in which normative reasons can interact and produce unexpected outcomes. Drawing on our own work, we have shown how people reason in light of context. In practice, potential conflicts and distinctions can dissolve so that utility and objectification can inform attempts to ensure dignity and respect for subjectivity.

Often policy makers define organ donation issues as 'ethical' and include recommendations from ethicists, philosophers, or as in Denmark, an Ethics Council that advises parliament or ministries. While policymaking can benefit from the reasoning developed in normative ethics, we believe that policymaking on organ donation can also benefit from empirical insights into donation reasoning. For instance, Jensen was invited to talk about her research on donor family experiences by the Danish Secretary of Health, when politicians debated whether or not to implement presumed consent.

Insights on family decision-making and grief, topics that politicians usually have no access to explore, might not change political attitudes, but they provide empirically based argumentation to build more socially robust policies. A better understanding of how people in different contexts make sense of organ donation – and sometimes use organ donation to make sense of death – can help build socially sustainable institutions. Sustainability involves trustworthiness and sensitivity towards core values among the citizens affected by the adopted policies. We cannot assume that people weigh up options in uniform ways irrespective of context, and therefore we need to invest in studies of donor reasoning locally to make policies that respect local values. Reasoning also changes over time. There is therefore a need for continuous studies of donor reasoning.

One policy area that might particularly benefit from a deeper empirical engagement is the discussion about presumed consent. Presumed consent policies are associated with increasing donor rates, though it is debatable whether this effect stems from the investment in public campaigns and increased national attention rather than the policy per se (Albertsen 2018; Rhitalia et al. 2009; Sharif 2018; Shaw 2018). Generally, a national policy of presumed consent raises questions regarding the role of the family of the potential organ donor in the organ donation decision (Delgado et al. 2019; Shaw 2017). Should the donor's opinion be overruled? How does this comply with family communication and end-of-life-care in organ donation? Across Europe, presumed consent legislation is organized and practiced in different ways ranging from soft opt-out, where the family is included in decision-making, to hard opt-out, where families cannot veto a donation (Noyes et al. 2019; Prabhu 2019). The same policy, presumed consent, interacts with different values and organizational infrastructures in different countries, and therefore may have different effects. We believe that it is important to study dominant forms of reasoning in local contexts before adopting such policy changes. Policy developments benefit from both prescriptive and descriptive perspectives. It can also help policymakers to articulate criteria of success for a policy change: Is it the number of donations? Or the level of care for relatives? Or, perhaps, sustained public trust and legitimacy?

If national policies consider appropriately how people make sense of death and donation, donor rates can develop in balance with family care and public legitimacy. We believe that this balance cannot be found without a strong empirical engagement. A key task therefore remains to explore how the decision to donate can be made meaningful for those who have to live with it.

Acknowledgements

We would like to thank our informants for participating in the research, and we would like to thank the anonymous reviewers, as well as the editors of the book, for helpful comments and suggestions for improving the chapter.

References

Albertsen, Andreas (2018): "Deemed Consent: Assessing the New Opt-Out Approach to Organ Procurement in Wales." In: Journal of Medical Ethics 44/5, pp. 314–318.

Almassi, Ben (2014): "Trust and the Duty of Organ Donation." In: Bioethics 28/6, pp. 275–283.

Alnæs, Anne Hambro (2001): Minding Matter. Organ Donation and Medical Modernitys Difficult Decisions. Dissertation, University of Oslo.

Altman, Matthew C. (2011): Kant and Applied Ethics: The Uses and Limits of Kant's Practical Philosophy, Malden: Wiley-Blackwell.

Becker, Gary S./Elias, Julio J. (2007): "Introducing Incentives in the Market for Live and Cadaveric Organ Donations." In: Journal of Economic Perspectives 21/3, pp. 3–24.

Ben-David, Orit B. (2005): Organ Donation and Transplantation: Body Organs as an Exchangeable Socio–Cultural Resource, Westport: Praeger.

Berntzen, Helene/Bjørk, Ida T. (2014): "Experiences of Donor Families after Consenting to Organ Donation: A Qualitative Study." In: Intensive Critical Care Nursing 30/5, pp. 266–274.

Brecher, Bob (1994): "Organs for Transplant – Donation or Payment?" In: Raanan Gillion (ed.), Principles of Health Care Ethics, New York: Wiley, pp. 993–1002.

Bruzzone, Paolo (2008): "Religious Aspects of Organ Transplantation". In: Transplant Proceedings 40/4, pp. 1064–1067.

Burrows, Lewis (2004): "Selling Organs for Transplant". In: The Mount Sinai Journal of Medicine 71/4, pp. 251–254.

Cherry, Mark J. (2005): Kidney for Sale by Owner: Human Organs, Transplantation and the Market, Washington: Georgetown University Press.

Cooper, Jessie/Kierans, Ciara (2016): "Organ Donation, Ethnicity and the Negotiation of Death: Ethnographic Insights from the UK." In: Mortality 21/1, pp. 1–18.

DeCastro, Leonardo D. (2003): "Commodification and Exploitation: Arguments in Favour of Compensated Organ Donation." In: Journal of Medical Ethics 29, pp. 142–146.

Delgado, Janet/Molina-Pérez, Alberto/Shaw, David/Rodríguez-Arias, David (2019): "The Role of the Family in Deceased Organ Procurement." In: Transplantation 103/5, pp. 112–118.

Eaton, Stephanie (1998): "The Subtle Politics of Organ Donation: A Proposal." Journal of Medical Ethics 24/3, pp. 166–170.

Forsberg, Anna/Flodén, Anne/Lennerling, Anette/Karlsson, Veronika/Nilsson, Madeleine/Fridh, Isabell (2014): "The Core of after Death Care in Relation to Organ Donation – A Grounded Theory Study." In: Intensive Critical Care Nursing 30/5, pp. 275–282.

Fox, Renee C./Swazey, Judith P. (1992): Spare Parts: Organ Replacement in American Society, Oxford: Oxford University Press.

Gerrand, Nicole (1999): "The Misuse of Kant in the Debate about a Market for Human Body Parts." In: Journal of Applied Philosophy, 16/1, pp. 59–67.

Gill, Michael B. (2004): "Presumed Consent, Autonomy and Organ Donation." In: Journal of Medical Philosophy 29/1, pp. 37–59.

Goodwin, Michele (2006): Black Markets: the Supply and Demand of Body Parts, New York: Cambridge University Press.

Hamdy, Sherine (2012): Our Bodies Belong to God. Organ Transplants, Islam, and the Struggle for Human Dignity in Egypt, Berkeley: University of California Press.

Hansen, Solveig L./Eisner, Marthe I./Pfaller, Larissa/Schicktanz, Silke (2018): "'Are You in or are you out?!' Moral Appeals to the Public in Organ Donation Poster Campaigns: A Multimodal and Ethical Analysis." In: Health Communication 33/8, pp. 1020–1034.

Healy, Kieran (2006): Last Best Gifts. Altruism and the Market for Human Organs, Chicago/ London: University of Chicago Press.

Hester, D. Micah (2004): "Why we Must Leave our Organs to Others". In: American Journal of Bioethics 6/4: 23–28.

Hippen, Benjamin/Ross, Laine F./Sade, Robert M. (2009): "Saving Lives is More Important than Abstract Moral Concerns: Financial Incentives Should be Used to Increase Organ Donation." In: The Annals of Thoracic Surgery 88/4, 1053–1061.

Hoeyer, Klaus L. (2013): Exchanging Human Bodily Material: Rethinking Bodies and Markets, Dordrecht: Springer.

Hoeyer, Klaus L./Olejaz, Maria (2020): "Desire, Duty and Medical Gifting: how it Became Possible to Long for a Useful Death." In: Mortality, 25/4, 418-432.

Hoeyer, Klaus L./Schicktanz, Silke/Deleuran, Ida (2013): "Public Attitudes to Financial Incentive Models for Organs: a Literature Review Suggests that it is Time to Shift Focus from 'Financial Incentives' to 'Reciprocity'". In: Transplant International 26/4, pp. 350–357.

Hoeyer, Klaus/Jensen, Anja M. B./Olejaz, Maria (2015): "Transplantation as an Abstract Good: Practising Deliberate Ignorance in Deceased Organ Donation in Denmark". In: Sociology of Health and Illness, 37/4, pp. 578–593.

Hogle, Linda (1999): Recovering the Nation's Body: Cultural Memory, Medicine and the Politics of Redemption, New Brunswick, New Jersey/London: Rutgers University Press.

Jarvis, Rupert (1995): "Join the Club: A Modest Proposal to Increase Availability of Donor Organs." In: Journal of Medical Ethics 21: 199–204.

Jensen, Anja M. B. (2007): 'Those Who Give and Grieve' – an Anthropological Study of American Donor Families. Master Thesis, Vol. 430, University of Copenhagen.

Jensen, Anja M. B. (2010): "A Sense of Absence: The Staging of Heroic Deaths and Ongoing Lives among American Organ Donor Families." In: Mikkel Bille/Frida Hastrup/ Tim Flohr Sørensen (eds.), An Anthropology of Absence: Materialisations of Transcendence and Loss, London: Springer, pp. 63–81.

Jensen, Anja M. B. (2011a): Orchestrating an Exceptional Death: Donor Family Experiences and Organ Donation in Denmark. PhD Thesis, Vol. 69, University of Copenhagen.

Jensen, Anja M. B. (2011b): "Searching for Meaningful Aftermaths: Donor Family Experiences and Expressions in New York and Denmark." In: Sites: A Journal of Social Anthropology and Cultural Studies 8/1, pp. 129–148.

Jensen, Anja M. B. (2016): "Make Sure Somebody Will Survive from this: Transformative Practices of Hope among Danish Organ Donor Families." In: Medical Anthropology Quarterly 30/3, pp. 378–394.

Jensen, A. M. B. (2017). Guardians of 'the gift': the emotional challenges of heart and lung transplant professionals in Denmark. *Anthropology & medicine*, 24(1), 111-126.

Jensen, Anja M. B./Larsen, Johanne B. (2020): "The Public Debate on Organ Donation and Presumed Consent in Denmark: Are the Right Issues being Addressed?" In: *Scandinavian Journal of Public Health*, 48(5), 480–485. https://doi.org/10.1177/1403494819833797

Joralemon, Donald (1995): "Organ Wars: the Battle for Body Parts." In: Medical Anthropology Quarterly 9, pp. 335–356.

Kant, Immanuel (1997): Lectures on Ethics, Cambridge: Cambridge University Press.

Kierans, Ciara/Cooper, Jessie (2013): "The Emergence of the 'Ethnic Donor': the Cultural Production and Relocation of Organ Donation in the UK." In: Anthropology & Medicine 20/3, pp. 221–231.

Levy, Mélanie (2018): "State Incentives to Promote Organ Donation: Honoring the Principles of Reciprocity and Solidarity Inherent in the Gift Relationship." In: Journal of Law and the Biosciences 5/2, pp. 398–435.

Li, Danyang/Hawley, Zackary/Schnier, Kurt (2013): "Increasing Organ Donation via Changes in the Default Choice or Allocation Rule." In: Journal of Health Economics 32/6, pp. 1117–1129.

Lock, Margaret (1996): "Death in Technological Times: Locating the End of Meaningful Life." In: Medical Anthropology Quarterly 10/4, pp. 575–600.

Lock, Margaret (2002): Twice Dead: Organ Transplantation and the Reinvention of Death, Berkeley: University of California Press.

Mauss, Marcel (1990) [1950]: The Gift: The Form and Reason for Exchange in Archaic Societies, London and New York: Routledge.

Merle, Jean-Christophe (2000): "A Kantian Argument for a Duty to Donate One's Own Organs. A Reply to Nicole Gerrand." In: Journal of Applied Philosophy 17/1, pp. 93–101.

Molina-Pérez, Alberto/Rodriquez-Arias David/Delgado-Rodriquez, Janet/Morgan, Myfanwy/ Frunza, Mihaela/Randhawa, Gurch/Reiger-Van de Wijdeven, Jeantine/ Schiks, Eline/Wöhlke, Sabine/Schicktanz, Silke (2019): "Public Knowledge and Attitudes towards Consent Policies for Organ Donation in Europe. A Systematic Review." In: Transplantation Reviews 33/1, pp. 1–8.

Monroe, Kristen R (1996): The Heart of Altruism: Perceptions of a Common Humanity, Princeton/New Jersey: Princeton University Press.

Moore, George E. (1903): Principia Ethica, Cambridge: Cambridge University Press.

Moorlock, Greg/Jonathan, Ives/Draper, Heather (2014): "Altruism in Organ Donation: an Unnecessary Requirement?" In: Journal of Medical Ethics 40, pp. 134–138.

Murray, Thomas (1996): "Organ Vendors, Families and the Gift of Life." In: Stuart J. Younger/Renée Fox/Laurence J. O'Connell (eds.), Organ Transplantation: Meanings and Realities, Madison: University of Wisconsin Press, pp. 101–125.

Nordfalk, Francisca/Olejaz, Maria/Jensen, Anja M. B./Skovgaard, Lea L./Hoeyer, Klaus (2016): "From Motivation to Acceptability: a Survey of Public Attitudes towards Organ Donation in Denmark". In: Transplantation Research 5/5, pp. 1–8.

Nuffield Council on Bioethics (2011): Human Bodies: Donation for Medicine and Research, London.

Olejaz, Maria/Hoeyer, Klaus (2016): "Meet the Donors: a Qualitative Analysis of what Donation Means to Danish Whole Body Donors." In: European Journal of Anatomy 20/1, 19–29.

Piliavin, Jane A. (2001): "The Sociology of Altruism and Prosocial Behavior." In: Neil Smelser/Peter Bates (eds), International Encyclopedia of the Social & Behavioral Sciences, Oxford: Pergamon, pp. 411–415.

Prabhu, Pradeep K. (2019): "Is Presumed Consent an Ethically Acceptable Way of Obtaining Organs for Transplant?" In: Journal of the Intensive Care Society 20/2, pp. 92–97.

Randhawa, Gurch/Neuberger James M. (2016): "The Role of Religion in Organ Donation –Development of the UK Faith and Organ Donation Action." In: Transplantation Proceedings 48/3, pp. 689–694.

Rawls, John (1999): A Theory of Justice, Oxford: Oxford University Press.

Richardson, Ruth (1996): "Fearful Symmetry: Corpses for Anatomy, Organs for Transplantation." In: Stuart J. Younger/Renée Fox/Laurence J. O'Connell (eds.), Organ Transplantation: Meanings and Realities, Madison: University of Wisconsin Press, pp. 66–100.

Richardson, Ruth (2007): "Human Dissection and Organ Transplantation in Historical Context." In: Magi Sque/Sheila Payne (eds), Organ and Tissue Donation: An Evidence Base for Practice, Maidenhead: Open University Press.

Rithalia, Amber/McDaid, Catriona/Suekarran, Sara/Myers, Lindsey/Sowden, Amanda (2009): "Impact of Presumed Consent for Organ Donation on Donation Rates: a Systematic Review." In: British Medical Journal, pp. 338. DOI: 10.1136/bmj.a3162.

Rix, Bo A (1999): "Brain Death, Ethics and Politics in Denmark". In: Stuart J. Younger/ Robert M. Arnold/Renie Schapiro (eds), The Definition of Death: Contemporary controversies, Baltimore: Johns Hopkins University Press, pp. 227–238.

Sanal, Aslihan (2011): New Organs within Us: Transplants and the Moral Economy. Durham/ London: Duke University Press.

Sanner, Margareta (1994): "A Comparison of Public Attitudes toward Autopsy, Organ Donation and Anatomic Dissection. A Swedish Survey." In: Journal of the American Medical Association 271/4, pp. 284–288.

Satel, Sally (2008): When Altruism isn't Enough. The Case for Compensating Kidney Donors, Washington: AEI Press.

Saunders, Ben (2012): "Altruism or Solidarity? The Motives for Organ Donation and two Proposals." In: Bioethics 26/7, pp. 376–381.

Scheper-Hughes, Nancy (1996): "Theft of Life: Organ Stealing Rumours." In: Anthropology Today 12/3, pp. 3–11.

Scheper-Hughes, Nancy (2004): "Parts Unknown." In: Ethnography 5/1, pp. 29–73.

Schicktanz, Silke/Wiesemann, Claudia/Wöhlke, Sabine (2010) (eds): Teaching Ethics in Organ Transplantation and Tissue Donation, Göttingen: Universitätsverlag.

Schweda, Mark/Schicktanz, Silke (2008): "Public Moralities Concerning Donation and Disposition of Organs: Results from a Cross-European Study." In: Cambridge Quarterly of Healthcare Ethics 17/3, 308–317.

Schweda, Mark/Schicktanz, Silke (2009): "The 'Spare Parts Person'? Conceptions of the Human Body and their Implications for Public Attitudes towards Organ Donation and Organ Sale" In: Philosophy, Ethics, and Humanities in Medicine 4/4. DOI: 10.1186/1747-5341-4-4

Sharif, Adnan (2018): "Presumed Consent will not automatically Lead to Increased Organ Donation". In: Kidney International 94/2, pp. 249–251.

Sharp, Chloe/Randhawa, Gurch (2014): "Altruism, Gift Giving and Reciprocity in Organ Donation: A Review of Cultural Perspectives and Challenges of the Concepts." In: Transplantation Reviews 28/4, pp. 163–168.

Sharp, Chloe/Randhawa, Gurch (2016): "Death Practices, Attitudes toward the Body after Death and Life after Death in Deceased Organ Donation: A UK Polish Migrant Perspective." In: Journal of Palliative Care and Medicine 6/3. DOI: 10.4172/2165-7386.1000262

Sharp, Lesley A. (2000): "The Commodification of the Body and its Parts." In: Annual Review of Anthropology 29/1, pp. 287–328.

Sharp, Lesley A. (2001): "Commodified Kin: Death, Mourning and Competing Claims on the bodies of Organ Donors in the United States." In: American Anthropologist 103/1, pp. 112–133.

Sharp, Lesley A. (2006): Strange Harvest: Organ Transplants, Denatured Bodies and the Transformed Self, Berkeley: University of California Press.

Shaw, David (2017): "Presumed Consent to Organ Donation and the Family Over-rule". In: Journal of the Intensive Care Society 18/2, pp. 96–97.

Shaw, David (2018): "Presumed Evidence in Deemed Consent to Organ Donation." *In: Journal of the Intensive Care Society 19/1, pp. 2–3.*

Shaw, Rhonda M. (2015): "Expanding the Conceptual Toolkit of Organ Gifting". In: Sociology of Health and Illness 37/6, pp. 952–966.

Shepherd, Lee/O'Carroll, Ronan E./Ferguson, Eamonn (2014): "An International Comparison of Deceased and Living Organ Donation/Transplant Rates in Opt-In and Opt-Out Systems: a Panel Study." In: BMC 12/131. DOI: 10.1186/s12916-014-0131-4

Siminoff, Laura A./Chillag, Kate (1999): "The Fallacy of the Gift of Life." In: The Hastings Center Report 29/6, pp. 34–41.

Siminoff, Laura A./Burant, Christopher J./Ibrahim, Said A. (2006): "Racial Disparities in Preferences and Perceptions Regarding Organ Donation." In: Journal of General Internal Medicine 21/9, pp. 995–1000.

Sque, Magi/Galasinski, Dariusz (2013): "Keeping Her Whole." In: Cambridge Quarterly of Healthcare Ethics 22/1, pp. 55–63.

Sque, Magi/Payne, Sheila (1994): "Gift Exchange Theory: A Critique in Relation to Organ Transplantation." In: Journal of Advanced Nursing 19, pp. 45–51.

Sque, Magi/Payne, Sheila (1996): "Dissonant Loss: The Experience of Donor Relatives." In: Social Science & Medicine 43/9, pp. 1359–1370.

Steinberg, David (2004): "An 'Opting in' Paradigm for Kidney Transplantation." In: American Journal of Bioethics 4/4, pp. 4–14.

Stephenson, Michael T./Morgan, Susan E./Roberts-Perez, Samaria D./Harrison, Tyler/Afifi, Walid/Long, Shawn D. (2008): "The Role of Religiosity, Religious Norms, Subjective Norms, and Bodily Integrity in Signing an Organ Donor Card." In: Health Communication 23/5, pp. 436–447.

Stoler, Avraham/Kessler, Judd B./Ashkenazi, Tamar/Roth, Alvin E./Lavee, Jacob (2016): "Motivating Authorization for Deceased Organ Donation With Organ Allocation Priority: The First 5 Years." In: American Journal of Transplantation 16, pp. 2639–2645.

Taylor, James S. (2005): Stakes and Kidneys: Why Markets in Human Body Parts are Morally Imperative, Hampshire: Ashgate.

Thornton, Vicky (2019): "Lives and Choices, Give and Take: Altruism and Organ Procurement". In: Nursing Ethics 26/2, pp. 587–597.

Tontus, H. Omer (2020): "Educate, Re-educate, Then Re-educate: Organ Donation-centered Attitudes Should Be Established in Society." In: Transplantation Proceedings 52/1, pp. 3–11.

Wakefield, Claire E./Reid, John/Homewood, Judy (2011): "Religious and Ethnic Influences on Willingness to Donate Organs and Donor Behavior: An Australian Perspective." In: Progress in Transplantation 21/2, pp. 161–168.

2. Defining Consent
Autonomy and the Role of the Family

Alberto Molina Pérez, Janet Delgado & David Rodriguez-Arias

1. Introduction

> "[O]rgans may be removed from the bodies of deceased persons for the purpose of transplantation if: (a) any consent required by law is obtained, and (b) there is no reason to believe that the deceased person objected to such removal." (World Health Organization)

Consent is usually considered the ethical cornerstone of organ procurement (OP). The World Health Organisation's Guiding Principle 1 on human organ transplantation stresses its ethical importance and emphasizes that a valid indication of the deceased's objection to the removal of his or her organs must prevent such removal. In addition, it indicates that procurement programs under explicit consent (opt-in) policies "typically seek permission from the family even when the deceased gave pre-mortem consent", while programs under presumed consent (opt-out) "may be reluctant to proceed if the relatives oppose the donation" (WHO 2010, 2).

A trend towards presumed consent (according to which every deceased person is a potential donor) can be observed in Europe, where several countries have changed their legislation in that direction in recent years (England, Greece, Iceland, The Netherlands, Scotland, Wales) or considered doing so (Denmark, Germany, Romania, Switzerland). Beyond Europe, Chile and Japan switched to presumed consent in 2010, and Uruguay did so in 2013. Australia and several US states have also considered this but eventually decided against it.

A tendency towards lessening the role families have in the decision about OP is also evident. In 2006, the USA amended the Uniform Anatomical Gift Act to restrict the family's authority to veto the deceased's first-person authorization. France amended its law in 2017 to "reinforce" presumed consent so that families can no longer oppose nor veto OP. Argentina updated its opt-out law in 2018 so that relatives are not even required to inform the medical team about the deceased's wishes, thus removing any family involvement. Uruguay enacted a similar law in 2013. Prior to this, only Austria was known to have such a 'hard' opt-out legislation.

While consent is considered a key element for acceptable OP, how it is understood varies widely. In the first section, we attempt to systematically classify all different models of consent in that field. We claim that these models can vary widely depending on whether decisional authority is given only to living prospective donors, to donors and their relatives, or exclusively to the family. In the second section, we examine the concepts of autonomy underlying these models: individual, relational, and family autonomy. In the third section, we discuss some ethical issues derived from presumed consent and family veto.

2.   Consent Models for Organ Procurement

There are three main kinds of systems for deceased organ procurement (OP): altruistic, commercial, and compulsory. *Altruistic* systems are the most common worldwide, based on the idea that organ donation is a free gift that relies upon individual autonomy. *Commercial* or *market-based* systems are based on incentives (financial or not) and on the idea that organs are commodities subject to supply and demand. Finally, *compulsory* systems do not depend on the individual's autonomous decision to donate or to sell their organs but on national or local regulations. Compulsory systems can take two opposite forms: conscription (or confiscation), under which OP is mandatory; and prohibition, under which OP is illegal. In the following, we will only focus on altruistic and compulsory systems.

Altruistic models of consent for deceased OP can be classified according to the relative authority they grant to three main variables: (1) the preferences expressed by the deceased, if any; (2) the preferences expressed by the family, if any; and (3) the default policy when no preference has been expressed by either the deceased or the family (Delgado et al. 2019).[1]

2.1   Definition of Terms

2.1.1   Preferences of the Deceased
Individuals can either consent or refuse to donate their organs after death. 'Consent' is understood here as explicit permission granted by the deceased to the removal of his or her organs, while 'refusal' is an explicit objection by the deceased. We consider that the absence of an expressed refusal is not equivalent to the deceased's consent, and the absence of expressed consent is not equivalent to the deceased's refusal. In some countries, individuals also have the option to request a proxy or surrogate to make the decision on their behalf after they die.

---

1 Several other variables could have been taken into account, but they would have excessively complicated an already complex picture. For instance: the decisional capacity of the medical, legal or religious authorities; the role of community leaders; procedures to express preferences; incentives (e.g. prioritization in the waiting list of recipients, monetary rewards for survivors); directed post-mortem donation (e.g. family-oriented priority).

2.1.2 Role of the Family

The family[2] may be allowed to intervene in three incremental ways in the decision-making process:

1. *As a witness of the deceased's preferences*: The family can obtain and record the deceased's most recent expressions of consent or refusal and communicate them to the medical team.
2. *As a surrogate of the deceased*: The family can be allowed to decide on OP when the deceased has not. Depending on the default policy, they can *authorize* or *oppose* the removal, and their decision can be based either on their own views or on what they speculate the deceased may have wished.
3. *As the final decision-maker*: The family can be allowed to make the final decision on OP despite and against the wishes of the deceased. They can: a) *overrule* the deceased's *consent* by blocking (vetoing) the removal of organs, or b) *overrule* the deceased's *refusal* by allowing the doctors to proceed.

In some jurisdictions, the family may not be allowed to intervene at all in OP decision-making. Although they might be kept informed about what is going to be done with the organs, they are not consulted.

2.1.3 Default Policy

Organ procurement policies can be defined by the default option that applies when the deceased's wishes are unknown to the medical team. Opt-out policies allow organs to be automatically removed under such circumstances, while opt-in policies forbid it. A third option, known as 'mandatory choice', requires by law that all adults express their decision while executing state-regulated tasks, such as registering for a driver's license or applying for a renewal of their ID card.[3]

2.2 Clarifying the Complexity of Systems

The labels 'soft' and 'hard' are sometimes used in the literature to characterize opt-in and opt-out policies depending on whether or not families are involved in the decision-making process (cf. Rithalia et al. 2009a; Shepherd et al. 2013; Etheredge et al. 2018). However, these categories are unable to account for the complexity of a family's range of possible actions in different circumstances, and they may create more confusion.

For example, according to their laws Austria and Spain can both be called 'hard opt-out' countries, but their systems are actually quite dissimilar. In Spain, because there is no register of refusals, physicians are required by law to ask relatives about the

---

2   We use the word "family" throughout to refer to those involved in discussing OP with health care professionals: relatives, next-of-kin, and friends of the deceased, who may have different knowledge and opinions regarding both the patient's donation preferences and OP in general, and who may disagree about what the deceased would have wanted, and whether to obey his or her wishes. In some countries, such as the UK and Chile, the decision-making person within the family is determined by law according to a hierarchical list of relatives.

3   To our knowledge, New Zealand is the only country worldwide to implement a true mandatory choice system.

deceased's preferences. In addition, physicians are required by practical guidelines to ask for an authorization from the family to proceed with organ removal. In Austria, by contrast, individuals can register their refusal to donate, and relatives have no legal role whatsoever. In practice, the situation is less clear, and physicians may or may not consider the wishes of the family.

Decea-sed's wishes	Model of consent	Role of the family			
		No role (L0)	Witness (L1)	Surrogate (L2)	Full decisional authority (L3)
Unknown	Opt-out	—	Can *inform* about the deceased's wishes	Can oppose OP*	Can oppose OP*
	Opt-in	—	Can *inform* about the deceased's wishes	Can authorize OP*	Can authorize OP*
Consent	Opt-in, Opt-out	—	Can *update* the deceased's wishes	Can *update* the deceased's wishes	Can overrule consent
Refusal	Opt-in, Opt-out	—	Can *update* the deceased's wishes	Can *update* the deceased's wishes	Can overrule refusal**

Table 1: Levels of involvement of the family by columns in increasing order. Each level specifies what relatives can do under three different situations ordered by rows: when the medical team does not know the wishes of the deceased ("Unknown"), when the deceased had explicitly consented to becoming a donor ("Consent"), and when the deceased had explicitly objected to becoming a donor ("Refusal"). The table also takes into account the model of consent (opt-in, opt-out), although this variable is relevant only when the deceased's wishes are unknown. Source: Delgado et al. (2019).
* The family can be asked to make a decision either on behalf of the deceased or according to their own views.
** This option is theoretically possible but unlikely in practice.

For clarification and standardization purposes, we have proposed a simple but comprehensive framework that systematically categorizes the role of the family in relation to the deceased's preferences and the systems' default policy (Delgado et al. 2019).

Table 1 shows four possible incremental levels of family involvement. Each level includes actions families can do, depending on the deceased's wishes and the default system:

1. At the lowest level (L0, *no role*), the family has no involvement whatsoever. They may be informed about what will happen to their loved one's organs, but they are not consulted.
2. At the next level (L1, *witness*), relatives are considered as mere witnesses of the deceased's preferences. They may be asked for information about the deceased's last wishes, if any, but they are not allowed to make any decision on their own.

3. At the subsequent level (L2, *surrogate*), in addition to being witnesses, relatives may be allowed to make a decision *if the deceased has not*. This decision may be made on behalf of the deceased or according to their own views. At this level of involvement, the family can overrule the system's default, but not the deceased's wishes.

4. At the highest level (L3, *full decisional authority*), the family may be granted a full decisional capacity, even when the deceased had expressed a preference. They may be allowed to overrule the deceased's decision and, therefore, be given the last word regarding OP.

2.3   Taxonomy of Consent Models

Building on Table 1, we propose a comprehensive and fine-grained taxonomy of all justifiable models of consent, either actual or theoretical, that take into account the three variables: the deceased's preferences, family preferences, and the default policy. This taxonomy results in the following ten categories (Table 2, Fig. 1):

#	Model	Description	Default	
			a (opt-out)	**b** (opt-in)
1	Deceased's wishes only	If the deceased expressed a preference, it is respected; otherwise, the default policy applies. The family may or may not be allowed to inform/update the medical team about the wishes of the deceased, but they cannot decide under any circumstance.	**1a.** Organs procured, unless the deceased had refused OP.	**1b.** Organs *not* procured, unless the deceased had consented to OP.
2	Deceased's wishes mostly	If only the deceased expressed a preference, it is respected; if only the family expresses a preference (the deceased did not), it is also respected; if both have expressed a preference, the deceased's prevails; and if neither party has expressed a preference, the default policy applies.	**2a.** Organs procured, unless the deceased refused OP or, if the deceased's wishes are unknown, when the family opposes OP.	**2b.** Organs *not* procured, unless the deceased consented to OP, or if the deceased's wishes are unknown, when the family authorizes OP.
3	Deceased's wishes or agreement	If the deceased expressed a preference, it is respected, unless the family disagrees; in that case and all other cases, the default policy applies.	**3a.** Organs procured, unless the deceased refused OP AND the family either opposes OP or expresses no preference.	**3b.** Organs *not* procured, unless the deceased consented to OP AND the family either authorizes OP or expresses no preference.
4	Agreement only	If both the deceased and the family agree, their shared preference is respected. In all other cases, the default policy applies.	**4a.** Organs procured, unless the deceased refused OP AND family opposes OP.	**4b.** Organs *not* procured, unless the deceased consented to OP AND the family authorizes OP.

#	Model	Description	Default	
5	Family wishes or agreement	If the family has expressed a preference, it is respected, unless it contradicts the deceased's expressed preferences; in that case and all other cases, the default policy applies.	**5a.** Organs procured, unless the family opposes OP AND the deceased had either also refused OP or had expressed no preference.	**5b.** Organs *not* procured, unless the family authorizes OP AND the deceased either had also consented to OP or had expressed no preference.
6	Family wishes mostly	If only the deceased expressed a preference, it is respected; if only the family has expressed a preference (the deceased did not), it is also respected; when both have expressed a preference, the family's prevails; and when neither party have expressed a preference, the default policy applies.	**6a.** Organs procured, unless the family opposes OP or, if the family wishes are unknown, when the deceased had refused OP	**6b.** Organs *not* procured, unless the family authorizes OP or, if family wishes are unknown, when the deceased had consented to OP
7	Family wishes only	If the family has expressed a preference, it is respected; otherwise, the default policy applies.	**7a.** Organs procured, unless the family opposes OP	**7b.** Organs *not* procured, unless the family authorizes OP
8	Refusal prevails	If only the deceased expressed a preference, it is respected; if only the family has expressed a preference (the deceased did not), it is also respected; and when the deceased and the family have conflicting preferences, refusal/opposition (whoever has expressed it) prevails.	**8a.** Organs procured, unless the deceased had refused OP and/or the family opposes OP	**8b.** Organs *not* procured, unless the deceased and the family both agreed with OP, or at least one has consented or authorized OP while the other party has expressed no preference.
9	Consent prevails	If only the deceased expressed a preference, it is respected; If only the family has expressed a preference (the deceased did not), it is also respected; if the deceased and the family have conflicting preferences, consent/authorization (whoever has expressed it) prevails.	**9a.** Organs procured, unless the deceased and the family both objected to OP, or at least one has refused or opposed OP while the other party has expressed no preference.	**9b.** Organs *not* procured, unless the deceased consented OP and/or the family authorizes OP.
10	Default only	The default policy always applies, irrespective of the deceased's and the family's preferences.	**10a.** Organs always procured	**10b.** Organs never procured

Table 2: Taxonomy of models of consent for organ procurement according to three variables: (1) deceased's wishes, if any; (2) family wishes, if any; and (3) default policies. Several of these models (3a, 4, 5, 7, 9, 10a) are theoretically possible but may not have been implemented so far.

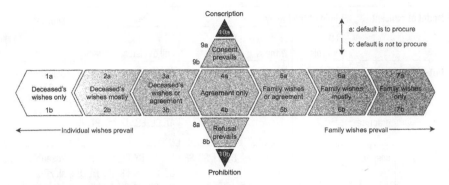

Fig. 1. Consent models for organ procurement organized in a cross diagram. On the horizontal scale, models that prioritize the wishes of the deceased on the left (#1 to #3) or those of the family on the right (#5 to #7). On the vertical scale, models that do not prioritize one party over the other but favor the objection to OP (#9a, #8b), whoever it comes from, over consent or authorization (#8a, #8b). On the edges of the vertical line are two models that do not take any preferences into account: organ conscription (#10a) and prohibition (#10b). At the center of the cross are the two models (#4a, #4b) that do not prioritize one party nor one decision over the other

2.4   Distribution of Consent Models around the World

Descriptive information regarding the existing policies for OP around the world is scarce, incomplete, and quickly outdated, because countries change their legislation from time to time. Additionally, there are differences between law and practice (Delgado et al. 2019). For instance, under Australian *law* (opt-in), prior consent by the deceased person is sufficient to authorize organ recovery. However, according to Government's Guidelines for Ethical Practice, the deceased's family needs also to be consulted and its agreement sought (National Health and Medical Research Council 2007).

Comparative international studies (Gimbel et al. 2003; Gevers et al. 2004; Bagheri 2005; Abadie/Gay 2006; Rithalia et al. 2009a; Horvat et al. 2010) often include incomplete information on the role of the family within a given nation, making it impossible to classify consent models according to the taxonomy above (Table 2). The most comprehensive data available to date regarding the level of involvement of the family in OP is summarized in Table 3.

Model of consent		Role of the family				Source[a]
		L0 No role	L1 Witness	L2 Surrogate	L3 Full decisional capacity	
Opt-out	law	AR, AT, PT, UY	BE, CL, ES, FR, SG, WA	SE, NO	JP	Delgado et al. 2019
	practice			BE, FR, SE, SG	AT, CL, ES, JP, NO, PT, WA	
	unspec.			BE, FI, SG, SE	AM, AT, BY, CL, CO, CR, CZ, EC, ES, FR, HR, IT, LU, NO, PL, PY, RU, SI, SK, TN, TR	Rosenblum et al. 2012
	unspec.	AT, CZ, LU		GR, PT, SK	BE, ES, FI, FR, HR, HU, IT, NO, PO, SE, SI	Bilgel et al. 2012
Opt-in	law			AU, CA, DE, NL[a], UK[a], USA	IN	Delgado et al. 2019
	practice			DE	AU, CA, IN, NL[a], UK[a], USA	
	unspec.			NL, RO, UK, USA	AU, BR, CA, CH, CU, DE, DK, EE, IE, IL, IN, IS, JP, KR, KW, LT, MT, MX, MY, NZ, PH, SA, TH, VE, ZA	Rosenblum et al. 2012
	unspec.	CA			AU, CH, DE, DK, IE, IL, NL, NZ, UK, USA	Bilgel et al. 2012

Table 3: Role of the family in several opt-out and opt-in countries according to three independent sources. Delgado et al. (2019) differentiates family's involvement according to the law and in clinical practice. The other two sources are not specific enough about this difference.

[a] *Data from Delgado et al. (2019) has been completed and updated for this chapter. Data from the two other sources may be outdated.*

[b] *The Netherlands, England and Scotland have implemented opt-out systems by 2020.*

Legend: AM: Armenia; AR: Argentina; AT: Austria; AU: Australia; BE: Belgium; BR: Brazil; BY: Belarus; CA: Canada; CH: Switzerland; CL: Chile; CO: Colombia; CR: Costa Rica; CU: Cuba; CZ: Czech Republic; DE: Germany; DK: Denmark; EC: Ecuador; EE: Estonia; ES: Spain; FI: Finland, FR: France; HR: Croatia; HU: Hungary; IE: Ireland; IL: Israel; IN: India; IS: Iceland; IT: Italy; JP: Japan; KR: South Korea; KW: Kuwait; LT: Lithuania; LU: Luxemburg; MT: Malta; MX: Mexico; MY: Malaysia; NL: The Netherlands; NO: Norway; NZ: New Zealand; PH: Philippines; PL: Poland; PT: Portugal; PY: Paraguay; RO: Romania; RU: Russia; SA: Saudi Arabia; SE: Sweden; SG: Singapore; SI: Slovenia; SK: Slovakia; TH: Thailand; TN: Tunisia; TR: Turkey; UK: United Kingdom (Wales excepted); USA: United States of America; UY: Uruguay; VE: Venezuela; WA: Wales; ZA: South Africa.

Each country's policy could be more accurately classified if enough information was available. Here are some examples: Germany's legal policy for OP corresponds to the consent model #2b ("Deceased's preferences mostly"); it is an opt-in model where the wishes of the deceased are always respected, and where the family can make a decision if the deceased did not. Wales' legal policy is similar to Germany's but operates under presumed consent, thus being classified as #2a. Spain's legal policy corresponds to model #1a ("Deceased's preferences only") because the family is legally granted a witness role. However, according to clinical guidelines, it operates in practice as model #8a ("Refusal prevails"), because refusals are always respected, whomever they come from – the deceased or the family – and they prevail over the other party's explicit consent or authorization (Caballero/Matesanz 2015).

Failing to understand these nuances not only leads to confusion but can also result in misconceptions on the part of transplant policymakers. For instance, in countries where the family has full decisional capacity, moving to opt-out might be ineffective. By focusing on changes from opt-in to opt-out, policymakers may be overestimating the limited effect of the consent system, and underestimating the importance of the family.

3.   Concepts of Autonomy Underlying the Consent Models

Consent in medicine is both an ethical requirement and a legal concept. Individual consent is a key element of the Nuremberg Code (1947) and the Declaration of Helsinki (1964) that established ethical principles for protecting human subjects from clinical research malpractice. The term 'informed consent' in the context of medical care emerged in the USA in the 1950s through court decisions (Beauchamp 2011). As a legal tool present now in most jurisdictions, informed consent has the role of protecting a patient's rights, and also protecting medical practitioners from liability in case of harm to the patient.

In the context of deceased OP, the notion of consent should be used with some caveats, because deceased individuals are not patients, and the removal of their organs cannot cause them any sort of physical or psychological harm. Therefore, consent for organ procurement may be interpreted differently than informed consent for medical care or clinical research. This is the case in opt-out countries, where organs can be lawfully procured from a deceased individual without any evidence of informed and voluntary consent from that individual while alive.

In most countries, both opt-in and opt-out, individual consent for OP is neither necessary nor sufficient, and the family's decision may be more consequential than the deceased's preferences. To make sense of this, we propose to show how different models of consent may rely on different concepts of autonomy beyond the individual. Models #1 to #9 (Table 2, Fig. 1) may indeed be accounted for by a continuum of three forms of autonomy: individual autonomy, relational autonomy, and family autonomy. This proposal does not preclude other possible interpretations.

3.1   Individual Autonomy

The principle of autonomy in biomedical ethics (Beauchamp/Childress 1979) can be traced back to the moral philosophies of Immanuel Kant (1724–1804) and John Stuart Mill (1806–1873). For Kant, autonomy should not only be understood as the possibility of choosing between one option or the other, but also as the capacity and even the obligation to know for ourselves, as rational agents, what we should do. This means that our choices and actions must obey self-imposed norms dictated solely by our rationality, without influence from social and moral conventions, or from political, legal, and religious authority, or even from our own inclinations and desires (Kant 1785).

By contrast, Mill considers that individuals are autonomous when their choices and actions rely on their personal values, desires, and inclinations. For Mill, personal freedom is the absence of impositions and external interventions. Hence, paternalism should be limited to situations in which it is clearly justified: "the only purpose for which power can be rightfully exercised over any member of a civilised community, against his will, is to prevent harm to others. His own good, either physical or moral, is not a sufficient warrant [...]. Over himself, over his own body and mind, the individual is sovereign" (Mill 1856: 13).

Individual autonomy in liberal bioethics reflects Mill's understanding of the individual's freedom to develop his or her own life according to personal choices, without any kind of undue interference from others (Charlesworth 1993). Nobody else's preferences, including those of health care professionals and relatives, should prevail over the preferences of a patient. Hence, any intervention by the family or others could be interpreted as a disruption of individual autonomy.

In the context of OP, the requirement of consent, either explicit (opt-in) or presumed (opt-out), would somehow imply that individual autonomy should be respected after the individual's death. The fact that the organ donor is dead raises doubts about the applicability of this interpretation of freedom to this context. A proper analysis would need to address the topic of the legal and moral existence of posthumous rights and interests (cf. Sperling 2008). This important topic is however quite speculative and falls beyond the scope of this chapter.

Assuming that an individual's interests and rights survive after death, individual autonomy would be respected, according to our classification, in consent models where the deceased person is the sole decision-maker. This corresponds to the first column (L0) in Table 1, and to models #1a and #1b ('Deceased's preferences only') described in Table 2.

3.2   Relational Autonomy

Individual autonomy is supported by the individualistic paradigm: the idea that people are independent, self-interested and rational decision-makers. In the context of Feminist Theory, the term of *relational autonomy* has emerged to better explain the fact that people's autonomy, needs, and interests are shaped by their relations to others (Dove et al. 2017; Delgado 2019). We contend that, in the context of organ procurement, relational autonomy can better account for the connection between individual choice and family decisions as guardians of the deceased´s beliefs and values.

Over the last decades, an increasing amount of literature in Bioethics advocates that human beings are socially embedded and that, consequently, personal decisions take place in a context of social relationships (Nedelsky 1989; Mackenzie/Stoljar 2000; Rogers et al. 2012; Mackenzie et al. 2014; Straehle 2017). Relationships, responsibility, care and interdependence are key attributes of relational autonomy, for "people develop their sense of self and form capacities and life plans through the relationships they forge on a daily and long-term basis" (Dove et al. 2017: 153).

Relational autonomy does not reject the notion of the self but reflects on how individuals develop the capacity to make autonomous decisions with the support of family and friends (Herrings 2014). The development of the capacity of autonomy requires an appropriate environment to make it possible. This requires a change in our understanding of rights, shifting the attention from the protection from the interference of others towards the construction of relations which nurture autonomous decisions (Nedelsky 1993, 2011). What really makes autonomy possible is not separation from others but relationships with others (Nedelsky 1989). Relational autonomy is not seen as a static attribute but as a capacity that is continuously developing throughout our lives. What makes it possible is the context of social relations that supports it (ibid.). In the clinical context, the development of this capacity requires the contribution of health care professionals (Delgado 2019).

Some critics of the concept of relational autonomy acknowledge that autonomy is socially constituted, but they argue that the influences of the social environment on the individual patient are too unpredictable to be considered by health care professionals. Furthermore, they raise the concern that prioritizing the decisions of other people over those of the patient, in the name of promoting the conditions that improve autonomy, can be a form of paternalism (Wardrope 2015).

In this chapter we assume that people need the support of others to make autonomous decisions and, ultimately, to fulfil their autonomy. As such, relational autonomy supports the claim that consensus between the patient and the family is a sign of autonomous decisions. In our classification, this understanding of autonomy underlies all models where relatives participate in the decision-making process – models #3 to #5, as well as #8 and #9 (see Table 2) – provided that they do not contradict the preferences of their loved ones. When they contradict each other, neither of them prevails over the other, and the decision to procure or not depends on the system's architecture (the default option established by opt-in or opt-out).

Model #3 ('Deceased's preferences or agreement') requires consensus, but the wishes of the deceased are respected and suffice when the family has not expressed any preference. To the extent that family preferences are taken into account, we cannot consider it as a purely individual autonomy system.

Model #4 ('Agreement only') requires consensus, which means that neither the deceased nor the family can decide alone. One of the aspects that underlies OP decision-making is the communication that has previously taken place between the deceased and the family about their preferences. In this regard, this is the model that best represents relational autonomy in the context of OP.

Model #5 ('Family preferences or agreement') requires consensus, although the wishes of the family are respected when the deceased failed to express his or her preferences.

Models #8 ('Refusal prevails') and #9 ('Consent prevails') require consensus too, but both deceased and family may decide alone when the other party has not.

3.3   Family Autonomy

Families come in different shapes and sizes. In the context of health care and OP, the family can be understood as a 'collective actor' with 'collective autonomy' (Beier et al. 2016). The expression *family autonomy*, developed in American Law, refers to the assumption that a family unit should be governed by the private decisions of some or all of its members (McMullen 1992). Ann Elliot (2001) argues that in the family-centred model of care it is the sole responsibility of the family to hear bad news about a patient's diagnosis and prognosis and to make decisions regarding care and treatment, and what or whether the patient should be told. This model is related to some cultural and health care aspects in which individual autonomy is viewed as a reflection of isolation and burdensome to patients who are too sick to make meaningful decisions.

The notion of family autonomy has also been developed by East Asian bioethics. According to Ruiping Fan (1997), the East Asian principle of autonomy requires family-determination, presupposes an objective conception of the good, and upholds the value of harmonious dependence of the individual upon his or her family. This means that the family itself is an autonomous social unit, and that, although both the patient and family members must reach an agreement before a clinical decision can be made, it is the family that has the final authority to make clinical decisions in accordance with this principle.

In our classification, this concept of autonomy corresponds to consent models where the family is the sole decision-maker. This corresponds to the fourth column (L3) in Table 1, and to models #7a and #7b ('Family preferences only') described in Table 2.

3.4   Mixed Types of Autonomy

Some models take into account the preferences of both the deceased and their family, but they eventually give priority to one party over the other in case of contradiction. Models #2 and #6 are transitional models that represent the pathway from individual autonomy (#1) to relational autonomy (#3, 4, 5, 8, 9), and from relational autonomy to family autonomy (#7).

Model #2 ('Deceased's preferences mostly') respects the deceased's preferences and allows the family to decide when the deceased has not. Both deceased and family may decide alone, but the deceased's preferences prevail in case of conflict. A system based on individual autonomy alone would not allow the family to decide. At the same time, it may be supposed that the decision of the family represents the wishes of the deceased.

Model #6 ('Family preferences mostly') is symmetrical to model #2. It allows both deceased and family to decide alone (when the other party has not), but relatives have the final say in case of conflict.

3.5   Models in Which Autonomy Plays No Role

Organ procurement policies may disregard autonomy entirely. In our classification, model #10a ('Default only') corresponds to theoretical policies in which deceased OP would be mandatory. For example, a system of *organ conscription* would require organs to be automatically procured from every person who dies under the circumstances enabling organ transplantation, regardless of people's (the deceased and family) objections. Some have argued that such system would save lives by increasing the number of transplants (Hershenov/Delaney 2009) without thereby violating the autonomy of the deceased or harming their interests, because a person's autonomy is lost after death and the concept of posthumous harm is a fallacy (Spital/Taylor 2007). This system would still violate family autonomy.

Model #10b ('Default only') corresponds to policies in which cadaveric OP is forbidden or not legally permitted for some reason, including the absence of organ transplantation programs in the country. This is the case of several Islamic countries of sub-Saharan Africa (Ghods 2015).

4.   Ethical Issues

Transplantation policymaking seeks to govern competing interests in ways that foster the interests of patients on the waiting list while minimally compromising the interests of potential donors and their relatives. These trade-offs need to be made without upsetting the public, whose trust in the organ procurement and transplantation system is essential for achieving high organ donation rates (Rodríguez-Arias 2018). Yet, these trade-offs are ethically challenging and may be negatively perceived by one party or the other.

For example, allowing the family to overrule the deceased's wishes to donate may prevent litigation and bad publicity, and thus help preserve people's trust in the organ procurement system. However, this implies violating freedom of choice and respect for individual autonomy, which is a central value our modern societies cherish. Paradoxically, open violations of such a core value could easily undermine the very trust policymaking intends to protect.

This poses a strategic dilemma: should morally contentious policies be disclosed to, discussed with, and deliberated on by the public, or should they be kept in the relative concealment of political and academic debates? That is, do openness and transparency contribute to or threaten public trust? (Racine et al. 2015)

This could also be seen as a dilemma between short-term vs long-term benefits. On the one hand, full information about the model of consent and the role families play may result in fewer donors in the short term but increased donation rates in the long term due to the perception that the system is honest and trustworthy. Indeed, the public perception of transparency seems to be related to higher willingness to donate organs (Boulware et al. 2007). On the other hand, lack of communication about specific policy choices may result in more donors in the short term but can also be a breeding ground for scandals and decreased donation rates in the future. As Dan Brock (1987, 1999) brilliantly put it, bioethics scholarship and bioethics policymaking, especially in the field of organ transplantation, often rest on a choice between truth and consequences.

These notions seem to be particularly relevant for two ethically challenging policy choices: presumed consent and family veto. Any decision made on these issues may result in higher or lower donation rates, and be more or less respectful for individual or family autonomy. We will show in the next paragraphs that compelling moral arguments have been made in favour and against each option. Our own general position is that the ethical acceptability of any organ procurement policy should not be assessed in isolation from its efficacy, its social acceptability, and the transparency of the means they employ.

4.1   Presuming Consent

Policy changes towards presumed consent (opt-out) seek to increase donation rates by widening the pool of donors and by removing one of the main obstacles to OP, namely people's bias to choose the status quo – their tendency to stick with the current state of affairs or choose default options (Mackay/Robinson 2016; see also chapter 3 in this book). Opt-out policies are intended to act as a nudge: a way of designing the choice architecture that "alters people's behaviour in a predictable way without forbidding any options or significantly changing their economic incentives" (Thaler/Sunstein 2008: 6).

Even though nudges are a form of manipulation, opt-out advocates insist that they preserve people's autonomy, because individuals can still consent or refuse to donate their organs by expressing their wish. In addition, since most people, when asked, express a willingness to donate, the presumption in favour of donation is more likely to honour the autonomy of the deceased person than a presumption against (Cohen 1992; English/Sommerville 2003).

To be sure, the risk exists that surgeons could remove organs from the bodies of people who did not want their organs removed (Cantrell 2019). However, some would argue that it is morally no worse than *not* removing organs from people who wanted them removed (Gill 2004). On the contrary, mistaken presumptions of consent can save and improve the lives of many organ recipients, while mistaken presumptions of refusal cannot. Besides, opt-out systems may produce fewer mistakes than opt-in systems if objectors are more likely to register their opposition than supporters are to sign up as donors (Gill 2004).

Opt-out advocates also claim that it is morally permissible to use the organs of someone who did not opt out, because they have by their silence actually consented (Saunders 2011). However, proper consent requires that the consenting person is at least aware of the consequences of both expressing and not expressing a preference (Rodríguez-Arias/Morgan 2016). Consistently, opt-out advocates emphasize two essential conditions for its ethical acceptability: it must be clearly communicated to all involved that this is how their silence will be interpreted, and it must be possible for people to opt out without facing unreasonable costs for doing so (Saunders 2011). In other words, everybody must be aware of, and understand, the opt-out system, and they must be given a genuine opportunity to object (English/Sommerville 2003). Therefore, widespread public information campaigns should target sections of society that are hard to reach, and mechanisms must be in place to ensure all members of the public are informed of their choices and can register an objection quickly and easily (Hamm/Tizzard 2008; see also chapter 4 in this book).

Are these conditions fulfilled in practice? Empirical evidence suggests that they are usually not. On the one hand, people's awareness of the consent model in their own country, as well as people's knowledge of the procedures to express their preferences regarding OP is much lower in opt-out countries than in opt-in countries (Molina-Pérez et al. 2018). On the other hand, some opt-out countries, including Croatia, Norway and Spain, do not have refusal registries or a standard card enabling people to refuse to donate, making it more difficult for individuals to choose against the default status quo (Rodríguez-Arias/Morgan 2016).

Regarding effectiveness, the relative impact of consent policies on organ donation rates remains controversial. Some have argued that opt-out laws lead straight to larger pools of organs for transplantation (Mossialos et al. 2008; Bendorf et al. 2013; Shepherd et al. 2014; Ugur 2015), while others dispute this claim (Coppen et al. 2008; Bilgel 2012; Fabre et al. 2010; Boyarsky et al. 2012; Arshad 2019). Part of the difficulty resides in the fact that this model has rarely been implemented in isolation from other strategies aimed at fostering OP. One systematic review concluded that, while opt-out policies seem to be associated with increased organ donation rates,

> "it cannot be inferred from this that the introduction of presumed consent legislation per se will lead to an increase in organ donation rates. The availability of potential donors, the underpinning infrastructure for transplantation, wealth and investment in health care, and underlying public attitudes may all have a role" (Rithalia et al. 2009b: 7).

4.2   Family Veto

In most opt-in and opt-out countries, organs cannot be procured without family authorization, even when the deceased explicitly consented (Delgado et al. 2019; Rosenblum et al. 2012). We have suggested that a relational autonomy approach may justify honouring family preferences in the absence of any wish expressed by the deceased (but not when the family opposes the explicit preferences of the deceased). Individual autonomy does not suffice, but relational autonomy applies when there is no contradiction between family and the deceased´s preferences. Family veto to OP can only be justified by absolutely embracing the family autonomy model, at the cost of individual autonomy.

Arguments in support of family veto capacity include the following: (1) it reduces family distress (while the deceased cannot be harmed and holds no relevant interest anymore); (2) it reduces health professionals' stress; (3) it preserves family and public trust by reducing conflict and scandal; (4) it ensures long-term OP rates (as a consequence of 3); (5) families need to cooperate for donation to take place; and (6) families might have evidence regarding refusal (Wilkinson 2005; Shaw 2017).

Arguments against family veto include the following: (1) it violates the deceased's wishes; (2) it reduces organ supply and costs lives; (3) it discourages people from registering as donors, because they know their family may eventually overrule their wishes anyway; and (4) families will regret the decision, resulting in more complicated grief[4] (Cronin 2005; Shaw 2017).

Importantly, in cases of disagreement between the preferences of the deceased and those of their families, family *opposition* seems to be more stringent than family *acceptance* of OP. In other words, family autonomy, *when expressed via opposition*, prevails over the deceased's consent and the collective good represented by the interests of patients on the waiting list. However, *when expressed via a request for organs to be procured*, it does not. Similarly, while the deceased's *consent* does not guarantee compliance, their *refusal* is commonly considered sufficient to preclude OP.[5] Consequently, the deceased's refusal prevails over family preferences (to donate) and over recipients' interests.

An insight that follows from this analysis is that it is wrong to assume that, in cases where the individual and the family disagree among each other, respect for the autonomy of one party always prevails over respect for the autonomy of the other. In fact, this depends on the nature of such preferences. Martin Wilkinson accurately described the position of the UK and New Zealand on consent for OP as a 'double veto', in which each party has the power to withhold and override the other's desire to donate (Wilkinson 2005). However, in case of conflict, our taxonomy shows that models #3, #4, #5, #8 and #9 privilege one decision (to procure or not to procure) over the other, regardless of whether it is expressed by the deceased or by the family (Table 2 and Fig. 1). In other words, *objections* often prevail over *requests*, whoever they come from. This policy might find some theoretical grounding in a liberal bioethics tradition in which negative rights expressed through refusals are deemed more compelling than positive rights expressed via individual requests (Feinberg 1973; Gert et al. 1998).

This conclusion leads to an annoying question: If the deceased's consent to OP is virtually irrelevant (because it is commonly ignored when the family holds a different view), why is it required for deceased donation in the first place? Does the ethical acceptability of OP really require individual consent? Some might argue that the surgical removal of organs from the deceased actually does not require their consent (Emson 2003). At the end of the day, the deceased cannot be physically or psychologically harmed or wronged by organ removal because they no longer exist as persons. When compared with the common good and the public interest, any residual posthumous interest of the terminally ill or already-dead individuals who are candidates for OP fade (Harris 2003). Ultimately, this reasoning leads to a justification of organ conscription described by model #10a (Hershenov/Delaney 2009).

---

4 To the best of our knowledge, this last claim has never been empirically substantiated.

5 In Spain, a study on the effectiveness of targeted communication strategies to reverse family refusals by transplant coordinators shows that more than 40% of all family oppositions were attributed to and categorized by the authors as a "presumed refusal by the deceased". Among those, 25% could be reversed." (Gómez et al. 2001: 63, table 2).

5.   Conclusions

This systematic analysis of the different theoretical and practical models of consent points out the insufficiency of the distinction between opt-in and opt-out systems. We hope the taxonomy that we have provided constitutes a useful tool for researchers, policymakers and clinicians to understand current policy options and their clinical implications. Our analysis of the models of autonomy underlying each consent model may increase our understanding of the complex relationships between individual wishes, family preferences, and the interests of the recipients. Both clarifying the taxonomy of consent models and analysing the models of autonomy can underpin a proper discussion of the ethical problems that arise in the context of OP policymaking.

Acknowledgements

The authors would like to thank two anonymous reviewers, as well as the editors of this volume, for their useful comments. This research was supported by a postdoctoral fellowship from the Spanish Government (FJCI-2017-34286). It was conducted as part of Project INEDyTO [Investigation on the Ethics of Organ Donation and Transplantation], funded by the Spanish Government (MINECO FFI2017-88913-P).

References

Abadie, Alberto/Gay, Sebastien (2006): "The Impact of Presumed Consent Legislation on Cadaveric Organ Donation: A Cross-Country Study." In: Journal of Health Economics 25/4, pp. 599–620.

Arshad, Adam/Anderson, Benjamin/Sharif, Adnan (2019): "Comparison of Organ Donation and Transplantation Rates Between Opt-out and Opt-in Systems." In: Kidney International 95/6, pp. 1453–1460.

Bagheri, Alireza (2005): "Organ Transplantation Laws in Asian Countries: A Comparative Study." In: Transplantation Proceedings 37/10, pp. 4159–4162.

Beauchamp, Tom (2011): "Informed Consent: Its History, Meaning, and Present Challenges." In: Cambridge Quarterly of Healthcare Ethics 20/4, pp. 515–523.

Beauchamp, Tom/Childress, James (1979): Principles of Biomedical Ethics, New York: Oxford University Press.

Beier, Katharina/Jordan, Isabella/Wiesemann, Claudia/Schicktanz, Silke (2016): "Understanding Collective Agency in Bioethics." In: Medicine, Health Care and Philosophy 19/3, pp. 411–422.

Bendorf, Aric/Pussell, Bruce/Kelly, Patrick/Kerridge, Ian H. (2013): "Socioeconomic, Demographic and Policy Comparisons of Living and Deceased Kidney Transplantation Rates Across 53 Countries." In: Nephrology 18/9, pp. 633–640.

Bilgel, Fırat (2012): "The Impact of Presumed Consent Laws and Institutions on Deceased Organ Donation." In: The European Journal of Health Economics 13/1, pp. 29–38.

Boulware, L. Ebony/Troll, Misty U./Wang, Nae-Yuh/Powe, Neil R. (2007): "Perceived Transparency and Fairness of the Organ Allocation System and Willingness to

Donate Organs: A National Study." In: American Journal of Transplantation 7/7, pp. 1778–1787.

Boyarsky, Brian/Hall, Erin/Deshpande, Neha/Ros, R. Lorie/Montgomery, Robert/Steinwachs, Donald/Segev, Dorry (2012): "Potential Limitations of Presumed Consent Legislation." In: Transplantation 93/2, pp. 136–140.

Brock, Dan (1987): "Truth or Consequences: The Role of Philosophers in Policy-making." In: Ethics 97/4, pp. 786–791.

Brock, Dan (1999): "The Role of the Public in Public Policy on the Definition of Death." In: Stuart J. Youngner/Robert M. Arnold/Renie Schapiro (eds.), The Definition of Death: Contemporary Controversies, Baltimore: Johns Hopkins University Press, pp. 293–308.

Caballero, Francisco/Matesanz, Rafael (2015): Manual de Donación y Trasplante de Órganos Humanos, Madrid: Ministerio de Sanidad, Servicios Sociales e Igualdad.

Cantrell, Tobias (2019): "The 'Opt-out' Approach to Deceased Organ Donation in England: A Misconceived Policy Which May Precipitate Moral Harm." In: Clinical Ethics 14/2, pp. 63–69.

Charlesworth, Max (1993): Bioethics in a Liberal Society, Cambridge: Cambridge University Press.

Cohen, C. (1992): "The Case for Presumed Consent to Transplant Human Organs after Death." In: Transplantation Proceedings 24/5, pp. 2168–2172.

Coppen, Remco/Friele, Roland/Gevers, Sjef/Blok, Geke A./Zee, Jouke van der (2008): "The Impact of Donor Policies in Europe: A Steady Increase, but Not Everywhere." In: BMC Health Services Research 8/1, pp. 235.

Cronin, Antonia (2007): "Transplants Save Lives, Defending the Double Veto Does Not: A Reply to Wilkinson." In: Journal of Medical Ethics 33/4, pp. 219–220.

Delgado, Janet (2019) "Re-thinking Relational Autonomy: Challenging the Triumph of Autonomy through Vulnerability". In: Bioethics Update 5/1, pp. 50–65.

Delgado, Janet/Molina-Pérez, Alberto/Shaw, David/Rodríguez-Arias, David (2019): "The Role of the Family in Deceased Organ Procurement. A Guide for Clinicians and Policy Makers." In: Transplantation 103/5, pp. e112–118.

Dove, Edward/Kelly, Susan/Lucivero, Federica/Machirori, Mavis/Dheensa, Sandi/Prainsack, Barbara (2017): "Beyond Individualism: Is There a Place for Relational Autonomy in Clinical Practice and Research?" In: Clinical Ethics 12/3, pp. 150–165.

Elliott, Ann (2001): "Health Care Ethics: Cultural Relativity of Autonomy." In: Journal of Transcultural Nursing 124, pp. 326–330.

Emson, H. E. (2003): "It Is Immoral to Require Consent for Cadaver Organ Donation." In: Journal of Medical Ethics 29/3, pp. 125–127.

English, V./Sommerville, A. (2003): "Presumed Consent for Transplantation: A Dead Issue after Alder Hey?" In: Journal of Medical Ethics 29/3, pp. 147–52.

Etheredge, Harriet/Penn, Claire/Watermeyer, Jennifer (2018): "Opt-in or Opt-out to Increase Organ Donation in South Africa? Appraising Proposed Strategies Using an Empirical Ethics Analysis." In: Developing World Bioethics 18/2, pp. 119–125.

Fabre, John/Murphy, Paul/Matesanz, Rafael (2010): "Presumed Consent: A Distraction in the Quest for Increasing Rates of Organ Donation." In: British Medical Journal 341, p. c4973. DOI: 10.1136/bmj.c4973

Fan, Ruiping (1997): "Self-Determination vs. Family-Determination: Two Incommensurable Principles of Autonomy." In: Bioethics 11/3–4, pp. 309–322.

Feinberg, Joel (1973): Social Philosophy, Englewood Cliffs: Prentice Hall.

Gert, Bernard/Culver, Charles M./Clouser, K. Danner (1998): "An Alternative to Physician Assisted Suicide: A Conceptual and Moral Analysis." In: Margaret P. Battin/ Rosamond Rhodes/Anita Silvers (eds), Physician Assisted Suicide: Expanding the Debate, New York: Routledge, pp. 182–203.

Gevers, Sjef/Janssen, Anke/Friele, Roland (2004): "Consent Systems for Post Mortem Organ Donation in Europe." In: European Journal of Health Law 11/2, pp. 175–186.

Ghods, Ahad (2015): "Current Status of Organ Transplant in Islamic Countries." In: Experimental and Clinical Transplantation 13/1, pp. 13–17.

Gill, Michael (2004): "Presumed Consent, Autonomy, and Organ Donation." In: The Journal of Medicine and Philosophy 29/1, pp. 37–59.

Gimbel, Ronald/Strosberg, Martin/Lehrman, Susan/Gefenas, Eugenijus/Taft, Frank (2003): "Presumed Consent and Other Predictors of Cadaveric Organ Donation in Europe." In: Progress in Transplantation 13/1, pp. 17–23.

Gómez Marinero, Purificación/Santiago Guervos, Carlos de/Getino Milan, Adela/ Moñino Martínez, Adela/Richart-Martínez, Miguel/Cabrero-García, Julio (2001): "La Entrevista Familiar: Enseñanza de las Técnicas de Comunicación." In: Nefrología 21/4, pp. 57–64.

Hamm, Danielle/Tizzard, Juliet (2008): "Presumed Consent for Organ Donation." In: British Medical Journal 336/7638, pp. 230.

Harris, John (2003): "Organ Procurement: Dead Interests, Living Needs." In: Journal of Medical Ethics 29/3, pp. 130–134.

Herring, Jonathan (2014): Relational Autonomy and Family Law, New York: Springer.

Hershenov, D. B./Delaney, J. J. (2009): "Mandatory Autopsies and Organ Conscription." In: Kennedy Institute of Ethics Journal 19/4, pp. 367–91.

Horvat, Lucy/Cuerden, Meaghan/Kim, S. Joseph/ Koval, John J./Young, Ann/Garg, Amit X. (2010): "Informing the Debate: Rates of Kidney Transplantation in Nations with Presumed Consent." In: Annals of Internal Medicine 153/10, pp. 641–649.

Kant, Immanuel (2002 [1785]): Groundwork for the Metaphysics of Morals, London: Oxford University Press.

MacKay, Douglas/Robinson, Alexandra (2016): "The Ethics of Organ Donor Registration Policies: Nudges and Respect for Autonomy." In: American Journal of Bioethics 16/11, pp. 3–12.

Mackenzie, Catriona/Stoljar, Natalie (2000) (eds.): Relational Autonomy: Feminist Perspectives on Autonomy, Agency, and the Social Self, New York: Oxford University Press.

Mackenzie, Catriona/Rogers, Wendy/Dodds, Susan (2014) (eds.): Vulnerability: New Essays in Ethics and Feminist Philosophy, New York: Oxford University Press.

McMullen, Judith (1992): "Privacy, Family Autonomy, and the Maltreated Child." In: Marquette Law Review 75/3, pp. 569–598.

Mill, John Stuart (2001 [1856]): On Liberty, Ontario: Batoche Books Limited.

Molina-Pérez, Alberto/Rodríguez-Arias, David/Delgado-Rodríguez, Janet/Morgan, Myfanwy/Frunza, Mihaela/Randhawa, Gurch/Reiger-van de Wijdeven, Jeantine/ Schiks, Eline/Wöhlke, Sabine/Schicktanz, Silke (2019): "Public Knowledge and Attitudes towards Consent Policies for Organ Donation in Europe. A Systematic Review." In: Transplantation Reviews 33/1, pp. 1–8.

Mossialos, Elias/Costa-Font, Joan/Rudisill, Caroline (2008): "Does Organ Donation Legislation Affect Individuals' Willingness to Donate Their Own or Their Relative's Organs?" In: BMC Health Services Research 8/48. DOI: 10.1186/1472-6963-8-48

National Health and Medical Research Council (Australia) (2007): Organ and Tissue Donation after Death, for Transplantation: Guidelines for Ethical Practice for Health Professionals, Canberra.

Nedelsky, Jennifer (1989): "Reconceiving Autonomy: Sources, Thoughts, and Possibilities." In: Yale Journal of Law and Feminism 1/1, pp. 8–36.

Nedelsky, Jennifer (1993): "Reconceiving Rights as Relationships." In: Review of Constitutional Studies 1/1, pp. 1–26.

Nedelsky, Jennifer (2011): Law's Relations. A Relational Theory of Self, Autonomy and Law, New York: Oxford University Press.

Racine, Eric/Jox, Ralf/Bernat, James/Dabrock, Peter/Gardiner, Dale/Marckmann, Georg/Rid, Annette/Rodriguez-Arias, David/In Schmitten, Rgen/Schöne-Seifert, Bettina (2015): "Determination of Death: A Discussion on Responsible Scholarship, Clinical Practices, and Public Engagement." In: Perspectives in Biology and Medicine 58/4, pp. 444–465.

Rithalia, Amber/McDaid, Catriona/Suekarran, Sara/Norman, Gill/Myers, Lindsey/Sowden, Amanda (2009a): "A Systematic Review of Presumed Consent Systems for Deceased Organ Donation." In: Health Technology Assessment 13/26, pp. 1–95.

Rithalia, Amber/McDaid, Catriona/Suekarran, Sara/Myers, Lindsey/Sowden, Amanda (2009b): "Impact of Presumed Consent for Organ Donation on Donation Rates: A Systematic Review." In: British Medical Journal 338, p. a3162. DOI: 10.1136/bmj.a3162

Rodríguez-Arias, David (2018): "The Dead Donor Rule as Policy Indoctrination." In: The Hastings Center Report 48/4, pp. S39–S42.

Rodriguez-Arias, David/Morgan, Myfanwy (2016): "'Nudging' Deceased Donation through an Opt-Out System: A Libertarian Approach or Manipulation?" American Journal of Bioethics 16/11, pp. 25–28.

Rogers, Wendy/Mackenzie, Catriona/Dodds, Susan (2012): "Why Bioethics Needs a Concept of Vulnerability." In: International Journal of Feminist Approaches to Bioethics 5/2, pp. 11–38.

Rosenblum, Amanda/Horvat, Lucy/Siminoff, Laura/Prakash, Versha/Beitel, Janice/Garg, Amit X. (2012): "The Authority of Next-of-kin in Explicit and Presumed Consent Systems for Deceased Organ Donation" In: Nephrology Dialysis Transplantation 27/6, pp. 2533–2546.

Saunders, John (2008): "No Such Thing." In: British Medical Journal 336/7640, p. 345.

Saunders, Ben (2011): "Opt-out Organ Donation without Presumptions." In: Journal of Medical Ethics 38/2, pp. 69–72.

Shaw, David/Georgieva, Denie/Haase, Bernadette/Gardiner, Dale/Lewis, Penney/Jansen, Nichon/Wind, Tineke/Samuel, Undine/McDonald, Maryon/Ploeg, Rutger (2017): "Family Over Rules? An Ethical Analysis of Allowing Families to Overrule Donation Intentions." In: Transplantation 101/3, pp. 482–487.

Shepherd, Lee/O'Carroll, Ronan/Ferguson, Eamonn (2014): "An International Comparison of Deceased and Living Organ Donation/Transplant Rates in Opt-in and Opt-out Systems: a Panel Study." In: BMC Medicine 12, p. 131.

Sperling, Daniel (2008): Posthumous Interests: Legal and Ethical Perspectives, Cambridge/New York: Cambridge University Press.

Spital, Aaron/Taylor, James Stuart (2007): "Routine Recovery of Cadaveric Organs for Transplantation." In: Clinical Journal of the American Society of Nephrology 2/2, pp. 300–303.

Straehle, Christine (2017) (ed.): Vulnerability, Autonomy and Applied Ethics, London: Routledge.

Thaler, Richard/Sunstein, Cass (2008): Nudge: Improving Decisions about Health, Wealth, and Happiness, New Haven: Yale University Press.

Ugur, Zeynep (2015): "Does Presumed Consent Save Lives? Evidence from Europe." In: Health Economics 24/12, pp. 1560–1572.

Wardrope, Alistair (2015): "Liberal Individualism, Relational Autonomy, and the Social Dimension of Respect." In: The International Journal of Feminist Approaches to Bioethics 8/1, pp. 37–66.

WHO (2010): "WHO Guiding Principles on Human Cell, Tissue and Organ Transplantation." In: Cell and Tissue Banking 11/4, pp. 413–419.

Wilkinson, T. Martin (2005): "Individual and Family Consent to Organ and Tissue Donation: Is the Current Position Coherent?" In: Journal of Medical Ethics 31/10, pp. 587–590

3. Nudging in Donation Policies
Registration and Decision-Making

Douglas MacKay & Katherine Saylor

1. Introduction

Suppose you are a policymaker responsible for addressing the shortage of donated organs in your jurisdiction. What types of policies might you implement to increase the number of organs available for transplantation? You might first consider coercive measures, for example, requiring all competent adults to register as organ donors, or simply laying claim to the organs of deceased citizens, regardless of their objections or the objections of their family members. You could also introduce incentives, permitting people to sell their kidneys while alive, and perhaps also permitting the buying and selling of the organs of the deceased. Finally, you could mount an information campaign, informing people of the benefits to others of organ donation with the aim of persuading them to register as donors.

Unfortunately, each of these strategies faces significant problems. Coercive policies would limit people's liberty, preventing them from deciding not to donate their organs, for example for religious reasons or because they are skeptical of the concept of brain death. A system of incentives threatens to commodify people's bodies and exacerbate inequality between the rich and the poor. Finally, while there are no ethical objections to information campaigns, they are unlikely to move the needle on the problem at hand. If only there were a type of intervention that was more effective than an information campaign but also avoided the ethical objections to policies that employ coercion and incentives.[1]

Nudges would seem to fit the bill, promising to influence people's actions in predictable directions without limiting their choices – i.e. employing coercion – or significantly changing their incentives (Thaler/Sunstein 2008: 6). It is thus not surprising that scholars have strongly advocated the use of nudges to increase the number of organs available for transplantation, and that policymakers have listened, for example by implementing opt-out donor registration systems. Nudges are not without their critics though. Although nudges are respectful of people's liberty, some argue that

---

1 We recognize of course that these are not the only policy options on the table. Policymakers can no doubt increase the number of organs available for donation by reforming the processes by which potential donors are identified and assessed by organ procurement organizations.

they are not respectful of people's autonomy, instead influencing people's choices through nonrational means.

In this chapter, we provide an overview of the ethical considerations relevant to the use of nudges in organ donation policy. We do not defend a position on the permissibility of nudging in this context. Instead, we aim to clearly outline the most prominent arguments on the different sides of this issue that have been presented in the English-language scholarly bioethics literature. We also highlight the questions that are in need of further investigation.

In part 1, we briefly discuss nudging before considering proposals to use nudges to increase the number of registered organ donors, including opt-out donor registration systems and the use of 'nudge statements'. In part 2, we discuss the use of nudges to influence the decision-making of family members in circumstances where they have a veto over the donation of their loved one's organs.

2.   Nudges and Organ Donor Registration Policy

Nudges would not be possible if people were "Econs," that is, agents with full information, unlimited cognitive abilities, a complete and consistent set of preferences, and perfect self-control (Thaler/Sunstein 2008: 6–7). But people are Humans, not Econs, and while Humans are like Econs in some respects, they are unlike them in important ways. Humans approach the world with two cognitive systems. System 1 is the Automatic System: the system of gut reactions. It is intuitive, fast, effortless, associative, unconscious, and skilled (ibid.). System 2 is the Reflective System: the system of conscious thought. It is the system Humans share with Econs and is deliberate, controlled, effortful, deductive, slow, self-aware, and rule-following (Thaler/Sunstein 2008: 20). We use System 2 to solve a math or logic problem; we use System 1 to make a snap judgment.

Since nudges influence us to act in predictable ways, they would also not be possible if System 1 were unstructured. However, System 1 biases our decision-making in consistent ways. As Dan Ariely puts it, "we are not only irrational, but *predictably irrational* [...] our irrationality happens the same way, again and again" (2008: xx). Choice architects – those who design the environments within which people make choices – can thus significantly influence the choices people make. As such, choice architects can nudge people, influencing their choices in predictable ways without limiting their options through coercion or making certain options costlier than others (Thaler/Sunstein 2008: 3).

System 1 has a number of features that are directly relevant to the registration of organ donors. In this part of the chapter, we consider two nudges in the context of organ donor registration policy: 'opt-out' registration policies and 'nudge statements'. In exploring the ethics of nudges in this context, we accept an assumption made by scholars working on this question – namely, that people have a moral right to determine what happens to their organs after they die.[2] People therefore have a right to decide whether they wish to register as an organ donor, and their decisions and preferences regarding the donation of their organs should be given great weight by deci-

2 Wilkinson (2011: 11–62) offers what we take to be the strongest defense of this claim.

sion-makers. The central ethical question in this context concerns the permissibility of using nudges to influence people's registration choices, a question that is ethically challenging only if these choices are deserving of respect.

2.1   Opt-Out Donor Registration Systems

Humans exhibit status quo bias, a tendency to stick with the current state of affairs (Thaler/Sunstein 2008: 34). Humans are thus more likely to choose the option that choice architects have presented as the default – that is, the option choosers are left with if they take no positive action (ibid.: 35). With respect to the design of organ donor registration policy, a number of commentators argue that policymakers should nudge people to register as organ donors by making donor registration the default option (ibid.: 177–179; Rippon 2012; Whyte et al. 2012; Saunders 2012). Such policies are typically referred to as 'opt-out' policies since they register all citizens as donors, putting the onus on individuals to opt out of this status if they so choose. Proponents argue that because people exhibit status quo bias, such a policy will increase the number of registered donors and so lead to a greater number of donated organs. Because people have the option to easily opt-out of being registered, proponents argue, such systems do not coercively limit people's choices and so adequately respect their liberty.[3]

Opt-out systems raise a number of interesting questions that we cannot fully address here. First, will such systems actually lead to an increase in the number of donated organs? A good deal of the evidence regarding the importance of defaults in this context has been provided by lab experiments (Johnson/Goldstein 2003; van Dalen/Henkens 2014). Furthermore, some scholars are skeptical that transitioning to an opt-out system alone will significantly raise the number of donated organs in a jurisdiction, for example because of the role played by families in deciding whether or not to authorize donation, and the crucial importance of an effective procurement system (Wilkinson 2011: 94–95; Willis/Quigley 2014). Second, do opt-out systems adequately secure people's consent to donation? Some scholars defend the claim that such systems do so, where this consent is understood as presumed (Cohen 1992), normative (Saunders 2010), or implicit (Saunders 2012). Others, by contrast, are skeptical of such claims (Veatch 2000: 167–174; Kluge 2000; den Hartogh 2011a; den Hartogh 2011b; MacKay 2015). Still others argue that consent is not necessary for the ethical removal

---

3   Whyte et al. (2012: 33–34) also suggest that mandated active choice policies would nudge people to register as organ donors. Such policies do not present one with a default, but instead ask them whether they would like to be registered as an organ donor or not and require them to answer the question or face a sanction, for example not receiving their driver's license or identification card (Thaler/Sunstein 2008: 180). We suggest however that mandated active choice policies are not best characterized as nudges. The justification for these policies is that they do not present people with a default option and so do not influence their choices by engaging their status quo bias (MacKay/Robinson 2016: 6 fn 2). It's possible that mandated active choice policies play upon other features of System 1 – e.g. a desire to conform to the beliefs of others (Thaler/Sunstein 2008: 53–55) – but we are aware of no empirical research that establishes this effect in this context. Also, even if mandated active choice policies do nudge potential donors in this way, the nudge is likely to be far less effective than the nudge employed by opt-out policies. Mandated active choice policies, unlike opt-out policies, employ no default, which we know has a strong effect on people's decision-making in the context of organ donor registration (MacKay/Robinson 2016: 7–8).

of people's organs (Gill 2004; Zambrano 2018). Our focus here, however, is whether it is permissible for policymakers to nudge people to register as organ donors by taking advantage of their status quo bias.[4]

A common objection to the use of nudges is that they are disrespectful of people's autonomy (Bovens 2008; Hausman/Welch 2010; Wilkinson 2013; White 2013; Guldborg/Jespersen 2013; Rebonato 2014). While nudges do not change people's incentives or limit their choices, critics argue that they do interfere with people's decision-making, namely the exercise of their rational capacities. Douglas MacKay and Alexandra Robinson (2016) raise this objection against the use of nudges in the context of organ donor registration policy. Following Jennifer Blumenthal-Barby (2012), they argue that opt-out systems are a form of *reason-bypassing nonargumentative influence* – that is, influence that bypasses or works around people's rational capacities, often without their knowledge (MacKay/Robinson 2016: 4). Opt-out systems employ this form of influence since they use a default rule to influence people to register as donors.

MacKay and Robinson further argue that the use of a default rule in opt-out systems is disrespectful of people's autonomy (2016: 6). People are autonomous if they have the capacity to govern their lives on the basis of reasons; and people exercise their autonomy by "deciding what to do with their bodies and minds on the basis of their values and preferences, and the reasons they take to be binding on them" (ibid.). The use of a default rule is disrespectful of people's autonomy, MacKay and Robinson claim, since it involves working around rather than engaging with people's rational capacities. To respect people's autonomy, they write, agents must recognize the value of people governing their lives based on their values and preferences. This involves "engaging people's rational capacities through rational persuasion, not (1) restricting their options or (2) corrupting the deliberative processes by which they make decisions" (ibid.).

MacKay and Robinson do not conclude from this that it is wrong on balance for policymakers to employ default rules to register donors, only that it is *pro tanto* wrong. They also provide a framework for evaluating the degree of pro tanto wrongness of opt-out systems and their principal alternatives: opt-in, mandated active choice (MAC), and voluntary active choice (VAC) (ibid.: 10–11). MacKay (2017) refines this framework in a later paper (see Table 1):

---

4 If opt-out systems cannot be said to secure people's consent, one might argue that it is a mistake to speak of organ 'donation' in the context of such systems. This is a good point; however, we will continue to the use the term 'donation' throughout this chapter since it is common practice to do so within the existing literature, and the most plausible replacement term – 'procurement' – may confuse some readers.

	Coercion?	Reason-bypassing nonargumentative influence?	Pro tanto wrong?	Value of Choice	Degree of influence	Degree of Wrongness
Opt-in	No	Yes	Yes	High	Very low – moderate	Low - high
Opt-out	No	Yes	Yes	High	Very low – moderate	Low - high
MAC	Yes	No	Yes	Very low	High	Low
VAC	No	Yes	Yes	High	Very low – low	Low - mo- derate

Table 1: Evaluating Pro Tanto Wrongness

Each option's degree of pro tanto wrongness, MacKay claims, is a function of the value of the choice that is the target of the policy, and the degree to which the policy influences this choice. In cases where an opt-out system is expected to significantly influence this choice, MAC may be less pro tanto wrong since although it employs coercion, it targets a very low-value choice – namely, people's choice to state their preference regarding the donation of their organs. More generally, MacKay and Robinson (2016) conclude that the question of which system is, on balance, morally preferable depends on each system's degree of pro tanto wrongness, whether it secures people's valid consent to donation, and the number of donated organs it is likely to yield.

A number of scholars dispute MacKay and Robinson's claim that opt-out systems of organ donor registration are pro tanto wrong because they employ a default rule. Responding directly to MacKay and Robinson, Cass R. Sunstein argues that opt-out systems might infringe people's autonomy because they do not secure people's explicit consent, but not because default rules "bypass people's rational capacities" (2016: 1). Instead, Sunstein argues, "default rules, taken as such, do not intrude on autonomy even if they influence people without persuading them" (ibid.). Because human beings have limited cognitive bandwidth to make choices, default rules, when they are carefully designed, promote people's "freedom to focus on their most pressing concerns" and improve their wellbeing (ibid.). Sunstein grants that it is wrong to use default rules in cases where "what is necessary is an explicit indication of people's values, wishes, and tastes," (2016: 2) not because default rules are a form of reason-bypassing nonargumentative influence but rather because in these cases we need people's explicit consent. In response, MacKay (2017) grants that default rules may *promote* people's autonomy in the way Sunstein suggests, but he argues that this does not entail that the use of such rules is *respectful* of people's autonomy – i.e. doesn't bypass or corrupt their deliberative processes.

Daniel Kelly and Nicolae Morar (2016) raise a different objection against MacKay and Robinson's analysis, arguing that it depends on a conception of autonomy and rationality that is too individualistic. Once we understand autonomy and rationality as social and embedded, they suggest, we will cease to see the use of defaults in opt-out systems as a corruption of people's autonomous decision-making.

Andreas T. Schmidt (2019) develops this argument in a more systematic fashion, arguing that not only is nudging compatible with treating people as rational agents, it also facilitates rational decision-making.[5] Schmidt first argues that objections to nudging such as MacKay and Robinson's, which focus on how nudges disrespect people as autonomous and rational agents, presuppose what he calls "heroic rationality" (ibid.: 518). According to this view, people make rational decisions by employing System 2 – i.e. considering all of the relevant information, performing correct probabilistic judgments, working through the various considerations in support of each option, and choosing the option for which one has the strongest reasons (Schmidt 2019: 519–520).

Second, Schmidt argues that heroic rationality, as a normative ideal, is implausible, and defends an alternative theory of rationality: "ecological rationality" (ibid.: 520). Following Jennifer Morton (2011), Schmidt argues that "a person's decision is procedurally rational in an environment to the extent that, given her particular psychological make-up, the decision-making procedures she uses allow her to reliably achieve her ends in this type of environment" (2019: 521). While heroic rationality locates rationality in System 2, ecological rationality counts certain System 1 decision-making procedures as rational when they reliably further an agent's ends (ibid.: 522–523).

Third, Schmidt argues that even though nudges act on System 1, their use by policymakers does not necessarily treat people as irrational because System 1 processes might count as rational in certain environments (ibid.: 526–527). Schmidt argues further that nudges may even support rational decision-making since governments can adjust people's choice environments to better fit both the decision-making procedures they use as well as their psychological make-up, thus improving their procedural rationality (ibid.: 528). For example, given people's status quo bias, Schmidt argues, governments can improve people's procedural rationality by setting defaults that better align with their ends (ibid.: 529-530). In a jurisdiction where people prefer to be organ donors, governments can improve people's abilities to satisfy this preference by implementing an opt-out system.

To summarize, MacKay and Robinson argue that opt-out systems are pro tanto wrong because they nudge people to register to donate and therefore engage in reason-bypassing nonargumentative influence. By contrast, Sunstein and Schmidt hold that policymakers' use of defaults in the context of organ donor registration can in fact support people's rational decision-making. Future work is necessary to resolve this conflict. In particular, one interesting question requiring further exploration is whether, following Schmidt, policies that aim to minimize the effect of cognitive biases on people's decision-making – e.g. active choice frames – are more respectful of people's autonomy than policies that employ nudges that improve people's ability to realize their ends. Implementing an opt-out system may improve people's procedural rationality – compared to an opt-in system – in jurisdictions where most people prefer to be organ donors. But is it correct to say that an opt-out system is more respectful of people's autonomy than an active choice system which aims to minimize the effect of status quo bias on people's decisions?

---

5 Bart Engelen (2019), Neil Levy (2019), and Timothy Houk (2019) have similarly argued that nudges should not be understood as bypassing people's rational capacities.

2.2   Organ Donor Registration and Nudge Statements

There are other features of System 1 that are important for the design of organ donor registration policy. First, people tend to be loss averse, meaning that they are more likely to value a good they possess than one they do not. In other words, people attach greater weight to losses than to equivalent gains (Thaler/Sunstein 2008: 33–34). Second, people are more likely to respond to appeals or warnings that engage their emotions – a central feature of System 1. Finally, although no Econ would feel obliged to reciprocate or give back upon receiving a gift, Humans do. People can therefore be nudged to act in pro-social ways – e.g. giving to charity – if they are provided with a small gift (Behavioral Insights Team 2013a).

In two recent experiments, scholars found that people can be nudged to register as organ donors if exposed to statements that play upon these features of System 1. The U.K. Government's Behavioral Insights Team (2013b) conducted a randomized controlled trial in which they evaluated the effect on donor registration rates of including different messages on a high traffic government webpage that encourages people to join the National Health Service Organ Donor Register. The most successful messages were those that employed a loss frame and that appealed to people's sense of reciprocity (ibid.: 7).[6] The Ontario Ministry of Health and Long Term Care and its partners conducted a similar randomized controlled trial evaluating the effectiveness of placing different 'nudge statements' at the top of the organ donor registration form (Government of Ontario 2019). Investigators found that the use of nudge statements respectively appealing to reciprocity and to people's emotions each increased the likelihood of people registering by 2.1 times (ibid.).

To our knowledge, no one has directly addressed the ethical issues regarding the use of these nudge statements to increase organ donor registration. However, scholars have addressed the ethics of such statements in other contexts.

Consider the use of a 'loss frame' to nudge people to register as donors. Because people tend to be loss averse, they may be more responsive to 'loss frames' compared to 'gain frames' that provide people with exactly the same information. To take the above example, it may be that people provided with the statement, 'three people die every day because there are not enough organ donors,' would be more likely to register as organ donors than people provided with the statement, 'three lives could be saved if

---

6   To explain the effectiveness of the loss frame, the U.K. Behavioral Insights Team (2013b: 5) appeals to loss aversion. However, the study's authors do not cite any evidence showing that people are loss averse not only with respect to their own wellbeing but also the wellbeing of others. It's possible therefore that loss aversion is not the driver of the effectiveness of the loss frame. An alternative explanation is that loss frames may better highlight gaps between people's intentions and actions because there is evidence that people can be spurred to action if differences between their intentions and actions are identified (Freijy/Kothe 2013). In addition, there is also good evidence showing that loss-framed messages in the context of organ donor registration can increase psychological reactance and so decrease people's intent to register (Reinhart et al. 2007). More research is therefore needed to determine whether loss frames can indeed be relied upon to increase donor registration rates, and if so, which psychological mechanism is responsible for this effect. Thanks to an anonymous reviewer for a helpful discussion of this issue.

there were enough organ donors.'[7] Supposing this is true, is there anything wrong with using the former frame?[8]

Consider first that MacKay and Robinson's objection to the use of defaults is relevant here. Employing a loss frame rather than a gain frame is also a form of reason-bypassing nonargumentative influence and is therefore arguably disrespectful of people's autonomy. However, scholars have argued that the use of framing effects to nudge people's choices is not problematic in similar contexts. For example, with respect to the clinical context, Gorin et al. (2017: 34–35), Cohen (2013), and Blumenthal-Barby et al. (2013) argue that nudges are permissible when (1) they are unavoidable, and (2) their direction is justifiable – for example, if they help patients to satisfy their deeply-held preferences or, where such preferences are lacking, to realize their best interests. In the context of registering organ donors, this position would imply that policymakers should employ the loss frame since (1) the information must be framed in some way, and (2) more people wish to register as organ donors than not.

In response to this line of argument, Søren Holm argues that while nudging may be inevitable – e.g. it is necessary to frame information in some way – it may be possible in certain contexts to minimize the impact of such nudges, either by designing choice situations to trigger System 2 or by designing "choice situations so that the nudges present in them cancel each other out" (Holm 2017: 39; cp. Miller/Gelinas 2013; cp. Chwang 2016; cp. Gelfand 2016; cp. Wilkinson 2017). Just as MacKay and Robinson argue that the use of an active choice policy rather than an opt-out policy is a way to avoid taking advantage of people's status quo bias, so too there may be ways for policymakers to provide people with information that minimizes the effect of nudges.

What about nudge statements that appeal to people's emotions or sense of reciprocity?

> "If you need a transplant, would you have one? If so, please help save lives and register today."

> "How would you feel if you or someone you love needed a transplant and couldn't get one? Please help save lives and register today" (Government of Ontario 2019).

Consider the latter nudge statement. Using Blumenthal-Barby's (2012) terminology, this statement would seem to employ reason-countering nonargumentative influence since it plays upon people's emotions. One might argue therefore that is objectionable. However, as Joshua Hobbs (2017: 41) argues regarding the use of similar types of nudge statements to facilitate charitable giving, emotion plays an important role in moral deliberation. Therefore, such nudge statements should not necessarily be understood as forms of reason-countering nonargumentative influence. Indeed, it seems reason-

---

7 Note that this is not what the U.K. study did. The various 'nudge statements' were compared against each other and a control of no statement (Behavioral Insights Team 2013b).

8 One additional potential problem with the phrasing of this statement – separate from the question of framing – is that it implies that three people die every day because of the actions of potential donors, not (primarily) because of illness. One might argue that this phrasing is somewhat manipulative. Thanks to an anonymous reviewer for identifying this potential problem.

able to think that the above statement need not be understood as a nudge at all but rather as a moral argument – presented in brief – with the following structure:

1. If you or a loved one needed an organ, you would want others to register as organ donors.
2. You should treat others as you would want them to treat you.
3. So, you should register as an organ donor.[9]

Once we reconstruct the statement in this way, it need not be understood as a nudge but rather as an act of rational persuasion, thus raising no problems regarding respect for autonomy. Indeed, we can also run the same analysis on the above statement in terms of its appeal to people's sense of reciprocity. In our view, more work is necessary to draw a boundary between moral argumentation and nudging. The latter, after all, certainly makes use of System 1 processes such as people's emotions and sense of reciprocity.

To sum up our discussion thus far, some scholars argue that the use of nudges to influence people to register as organ donors is pro tanto wrong when these nudges fail to engage people's rational capacities. The principal examples of such nudges include opt-out donor registration systems and the use of nudge statements that employ loss frames. With respect to opt-out donor registration systems, some respond that such systems promote people's autonomy by giving them the freedom to focus on their most pressing concerns, or that people's reliance on status quo bias is in fact rational, provided rationality is understood as ecological rationality. With respect to the use of loss frames in nudge statements, some respond that framing is inevitable and justifiable provided it leads people to make choices that align with their preferences. We have also seen that not all 'nudge statements' are normatively problematic. Some such statements can be reconstructed as moral arguments in brief, and so it is not clear that they are best understood as nudges in the first place.

Finally, it is important to note that even if the critics of nudges are right that it is pro tanto wrong to employ nudges to increase organ donor registration, this does not mean that policymakers should not use them. There may be competing considerations that render the use of nudges on balance permissible, even if it is the case that people have a moral right to determine what happens to their organs after they die. First, some scholars argue that people have a *duty* to register as organ donors, appealing either to notions of fairness (Steinberg 2004) or to the duty to easy rescue (Hester 2006; Fabre 2006: 72–97; Snyder 2009; Saunders 2010). If this view is right,[10] one might argue that although nudges are pro tanto wrong, they prevent people from committing a second wrong, namely failing to register as an organ donor, and so may be on balance justifiable for that reason (Blumenthal-Barby/Opel 2018).

Second, as MacKay and Robinson (2016) and Gelinas (2016) argue, if the use of nudges is expected to significantly increase the number of donated organs available for transplantation, the gains to people's wellbeing may be great enough to outweigh the pro tanto wrong in question. Importantly, these two competing considerations may work together to justify the use of nudges if (1) people have a duty to register

---

9   Steinberg (2004) offers a more systematic development of this argument.

10   For responses to these arguments, see Ben Almassi (2014).

as organ donors, and (2) such registration will significantly increase the number of donated organs (Navin 2017).

3.   Nudging and Next-of-Kin Clinical Decisions

In the effort to increase organ donation, next-of-kin decision-making at the end of life is another potential target for nudges. Many jurisdictions offer family members a de facto or de jure veto over organ donation. In the U.S., despite first-person authorization laws, a recent survey of all 58 organ procurement organizations found that 20 per cent would not proceed without the consent of the family (Chon et al. 2014). Limited international data show that an estimated 34–38 per cent of families refuse donation under both opt-in and opt-out systems (Rosenblum et al. 2012). Family members can thus pose an obstacle to donation, and, in some cases, may choose to frustrate the prior preferences of the decedent.

Organ donation requestors may wish to nudge family members to make one decision rather than another, relying on many features of System 1, including status quo bias and loss aversion. This type of case is different from that of registering organ donors, since the target of the nudge is not the potential donor but rather the potential donor's family members. For example, Sheldon Zink and Stacey Wertlieb suggest that rather than adopting a "value-neutral approach" (2006: 130) in which families are provided with information regarding donation in an unbiased manner, requestors should adopt a "presumptive approach" (ibid.) by presenting donation as the default option. With respect to the request for authorization in particular, Zink and Wertlieb (2006: 135) contrast the standard and presumptive approaches in the following way:

	Standard	Presumptive
The request	Would you like me to give you some time before you make your final decision?	If you do not have any more questions, I will now guide you through this process.

Table 2: Securing Familial Authorization (adapted from Zink and Wertlieb 2006)

Scholars disagree both about whether it is permissible to nudge family members and about what the goal of the nudge ought to be. First, Sharif and Moorlock (2018) argue that it is permissible to nudge family members in order to bring their decisions in alignment with the decedent's prior wishes. Accepting the premises that (1) people have a duty to donate their organs, and (2) people have a right to determine what happens to their organs after they die, Sharif and Moorlock present the following argument in support of the use of nudges:

"a) If a person wants, or would want, to do the right thing, and (b) it is important to respect that person's wishes in a given context, (c) it is prima facie ethically permissible to remove barriers to that person doing the right thing in the given context. (d) Donating organs is the morally right thing to do, so (e) it is therefore prima facie ethically permissible to remove barriers to organ donation." (2018: 157)

They therefore conclude that it is permissible to use nudges to remove barriers to donation, including the objections of family members.

Sharif and Moorlock (2018) recognize that nudging is a form of nonrational influence and so disrespectful of people's autonomy, but they argue that it is justifiable because it both benefits potential recipients and fulfills the decedent's prior preference to donate. Importantly, recognizing that people have a right to determine what happens to their organs after they die, Sharif and Moorlock (2018) argue that family members should not be nudged to authorize donation in cases where donation would compromise the decedent's prior wishes.

Other scholars reject Sharif and Moorlock's position, suggesting that family members should be nudged to authorize donation with the goal of benefiting recipients. Zink and Wertlieb (2006: 130) argue that requestors should adopt a presumptive approach to all families on the grounds that requestors have a responsibility to be advocates of donation, and that organ donation is the morally right thing to do. In contrast to Sharif and Moorlock, Zink and Wertlieb (2006) hold that the goal of the nudge is not to fulfill the preferences of the decedent but rather to benefit potential recipients.

A number of scholars are critical of this position, however. Some reject it on the grounds that people have a right to determine what happens to their organs after they die and therefore their preferences should take priority over benefits to recipients (Sharif/Moorlock 2018). Others argue that the presumptive approach is potentially manipulative and so may lead family members to make decisions that are not fully autonomous or in the best interests of family members and patients (Rippon 2012; Troug 2012). Nevertheless, if nudging family members is expected to significantly increase the supply of donated organs, one might argue that societal benefits outweigh the pro tanto wrongness of nudging family members (MacKay/Robinson 2016). Therefore, it may be justifiable to use pro-donation nudges even when the explicit motivation is societal benefit rather than aligning outcomes with decedent's preferences.

A third possibility, which is deserving of future research, is whether it is permissible to use nudges to help family members make the 'best' decision for both the family and patient, where this may involve donation under some circumstances and no donation under others. Thaler and Sunstein (2008) understand nudges as a way to help decision-makers make good decisions under sub-optimal conditions. Given that more family members regret refusals than authorizations, interventions that increase donation authorization may promote the realization of stable, considered preferences for many family members (Rodrigue et al. 2008). There may be some set of nudges requestors could use to aid family members in making the best decision for themselves and the patient under challenging end-of-life circumstances.

4. Conclusion

Our aim in this chapter has been to provide an overview of the ethical dimensions of the use of nudges in organ donation policy. We first explored the use of nudges to increase organ donor registration before turning to the use of nudges to influence the decision-making of family members in cases where they are asked to authorize the use of their loved one's organs.

We conclude by highlighting a number of ethical questions regarding the use of nudges in donation policy that require further research. First, regarding the use of opt-out systems of donor registration, more work is needed to determine if such systems should be understood as fully respectful of people's autonomy, following Schmidt's conception of ecological rationality, or whether systems that employ active choice frames – e.g. mandated active choice – are superior in this respect because they aim to minimize the effect of bias on people's decision-making. Second, should statements that can be understood to offer moral arguments in brief be considered nudges, even though they appeal to aspects of System 1? Third, nudges frequently support better choices for people who hold majority views but not those who hold minority views. Additional consideration is needed regarding how nudges can both reduce mistakes for the majority while also respecting the autonomy of people whose stable, considered preferences are minority views – i.e. those who prefer not to donate their organs.

Finally, even if it is in principle permissible to nudge potential donors and/or family members to increase donation rates, there are a number of further ethical issues policymakers must consider before implementing such a system. A number of scholars have argued that because, as Luc Bovens puts it, the features of System 1 exploited by nudges "work better in the dark," (2009: 209) policies that employ nudges must be implemented with transparency and accountability (Thaler/Sunstein 2008: 244–245; Bovens 2009; Farrell 2015). In addition, even if governments and organ procurement organizations implement nudges in a transparent way, there is always the difficult question of whether the use of nudges may undermine public trust in the organ transplantation and broader health care system. Although there is widespread scholarly agreement on the need for transparency and the potential detriment to public trust, further work is necessary to determine exactly how the principles of transparency and accountability should be understood in this context.

References

Almassi, Ben (2014): "Trust and the Duty of Organ Donation." In: Bioethics 28/6, pp. 275–283.

Ariely, Dan (2008): Predictably Irrational: The Hidden Forces That Shape Our Decisions, New York: Harper Collins.

Behavioral Insights Team (2013a): Applying Behavioral Insights to Charitable Giving, Cabinet Office.

Behavioral Insights Team (2013b): Applying Behavioral Insights to Organ Donation: Preliminary Results from a Randomised Controlled Trial, Cabinet Office.

Blumenthal-Barby, Jennifer S. (2012): "Between Reason and Coercion: Ethically Permissible Influence in Health Care and Health Policy Contexts." In: Kennedy Institute of Ethics Journal 22/4, pp. 345-366.

Blumenthal-Barby, Jennifer S./Cantor, Scott B./Russell, Heidi Voelker/ Naik, Aanand D./Volk, Robert J. (2013): "Decision Aids: When 'Nudging' Patients to Make A Particular Choice is More Ethical Than Balanced, Nondirective Content." In: Health Affairs 32/2, pp. 303–310.

Blumenthal-Barby, Jennifer S./Opel, Douglas J. (2018): "Nudge or Grudge? Choice Architecture and Parental Decision-Making." In: Hastings Center Report 48/2, pp. 33–39.

Bovens, Luc (2008): "The Ethics of Nudge." In: Mats J. Hansson/Till Grüne-Yanoff (eds.), *Preference Change: Approaches from Philosophy, Economics and Psychology*, Berlin: Springer, pp. 207–220.

Chon, W. J./Josephson, M. A./Gordon, E. J./Becker, Y. T./Witkowski, P./Arwindekar, D. J./ Naik, A./Thistlethwaite Jr., J. R./Liao, C./Ross, L. F. (2014): "When the Living and the Deceased Cannot Agree on Organ Donation: A Survey of US Organ Procurement Organizations (OPOs)." In: American Journal of Transplantation 14/1, pp. 172–177.

Chwang, Eric (2016): "Consent's Been Framed: When Framing Effects Invalidate Consent and How to Validate It Again." In: Journal of Applied Philosophy 33/3, pp. 270-285.

Cohen, Carl (1992): "The Case for Presumed Consent, to Transplant Human Organs after Death." In: Transplantation Proceedings 24/5, pp. 2168–2172.

Cohen, Shlomo (2013): "Nudging and Informed Consent." In: The American Journal of Bioethics 13/6, pp. 3–11.

Den Hartogh, Govert (2011a): "Can Consent be Presumed?" In: Journal of Applied Philosophy 28/3, pp. 295–307.

Den Hartogh, Govert (2011b): "Tacitly Consenting to Donate One's Organs." In: Journal of Medical Ethics 37/6, pp. 344–347.

Engelen, Bart (2019): "Nudging and Rationality: What is There to Worry?" In: Rationality and Society 31/2, pp. 204–232.

Fabre, Cécile (2006): Whose Body is it Anyway? Justice and the Integrity of the Person, New York: Oxford University Press.

Farrell, Anne-Maree (2015): "Addressing Organ Shortage: Are Nudges the Way Forward." In: Law, Innovation and Technology 7/2, pp. 253–282.

Freijy, Tanya/Kothe, Emily J. (2013): "Dissonance-based Interventions for Health Behavior Change: A Systematic Review." In: British Journal of Health Psychology 18/2, pp. 310–337.

Gelfand, Scott D. (2016): "The Meta-Nudge – A Response to the Claim that the Use of Nudges During the Informed Consent Process is Unavoidable." In: Bioethics 30/8, 601–608.

Gill, Michael B. (2004): "Presumed Consent, Autonomy, and Organ Donation." In: Journal of Medicine and Philosophy 29/1, pp. 37–59.

Gorin, Moti/Joffe, Steven/Dickert, Neal/Halpern, Scott (2017): "Justifying Clinical Nudges." In: Hastings Center Report 47/2, 34–35.

Gelinas, Luke (2016): "Rights, Nudging, and the Good of Others." In: The American Journal of Bioethics 16/11, 18–19.

Government of Ontario: "Behavioural Insights Pilot Project – Organ Donor Registration", April 30, 2019 (https://www.ontario.ca/page/behavioural-insights-pilot-project-organ-donor-registration).

Guldborg, Pelle/Jespersen, Andreas Maaløe (2013): "Nudge and the Manipulation of Choice: A Framework for the Responsible Use of the Nudge Approach to Behavior Change in Public Policy." In: European Journal of Risk Regulation 4/1, pp. 3–28.

Hausman, Daniel M./Welch, Brynn (2010): "To Nudge or Not to Nudge," Journal of Political Philosophy 18/1, pp. 123–136.

Hester, D. Micah (2006): "Why We Must Leave Our Organs to Others." In: The American Journal of Bioethics 6/4, pp. W23–W28.

Hobbs, Joshua (2017): "Nudging Charitable Giving: The Ethics of Nudge in International Poverty Reduction." In: Ethics & Global Politics 10/1, pp. 37–57.

Holm, Søren (2017): "Authenticity, Best Interest, and Clinical Nudging." In: Hastings Center Report 47/2, pp. 38–40.

Houk, Timothy (2019): "On Nudging's Supposed Threat to Rational Decision-Making." In: The Journal of Medicine and Philosophy 44/4, pp. 403–422.

Johnson, Eric J./Goldstein, Daniel (2003): "Do Defaults Save Lives?" In: Science 302, pp. 1338–1339.

Kelly, Daniel/Morar, Nicolae (2016): "Nudging and the Ecological and Social Roots of Human Agency." In: The American Journal of Bioethics 16/11, pp. 15–17.

Kluge, Eike-Henner W. (2000): "Improving Organ Retrieval Rates: Various Proposals and Their Ethical Validity." In: Health Care Analysis 8/3, pp. 285–287.

Levy, Neil (2019): "Nudge, Nudge, Wink, Wink: Nudging is Giving Reasons." In: Ergo 6/10, pp. 281–302.

MacKay, Douglas/Robinson, Alexandra (2016): "The Ethics of Organ Donor Registration Policies: Nudges and Respect for Autonomy." In: The American Journal of Bioethics 16/11, pp. 3–12.

MacKay, Douglas (2015): "Opt-out and Consent." In: Journal of Medical Ethics 41/10, pp. 832–835.

MacKay, Douglas (2017): "Nudges, Autonomy, and Organ Donor Registration Policies: Response to Critics." In: The American Journal of Bioethics 17/2, pp. W6–W8.

Miller, Franklin G./Gelinas, Luke (2013): "Nudging, Autonomy, and Valid Consent: Context Matters." In: The American Journal of Bioethics 13/6, pp. 12–13.

Morton, Jennifer (2011): "Toward an Ecological Theory of the Norms of Practical Deliberation," In: European Journal of Philosophy 19/4, pp. 561–584.

Navin, Mark (2017): "The Ethics of Vaccination Nudges in Pediatric Practice." In: HEC Forum 29/1, pp. 43–57.

Rebonato, Riccardo (2014): "A Critical Assessment of Libertarian Paternalism." In: Journal of Consumer Policy 37/3, pp. 357–396.

Reinhart, Amber Marie/Marshall, Heather M./Feeley, Thomas Hugh/Tutzauer, Frank (2007): "The Persuasive Effects of Message Framing in Organ Donation: The Mediating Role of Psychological Reactance." In: Communication Monographs 74/2, pp. 229–255.

Rippon, Simon (2012): "How to Reverse the Organ Shortage." In: Journal of Applied Philosophy 29/4, pp. 344–358.

Rodrigue, James/Cornell, Danielle/Howard, Richard (2008): "The Instability of Organ Donation Decisions by Next-of-kin and Factors that Predict it." In: American Journal of Transplantation 8/12, pp. 2661–2667.

Rosenblum, Amanda/Horvat, Lucy/Siminoff, Laura/Prakash, Versha/Beitel, Janice/Garg, Amit (2012): "The Authority of Next-of-kin in Explicit and Presumed Consent Systems for Deceased Organ Donation: an Analysis of 54 Nations." In: Nephrology Dialysis Transplantation 27/6, pp. 2533–2546.

Saunders, Ben (2010): "Normative Consent and Opt-out Organ Donation." In: Journal of Medical Ethics 36/2, pp. 84–87.

Saunders, Ben (2012): "Opt-out Organ Donation without Presumptions." In: Journal of Medical Ethics 38/2, pp. 69–72.

Schmidt, Andreas T. (2019): "Getting Real on Rationality – Behavioral Science, Nudging and Public Policy," In: Ethics 129/4, pp. 511–543.

Sharif, Adnan/Moorlock, Greg (2018): "Influencing Relatives to Respect Donor Autonomy: Should we Nudge Families to Consent to Organ Donation?" In: Bioethics 32/3, pp. 155–163.

Snyder, Jeremy (2009): "Easy Rescues and Organ Transplantation." In: HEC Forum 21/1, 27–53.

Steinberg, David (2004), "An 'Opting In' Paradigm for Kidney Transplantation." The American Journal of Bioethics 4/4, pp. 4–14.

Sunstein, Cass R. (2015): "The Ethics of Nudging." In: Yale Journal of Regulation 32/2, pp. 413–450.

Sunstein, Cass R. (2016): "Autonomy by Default." In: The American Journal of Bioethics 16/11, pp. 1–2.

Thaler, Richard H./Sunstein, Cass R. (2008): Nudge: Improving Decisions About Health, Wealth, and Happiness, New Haven: Yale University Press.

Taylor, James Stacey (2012): Death Posthumous Harm, and Bioethics, New York: Routledge.

Troug, Robert (2012): "When Does a Nudge Become a Shove in Seeking Consent for Organ Donation?" In: The American Journal of Bioethics 12/2, pp. 42–44.

Van Dalen, Hendrik P./Henkens, Kène (2014): "Comparing the Effects of Defaults in Organ Donation Systems" In: Social Science & Medicine 106/April, pp. 137–142.

Veatch, Robert M. (2000): Transplantation Ethics, Washington: Georgetown University Press.

White, Mark D. (2013): The Manipulation of Choice: Ethics and Libertarian Paternalism, New York: Palgrave Macmillan.

Whyte, Kyle Powys/Selinger, Evan/Caplan, Arthur L./Sadowski, Jathan (2012): "Nudge, Nudge or Shove, Shove – The Right Way for Nudges to Increase the Supply of Donated Cadaver Organs." In: The American Journal of Bioethics 12/2, pp. 32–39.

Wilkinson, T. M. (2011): Ethics and the Acquisition of Organs, New York: Oxford University Press.

Wilkinson, T. M. (2013): "Nudging and Manipulation" In: Political Studies 61/2, pp. 341–355.

Wilkinson, T. M. (2017): "Counter-Manipulation and Health Promotion." In: Public Health Ethics 10/3, pp. 257–266.

Willis, Brian H./Quigley, Muireann (2014): "Opt-out Organ Donation: On Evidence and Public Policy." In: Journal of the Royal Society of Medicine 107/2, pp. 56–60.

Zambrano, Alexander (2018): "Should Consent be Required for Organ Donation?" In: Bioethics 32/7, pp. 421–429.

Zink, Sheldon/Wertlieb, Stacey (2006): "A Study of the Presumptive Approach to Consent for Organ Donation: A New Solution to an Old Problem" In: Critical Care Nurse 26/2, pp. 129–136.

4. Appealing to Trust in Donation Contexts
Expectations and Commitments

Solveig Lena Hansen & Katharina Beier

1. Introduction

When the news reported on a German organ allocation scandal in 2012, transplantation medicine attracted significant attention in academic and political discourse. The media covered cases of manipulated data in the allocation of livers donated post-mortem in several German cities (Shaw 2013).[1] Even before those scandals, the absolute number of post-mortem donors had started to decrease, and continued to do so after those events. However, both media and research claimed that public distrust in the system had led to this decrease (Pondrom 2013).[2] This German case is not exceptional; other scandals have also caused international agitation. For example, the unauthorized retention of postmortem tissues/organs (mainly from children) from 1988 to 1995 at *Bristol Royal Infirmary* and *Liverpool Alder Hey Royal Infirmary* led to public outcry in the UK after a public inquiry in 1999. In the wake of this crisis, a new regulatory framework, the Human Tissue Act, together with the *Human Tissue Agency* as regulatory body, were established in 2004 in order to rebuild trust (Sheach Leith 2008).[3] Public debates on research with human tissues stored in biobanks were also triggered by the establishment of the Icelandic Health Sector Database and the exclusive license granted to the American enterprise deCODE for its commercial use. Consequently, there was rising awareness that abuse of samples and data might decrease people's trust in biobank research.[4] These examples indicate that "it is precisely non-routine contexts that generate the need to start talking about trust" (Simpson 2012: 560). References to trust are like an alarm, demonstrating that "the habitual assumption of cooperative behavior no longer applies" (ibid.).

---

1 This is not to deny that trust is also relevant in the context of organ donation after cardiac death or living donation. However, because trust may relate to different aspects here, this paper focuses, for reasons of scope, only on posthumous organ donation after brain death.

2 We use the term 'distrust' throughout the paper, also in cases where other authors speak of 'mistrust'. For us, mistrust and distrust are interchangeable terms.

3 In Germany, the Augsburg-Munich proposal for a distinct Biobank law has been solicited as a step for promoting the trustworthiness of biobanks (Gassner et al. 2015).

4 For an overview of the development of the Icelandic Health Sector Database see Beier (2019).

Trust therefore only becomes topical after scandals or other forms of disruptions. Typically, after such events, actions to rebuild trust are taken. In response to the German organ allocation scandal, for instance, the Medical Association (*Bundesärztekammer*) established a commission to which incidents of misuse or irregularities could be reported anonymously (*Vertrauensstelle Transplantationsmedizin*). Along with such actions, appeals to trust in both media and policy often seek to rebuild the belief that the institution is reliable, although a certain amount of damage took place and some risk or insecurity remains.

However, this does not mean that trust is irrelevant outside of disruptive events. Throughout their routine practices, institutions involved in the donation of human body parts, such as organ donation for transplantation and tissue donation for research, take active measures to ensure public trust in order to reach their specific goals.

In these routines, trust remains a necessary, yet implicit condition. Institutions and actors involved in bodily donations invest extensive resources into increasing trust, for instance through their self-presentation on websites and public involvement measures. In addition, the academic discourse that reflects such self-presentations and public involvement often argues that more trust potentially increases the willingness to donate (Brown 2018; Dabrock et al. 2012).

These discourses evoke a certain paradigm, which we will critically analyze in this chapter. This paradigm follows a logic in which the application of adequate practices and regulative frameworks leads to a well-informed public, thus leading to trusting donors who ultimately support donations in practice. As we will show, the emergence of trust is more complex than this paradigm suggests. In addition, the willingness to donate organs for transplantation and tissue for research depends not only on trust but also on other factors, such as concepts of the body, understandings of death, acceptance of research in general, as well as notions of altruism and solidarity. By comparing organ donation and tissue donation for research, our analysis will reveal these factors and their different relation to trust and distrust.

2.   Defining Trust

Trust is an essential precondition for human interaction. Without trust, many goals in personal life, such as friendship or cooperation at the working place, would not be achievable. Trust becomes particularly relevant in the face of irreducible uncertainty (Möllering 2006; Lahno 2001), e.g. when people lack information or, conversely, are overwhelmed with information. In both cases, they are limited in their ability to make a decision or act in a specific situation. By entrusting a decision to another person or institution, people can maintain their agency. In this regard, trust is essential for handling the complexities of modern life (Luhmann 1979). Although trust is an everyday concept, it is understood differently based on both divergent disciplinary perspectives as well as varying assumptions about its very nature.

2.1   Models of Trust

Broadly speaking, trust can be variously characterized as an expectation, an emotion, or a belief.[5] Early concepts of trust were inspired by rational choice models (Gambetta 1988). These explain "trust as a rational result of a self-interested actor's perceptions of another actor's trustworthiness" (Möllering 2006: 24). In particular, these models are concerned with calculating the probability that an expected action will be taken. In contrast, more recent approaches not only recognize the crucial role of affection for the emergence of trust but also stress its genuine moral dimension (Jones 1996; Lahno 2001; Wiesemann 2016). Our analysis of organ donation and tissue donation for research employs these more recent accounts, because both practices touch upon fundamental moral issues, e.g. using a person's body (parts) for the sake of others.

2.2   The Moral Dimension of Trust

Trust relationships play a crucial role in medical contexts. Therefore, it is important to look at accounts of trust that emphasize its relational and moral dimension. First, by trusting, a person ('trustor') exposes herself to another source of insecurity, when she assumes that the trusted person ('trustee') will act in accordance with her interests and values. Because there is no guarantee that the trustee will do so, the trustor makes herself vulnerable to the trustee. However, the trustor is optimistic that the trustee will live up to her expectations. In doing so, the trustor accepts her "vulnerability to another's possible but not expected ill will (or lack of good will)" (Baier 1986: 235). It is a constitutive aspect of trust that it grants the trustee considerable discretionary power (ibid.). Moreover, there is usually no predefined mode of action that the trustee must follow. While this gives the trustee some leeway to meet the trustor's expectations, this leeway is not unlimited. Rather, the trustee is morally bound by the trustor's expectation that she will use this power responsibly; if the trustee were to use his power irresponsibly, she would risk fostering distrust. For the trustor, the anticipation that the trustee is committed to her values or goals can strengthen trusting expectations (Lahno 2001).

2.3   Trust as Optimistic Expectation

Defining trust as an expectation illustrates its genuine moral dimension, distinguishing it from reliance.[6] When we rely on someone, we expect a predictable action or non-action by this person, but we are indifferent, unaware, or even critical of her

---

5   In contrast to the question of the 'nature of trust' is its social, moral or epistemic function in a complex, highly differentiated modern world.

6   Most of our favored approaches share the idea that reliance is a necessary but insufficient condition for trust. Other models of trust that we do not take up in detail understand trust as a belief (Hieronymi 2008). In these approaches to trust, someone needs to be convinced that he is acting according to one's expectations. Such beliefs influence someone's decision to trust. That way, the belief in one's own expectations becomes a sufficient condition for reliance.

underlying motivation (Mullin 2005: 324).[7] In contrast, by trusting we count on the personal motivation of the trustee[8] to be responsive towards our goals or values. When a person we rely on fails us, we feel disappointed, but we do not hold her morally accountable. In contrast, if our trust is broken we feel betrayed or let down (Baier 1986: 235). Because trust implies a genuine moral commitment to consider the others' concerns, failing to do so qualifies as moral failure (Hawley 2014; Wiesemann 2016).

As Möllering (2006) notes, trust does not emerge without reason (e.g. a belief in the other's competencies and integrity); however, such reasons alone are not sufficient to generate trust. Rather, there is a 'mystical' element that bridges the gap between our reasons to trust and trust itself. This element has been conceptualized as 'leap of faith' or 'suspension'; trust implies that the trustor temporarily treats uncertainty and vulnerability "*as if* they were favorably resolved" (ibid.: 111; original emphasis). Trustworthiness, thus, is not an intrinsic property of a trustee but an attribution from the side of the trustor. It is through trust-based interpretations that a trustor adopts a trusting attitude towards another person. In particular, the trustor's positive expectation builds on a selective perception of the world that is not primarily governed by objective facts but rather by subjective emotions or affections (Lahno 2001; Jones 1996). From the trustor's perspective, trust needs "to *feel* right, true, plausible, and so on in spite of inconclusive evidence" (Möllering 2006: 121). This feeling makes (dis)trusting attitudes quite resistant to contrary evidence. Both the trusting and distrusting person are inclined to emphasize reasons that support their attitudes and ignore those that could challenge their attitude towards the trustee (Jones 1996; Möllering 2006: 114). However, trust is not only "self-confirming" (Jones 1996:17) but also self-reinforcing insofar as it builds on the hope "that by trusting we will be able to bring about the very conditions that would justify our trust" (ibid.: 22). Trust has therefore been described as a performative act that brings about the desired disposition by the very act of trusting (Lahno 2001).

2.4   Trust and Distrust

Any examination of trust inevitably confronts us with the question of what differentiates trust from distrust. At first sight they appear to be opposites. However, recent approaches question this dichotomy by stressing the coexistence of trust, lack of trust, and distrust (Mühlfried 2018). In particular, the absence of trust does not automatically imply distrust; people may sometimes simply be indifferent or disengaged regarding a particular matter (Hawley 2014). Moreover, if trust is understood as a social practice (Hartmann 2011), distrust can form part of this practice. Specifically, distrust allows questioning of the underlying values of a specific practice and may thus contribute to its reformation without necessarily damaging the practice as a whole. This is very important for bodily donations because it also helps us to analyze which groups can be characterized as (dis)trustors: while trustors accept their vulnerability and expect that trustees will handle their power responsibly, distrustors expect (or have even experi-

---

7   If we rely on inanimate objects, it does not even make sense to assume any kind of positive or negative motivation if the expected result fails to materialize.

8   Current theories explain this motivation with reference to different factors, such as assumptions about the trustee's benevolence (Jones 1996) or moral integrity (McLeod 2000).

enced) the contrary. People who lack trust are indifferent here; they neither trust nor distrust.

2.5 Trust in Systems

Not only people but also abstract entities (e.g. institutions) can be the object of trust. We may plausibly assume, however, that trust in organizations or institutional procedures is always mediated via personal contacts with its representatives (Hartmann 2011). Within such systems trust is built via "access points", which connect "lay individuals or collectivities and the representatives of abstract systems" (Giddens 1990: 88). For example, in the context of bodily donations it is physicians and researchers who serve as access points for building trust in the medical system, or in research in general. Importantly, these personal contacts can be either "junctions at which trust can be maintained or built up" (ibid.) or, if doubts arise about the system representatives' moral integrity or their competence, gateways for the erosion of trust in the institution as whole.

Organ and tissue donations for research are beyond the donor's control and, therefore, require trust in the respective system and its actors. Donors in particular face irreducible uncertainty in both opt-in and opt-out contexts – though for different reasons. For example, in both systems, prospective organ donors can document and specify their preferences, but they must rely on the relevant actors in the system to respect their preferences. Many of the features of trust discussed above relate to the fields of organ donation (OD) for transplantation and tissue donation for biobank research (BR). In the following, we will analyze the role of trust in OD and tissue donation for research and highlight its ethical implications, especially regarding public communication.

3. The Ethical Relevance of Trust in Organ Donation

For various actors in the context of transplantation medicine, trust is needed to cope with multiple insecurities. By trusting, these actors become vulnerable, and are willing to accept their vulnerability. It is important to keep in mind, though, that trust is relevant in both opt-in and opt-out systems; transplantation medicine is always based on a dense network of trusting and distrusting relations. This becomes even more apparent in cases of successful transplantation, where we can observe the result of trusting relationships between different actors. Successful transplantations are joint accomplishments of "recipients, donors, surgeons and other medical professionals" (Almassi 2014: 275) that engage with each other through their knowledge, cooperativeness, and trust. This positive notion of trust, however, has gained very little attention. Rather, the debate's initial focus was – and still is – public *distrust* in OD (Newton 2011; Morgan et al. 2008); and this *distrust* is usually located in the unaffected, prospective organ donors (Brown 2018; Irving et al. 2012). Prospective donors need to trust that medical professionals and respective authorities will act according to their preferences. And in systems in which family members may have a say in the fate of the deceased's organs, prospective donors also need to trust their next of kin to decide according to their preferences. Moreover, given the pronounced need for organs in both opt-in and opt-out systems (Beard 2013), this focus on donors is unsurprising. It follows the logic already outlined in our introduction (see 1), which anticipates that providing information increases public trust. A trusting public, in turn, is likely to support organ donation, which would ideally lead to higher donation rates (Morgan et al. 2012). According to this logic, public distrust is one explanation for decreasing donation numbers (Morgan 2009). However, such a strong focus on public distrust might exclude some perspectives from analysis and risk overemphasizing the link between trust and willingness to OD while ignoring other reasons for non-willingness to donate.

3.1   Trustors, Trustees, Objects of Trust in Organ Donation

Successful donations remind us of the multiple dimensions of trust that transplantation medicine encompasses: not only prospective donors but also their families and organ recipients may count as trustors (Dicks et al. 2018). Trusting and distrusting attitudes amongst medical professionals have only recently begun to receive attention (Jawoniyi et al. 2017). At first blush, the idea that those involved in transplantation medicine might also trust or distrust the system seems very surprising. Because they are likely to be well-informed about transplantation matters, this idea complicates the assumed correlation between lack of information, public distrust, and low organ donation rates. Indeed, an attitude of trust is not limited to certain groups because "our varied experiences, perspectives, and social identities underwrite varied assessments of others' reliability, goodwill, and responsiveness in our interactions with them" (Almassi 2014: 279). This applies as much to experts as to laypeople.

However, aside from their moral expectations, there is still a difference between transplantation professionals and other groups involved, such as donors. As argued in section 2 above, a trustor exposes herself to insecurity when she assumes that the trustee will act in accordance with her interests and values and thus becomes dependent on the trustee's good will. Medical professionals who are involved in donations but are not themselves donors or recipients are unlikely to be vulnerable and dependent in the system. As access points to the transplantation system, they are very likely to be in the role of trustees.

Therefore, transplantation experts do not evaluate the transplantation system in terms of *trust* but rather in terms of its *reliability*. They expect predictable actions or non-actions (such as shared standards amongst colleagues), but they are indifferent, unaware or even critical of the underlying motivations. After disruptive events such as organ allocation scandals, experts try to ameliorate or increase the system's reliability (see also chapter 9 in this book).

Corresponding to the multitude of possible trustors and trustees is a broad range of objects of trust, namely those actions that constitute trusting relationships. As stated above, the debate has focused on donor autonomy and its relationship to donors' trust and distrust. However, even for donors there can be other objects of trust, such as careful diagnostics of brain death, respectful treatment of the body, and careful communication with the family of the deceased. A donor's relatives are likely to have the same objects of trust. For organ recipients, the conditions under which the explantation took place and the communication about risks and benefits of transplantations can be objects of trust. Another object of trust, however, which is central to all actors – donors, their families, and recipients – is the fair allocation of organs.

Just as the objects of trust in transplantation medicine vary, so do the objects of distrust. All the objects of trust mentioned here – donor autonomy, careful diagnostics of brain death, respectful treatment of the body, careful communication with donor families, and fair allocation of organs as a scarce resource – if being part of unfulfilled commitments, can also be objects of distrust. People who distrust OD feel that responsible actors or institutions did not honor their commitments. According to our understanding (see 2), trust and distrust are not dichotomous; some groups may neither trust nor distrust the system. Their 'lack of trust', therefore, must not be understood as distrust; they might simply be indifferent to trust because they have not taken the leap of faith.

3.2   Trust, Distrust, and the Willingness to Donate

It would seem logical to assume that those who trust systems of bodily donations are themselves likely to be donors. Conversely, distrust is commonly cited as a reason for low donation rates (see above). However, the situation is more complex than this. For example, distrust alone cannot explain negative attitudes towards organ donations. Rather, four factors, often intermingled, largely explain attitudes to OD: first, various social-psychological reasons (Falomir-Pichastor et al. 2013); second, cultural concepts of the body and/or death (Schicktanz et al. 2017); third, structural problems within the medical system (Jawoniyi et al. 2017); and, fourth, the legal model of consent (Molina-Pérez et al. 2018). There is no evidence that one factor alone can explain the differences in donation rates.

Moreover, there is a difference between people's support of organ or tissue donation in theory and actual donation rates (Caille-Brillet et al. 2019). Approaches that closely link trust, public information, and donation rates cannot explain why actual donations remain low despite increased regulation and information activities. Instead of arguing for even more information in order to increase trust, the debate could profit from a more complex model of OD-related decision making, taking into account concepts of the body, criteria of death, and preferences associated with dying (Pfaller et al. 2018). By trusting, a trustor adopts the attitude that trustees will respect their values regarding these issues. Therefore, a trustor is vulnerable, as she "allows another [person] to exercise a certain amount of control over matters that are of some importance" (Lahno 2001, 171). So, she accepts the risk of harm or an infringement of her values. On this understanding, trust is "to some extent, independent of objective information" (ibid.). This may be of only minor relevance to people who generally trust the system but need more information to make their decision. More transparency and correct information might indeed help this particular group to decide.

However, there are those that believe that the trustee will not respect their values or will not honor his commitments. They are the distrusting group. They do not see that trust in the medical system and the public institutions administrating OD will enhance their range of options. Rather, they expect harm from it: infringement of their interests, manipulation, prioritizing organ donation over preserving life, and much more. Thus, their distrust entails the expectation that transplantation medicine will violate its obligation to respect their preferences and vulnerability. False or misleading information might even trigger these forms of distrust (Hansen et al. 2020).

From a trust-based perspective, it thus follows that there is no need to closely link distrust and unwillingness to donate: people might be willing to be an organ donor *despite* distrusting the system. In such cases, other factors, such as solidarity with potential recipients or minimizing suffering, trump their distrust. Conversely, it is possible to find a system reliable and still *not* to support OD: for instance, if someone does not share the very core concepts of transplantation medicine, such as brain death or the replaceability of body parts, they are unlikely to be a willing donor. They have no reason for a 'leap of faith'. However, this does not automatically mean that they distrust the system in general. Rather, they do not identify with it at all. Consequently, trust is simply not applicable for those groups because they are not willing to make themselves vulnerable to the OD system. However, they can still value OD as a therapy. Such groups in particular feel ambivalent because they want to help others in need, and they do support OD systems, but they do not want to donate themselves (Pfaller et al. 2018). They might seek alternatives to support patients' needs (Dijker et al. 2019). Bodily donations for research might provide such an alternative because they might indirectly improve transplantation outcomes, immunosuppression or other drugs, or alternatives to organ donation.

4.   The Ethical Relevance of Trust in Tissue Donation for Research

Trust generally plays a crucial role in research involving human subjects. For example, research participants who subject themselves to potentially risky interventions must trust researchers' professional competencies as well as their ethical integrity. At the system level, trust in research oversight mechanisms, such as ethical review boards, is also crucial. But researchers must also be able to trust their potential research subjects, e.g. to provide correct information about their state of health or medication (Resnik 2018: 89f.). However, although trust is accepted as an important value in the context of research, its moral implications for medical research are far from clear (Kerasidou 2017). This inevitably raises questions for biobank research (BR). As BR research paradigmatically demonstrates, "*public trust* has become something of a buzzword: universally assumed to be crucial to biobank research, but rarely defined" (Johnsson 2013: 47, emphasis cited).

In order to better understand the role of trust and its ethical implications for BR, we will first discuss trust as an alternative ethical framework to informed consent (Hawkin/Doherty 2010) (see 4.1). Second, we will analyze the relevance and implications of trust/distrust for participation in BR. Trust is often presented as an empirically measurable indicator of people's actual willingness to donate their samples and data. However, just as in the case of OD, we will show that the relationship between trust/distrust and actual participation is not as straightforward as this rhetoric suggests (see 4.2).

4.1   Trust as Alternative Ethical Framework

The bioethical literature discusses various objects of trust in the context of BR. For example, people may place trust in biobank operators or researchers (Lipworth et al. 2009), in biomedical research in general (de Vries et al. 2016), or in governance mechanisms, such as independent oversight (Prainsack/Buyx 2013). Trust in BR may also derive from trust in the national health care system or the government in general (Gaskell et al. 2010). Not least, trust in BR may be mediated by physicians, who act as – following Giddens' terminology – "access points" (1999: 88) for patients' trust (see 2.5). It is worth noting that potential donors are typically approached by physicians in the clinical context, e.g. prior to surgery.

Just as in the case of OD, the debate on BR mainly focuses on donors' trust.[9] This can be explained by the open-ended purposes of BR, where, due to the rapid development of diagnostic tools and information technologies it impossible to foresee all future uses of donors' samples and data in research. This leaves potential donors in a situation of irreducible uncertainty which limits the possibility of truly informed consent. While it could be argued that the donation of tissue, blood, or other bodily fluids for research does not usually involve noteworthy physical risks (samples are often acquired during medical routines), there may still be immaterial dangers, e.g. disclosure of sensitive information to third parties.

By entrusting their samples and data to research, participants render themselves vulnerable to researchers' decisions. However, even though they are experts in their fields, researchers are no more able than donors to foresee all the possible future uses of tissue and data. Indeed, if they were able to predict this, it would be immoral for them to withhold this information from donors. Moreover, the fact that biobankers/researchers are entrusted with donor samples and data renders them morally obliged to use these materials in a way that respects the rights and values of donors, e.g. by promoting public health and protecting their privacy. Thus, far from sustaining a one-sided dependency, BR builds on a reciprocal relationship between donors and researchers. In fact, researchers or physicians that recruit tissue donors incur a moral responsibility towards the latter. Specifically, they are required, amongst other things, to avoid or at least to correct mistakenly assumed trust, e.g. if donors lack the respective competences or hold erroneous assumptions about the aims of research (Johnsson et al. 2013). In this way, the risk that donors become unilaterally dependent on researchers and thus disempowered is counterweighed by the moral obligation that their trust imposes on researchers.

Against this background, obtaining donor consent in BR, even though it is not fully informed, is at least symbolically important (O'Neill 2002). In particular, *the very act of being asked*, alongside the possibility of withdrawing from participation, respects donors as moral agents and allows researchers to present themselves and their institution as trustworthy (Allen/McNamara 2011). Boniolo et al. thus speak of a "trusted consent" (2012: 95) which requires that donors believe in the competence as well as moral integrity of researchers. Thus, from a trust-perspective, the design of (alternative) consent models is a sensitive issue: presumed and, to some extent, also open/blanket consent models[10] may not suffice to establish a relationship of mutual trust. In par-

---

9 Strictly speaking, however, trust is also relevant for biobank operators, and particularly researchers. Because BR may require repeated contributions by participants, banks and researchers must trust participants' ongoing willingness to support BR. In addition, when sharing their samples, researchers must trust that others also respect the donors' rights and values.

10 Although there is no uniform use of these terms, the different consent models can be roughly characterized as follows: Presumed consent implies that tissues/data are automatically taken (e.g. left-

ticular, the presumed consent model takes participation for granted and thus "lacks any symbolic act that enables individuals to declare their trust and their identity as moral actors in their community" (Allen/McNamara 2011: 165). In contrast, broad consent alongside mechanisms of independent ethical oversight can have a trust-ensuring effect. While researchers remain accountable to donors, the latter's trust grants them sufficient leeway to pursue research questions that are of general public interest. At the same time, donors are relieved of the time-consuming task of staying up to date about all relevant research aspects.

4.2   Trust, Distrust, and Participation

Empirical studies that examine people's willingness to participate in BR report concurrently on high participation rates. That patients but also healthy people are highly ready to donate their bodily materials – often leftovers from diagnostics or surgery but also samples specifically collected for research purposes – is often interpreted as an indication of public trust (Critchley et al. 2015). At the same time, there is a broad awareness that this trust can easily be lost, e.g. due to a mishandling of samples (Master et al. 2012). Reflecting this perception, ubiquitous appeals in both the media and also scientific discourse seek to build and sustain trust in BR (Sprecher 2017; German Ethics Council 2010; Hansson 2005). However, public solicitation for '(more) trust in biobank research' can be a strategic narrative in order to present biobanking in a favorable light and to encourage participation (Johnsson 2013; Snell/Tarkkala 2019). Simply calling for trust without corresponding action renders such appeals empty. In fact, trust cannot be forced; rather, it emerges subtly over time. For example, general trust in science may gradually grow into a personal trust-relationship with a specific researcher or research institution (Nobilé et al. 2016), but this process is not guaranteed.

Second, participation in BR is not a matter of donors' trust alone. Because perceptions of trustworthiness develop in the mind of the donor and are also influenced by social and cultural factors (Sheikh/Hoeyer 2018), it is not easy to determine what will tip the scale for an individual donor's decision to trust BR. Without deeper knowledge about donors' attitudes, it may be misleading to understand participation *per se* as a reflection of donors' trust in BR. Also, it need not necessarily be trust that motivates people to donate their samples and data to BR. For example, there is some evidence that people do not take much interest in what is happening to their samples (Hoeyer 2012). Beyond trust, participation in BR may be influenced by the personal predispositions of donors (Nobilé et al. 2016), reliance on the proper functioning of medical routines, or a sense of duty to support research. Furthermore, recruitment strategies employed by researchers are relevant here (Van Zon et al. 2016). For example, physicians may not be sufficiently motivated or prepared to inform their patients about the option of donating tissue to BR, e.g. due to time-pressure or discomfort to discuss the

---

overs from diagnostics or surgery) unless people file an objection. Open/blanket consent means that people are asked to agree to research in general, without any specification. Models of broad consent intend to use samples/data for a broad range of research purposes that cannot be specified in detail but at least narrowed down to certain fields. In addition, oversight by an independent ethical review board is typically foreseen.

donation of certain types of tissues, such as brain tissue (Beier/Frebel 2018). In this case, lack of participation cannot be attributed to a lack of donors' trust.

Even though participation in BR should not be framed as a matter of trust alone, it is still important to ask what promotes the trust of donors. In particular, the notion of trust as a moral commitment emphasizes the responsibility of researchers to live up to donors' expectations. A recurrent promise in the biobank discourse is to ensure this by strengthening ethical and legal governance mechanisms (e.g. with regard to information, control or transparency) (Hawkins/O'Doherty 2010). However, such measures may miss the point insofar as this increases *reliability* rather than trust per se (O'Neill 2002). For example, by insisting on strict informed consent rules – despite the public's broad support of biobank research – the public's trust may even be undermined by nourishing suspicion that had not previously existed (Ducournau/Strand 2009). In fact, in order to genuinely trust, potential donors to BR need a different kind of evidence, i.e. the commitment of researchers to respect their interests and values.

Empirical studies have shown that participants are predominantly motivated by the wish to help others and to improve the health of future generations (Kettis-Lindblad et al. 2006; Porteri et al. 2014). An important step for winning/maintaining potential donors' trust would thus be to respect "the spirit in which donations were made" (Hoeyer 2012: 36).[11] This could be done, for example, by delivering visible results for the common good (Zawati 2014) and by allowing for benefit-sharing and public involvement (Masui 2009). Against this background, donors' trust in BR would most likely be eroded if they came to realize that their interests and values had been disrespected or even misused, for example if donors learned that the samples they donated out of a sense of altruism and solidarity had been used for commercial purposes rather than to improve general health levels. In fact, the involvement of commercial actors and breaches of confidentiality, particularly regarding genetic information, have been identified as sources of distrust (Caulfield et al. 2014; Solum Steinsbekk et al. 2013a; Goddard et al. 2009).

At the same time, refusal to participate does not necessarily indicate a distrusting attitude; it may also be due to a lack of understanding regarding the relevance of BR, or simply a lack of time (Melas et al. 2010). Furthermore, people raising doubts about certain aspects of BR need not erode trust in BR in general. In fact, public deliberation and consultation on BR can be used to reflect on the underlying values of this practice in order to strengthen trust (De Vries et al. 2018). BR requires an ongoing relationship between donors and researchers: the former must repeatedly provide bodily materials and related data for research, while the latter regularly share the results of their research with donors as recognition of their contribution. This repeated mutual interaction can be conducive to the emergence of trust. However, since research is often closely related to medical treatment, there is also a risk that donors may (mistakenly) come to "understand the aim of research as serving them directly" (Solum Steinsbekk et al. 2013b: 899). Given that unfulfilled commitments can lead to distrust, the distinction between medical treatment and research participation must be made transparent to donors.

---

11   Patients' 'spirit of donation' may even be more pronounced than that of healthy donors. Although the motivation to contribute to biobank research is high in both groups, patients have a personal interest in promoting research. In particular, they trust the researchers to advance knowledge on their disease (Bochud et al. 2017).

5.   Trust and Public Communication

As our analysis shows, the role of trust in organ donation for transplantation and tissue donation for research is complex. It involves donors, patients, family members, health care professionals, and researchers in the roles of both trustors and trustees. Given this multitude of actors involved, there are various sources for error and uncertain outcomes, rendering both opt-in and opt-out systems fragile and highlighting the need for trust. Against this background, it is instructive to look at the role of communication. After all, what can establish, maintain, or increase trust if not communication?

According to our theoretical analysis, the role of communication for both reliance and trust must be considered here. One noticeable feature of our analysis is that we find references to 'trust' that follow a more instrumental logic: an increase of information leads to transparency, which leads to trust, which will then most likely increase people's willingness to donate/participate. This logic is reflected, for example, in the German Ethics Council's opinion on research biobanking: "To guarantee this trust [in BR], the procedure itself, the provisions governing it and the activities of the biobank must be transparent. Depending on the degree to which this transparency is guaranteed by law, it may be expected that donors are readier to cooperate and possibly also to accept a more extended use of samples and data" (German Ethics Council 2010: 21). However, ensuring transparency through communication does not increase *trust* but merely *reliance*.

Besides such official statements from public institutions, information campaigns are used to spread knowledge about bodily donations and – in many cases – to foster support for donations (Hansen et al. 2018). Again, the common wisdom here is that complete or accurate information maintains, protects, or even increases public trust: "The more accurate the information available, the more accurate the anticipation of future eventualities and the more appropriately directed the trust" (Brown 2018: 145). According to this logic, trust again becomes a synonym for mere reliance and is thus robbed of its dense moral implications. Speaking of reliance here seems more appropriate, as accurate information might indeed help the public to think of a system as reliable.

Against this background, it is striking that public campaigns also can have unintended counter effects when they are open to scrutiny. For example, early German organ donation campaigns introduced the idea that potential organ donors are given priority in organ allocation (Hansen et al. 2020). However, this implicit promise is, at least in the German system, false; no donor can rely on calculation to ensure that they will receive a needed organ. Research shows that skeptics are especially sensitive to such misleading claims, and reluctant persons even express that such information practices can lead to distrust (ibid.). These findings show that skeptical people are very sensitive to the ways OD issues are framed.

In the context of BR, donors are enticed to entrust their samples and data to research by more or less explicit references to solidarity, altruism, or notions of the common good. For example, in order to attract donors to an ongoing imaging study, the UK Biobank website features the slogan "Improving the health of future generations" above a counter that records the number of participants enrolled. The subtitle reads: "Participants scanned so far – help us to make it to 100.000!"[12] On the one hand, this can be seen as a way to present BR as a trustworthy endeavor; on the other hand, it is through this "normative recruitment" (Ursin and Solberg 2008: 109) that biobanks render themselves vulnerable to the public's critical eye. In order to deserve and maintain people's trust, they must show that they are seriously seeking to live up to these promises. This, however, may not always be easy in the context of BR. Due to its long-term nature, evidence of fulfilling specific promises may remain quite abstract. Also, researchers may not always be able to meet donors' expectations, e.g. regarding the effective use of samples due to the current underutilization of sample collections (Zika et al. 2011). In fact, the perception that notions of solidarity or the public good are being evoked instrumentally – e.g. to "sell science" (Johnsson 2013: 59) – could erode people's trust in BR, which may affect their willingness to participate in this strand of research.

In these cases, communication serves as a tool to strategically generate public understanding or even public acceptance, an aim that has been criticized by discourse ethicists, and by Habermas (1984) in particular. Indeed, this style of communication might increase the reliability of institutions and thus contribute to public acceptance. However, it will fail to increase trust if it does not invite people to make themselves vulnerable by taking a 'leap of faith' (Möllering 2006). In the analysis or creation of such communicational interventions, therefore, one should critically ask if the call for 'more trust' is a plea for ongoing dialogue or for the acknowledgement of both the vulnerabilities of trustors and the commitments of trustees? Or is it rather a strategic move to ensure more public acceptance by using 'trust' as a synonym for 'reliance'?

However, it is important to note that even communicational interventions that aim to increase public acceptance follow some "implicit expectations" (Johannesen et al. 2008: 12) of public discourse. Specifically, when such institutions are in need of moral support, e.g. from possible donors, they decide for campaigns or other interventions. These institutions take for granted that their goals are relevant to the public and cannot be solved by individual action or experts alone. Moreover, they consider their goal so important that they are willing to expose their practices to public scrutiny. It is precisely this fact that serves as a link between communication and trust, which goes beyond reliance.

Here, it is important to repeat that trust implies a 'leap of faith' (Möllering 2006). However, it is difficult to predict in specific cases which factors will generate public trust. There is no guarantee that people take the plunge into trust, especially if interventions mainly focus on rational aspects such as control, external surveillance, and formal procedures.

Nevertheless, we may still ask ourselves how we can strengthen trust. In other words, how can we invite potential donors to take a 'leap of faith' and to render themselves vulnerable? Even though trust includes a "mystical" element (ibid.: 118), we can still draw some lessons for public communication on OD/BR. First, it is important that the invitation to trust remains, due to the very nature of trust, an *invitation*. Trust can never be demanded or even enforced. On the contrary, attempts to enforce trust will most likely end in distrust. Second, it is important to examine what people require in order to perceive OD and BR systems as trustworthy. This is particularly important

---

12 UK Biobank: https://imaging.ukbiobank.ac.uk/#/ (accessed February 28, 2020).

because the objects of peoples' trust might be different from the objects that experts think they are entrusted with. Third, given that trust entails the trustor's belief that the trustee will respect her values and goals, OD and BR – as systems that are eager to win donors' trust – should remain aware of their moral responsibilities and critically reflect on whether their practices meet these obligations. This also implies a duty to correct unrealistic expectations. Fourth, it is important to acknowledge that the reasons for donating or refusing to donate vary due to cultural peculiarities, anxieties, and concepts of death that differ from the hegemonic discourse. A commitment to respect these concerns might do more to build trusting relationships than merely appealing for trust and strengthening governance ever can. This becomes even more apparent when we look at this issue from the perspective of distrust as unfulfilled commitment, and when we consider that distrustors might actually feel or experience that an institution does not fulfill its commitments. If distrust is the result of unfulfilled commitments, not only ameliorative strategies but also actions of moral repair (Urban Walker 2012), such as excuses, need to complete governance models and laws.

6.   Conclusion

As our examples illustrate, 'trust' is often used as an umbrella term to encompass obviously different circumstances. These circumstances can be analyzed in more detail if trust is differentiated from reliance, and if the moral dimension of trust is taken into account. As our analysis shows, non-participation in both OD and BR should not be equated with distrust. Distrust, as defined by Hawley, implies the expectation (or even experience) that the other party has a commitment but is expected not to honor it. This, however, is not the same as 'lack of trust', which can be characterized as an attitude of indifference or mere reliance. As we have argued, people may have a variety of reasons for not participating in OD and BR which have nothing to do with distrust. In particular, there are people who are unlikely to ever take the 'leap of faith' because they do not share the core principles of transplantation medicine or tissue donation for research. For these groups, the framework of trust is not applicable to explain their attitudes. In this way, our analysis contributes to a more analytical differentiation and clarification of the links between trust, lack of trust, distrust, and willingness/refusal to participation.

Consequently, our analysis helps both researchers and practitioners in the field of bodily donations to reflect more on their use of the term 'trust'. From our perspective, the critical point is that relying solely on factual information and transparency to ensure or increase trust will be of limited value. While we present some first ideas of how trust can be promoted, e.g. by respecting donors' values, communicative invitations and practices of moral repair, this is an issue that requires further research. Our analysis also shows that there are potential interactions between trust in organ donation for transplantation and tissue donation for research insofar as detrimental developments in one system may affect the other. Recent developments in, for instance, organ printing (see chapter 17 in this book) and organoids indicate this. Since there are crucial differences for why people are reluctant to engage with each of these fields, it might be worth treating these practices as alternatives and, thereby, opening up a broader discussion about supporting research that serves chronically sick patients.

Acknowledgements

This work is funded by the German Research Foundation (DFG) (SCHI 631/7-3). The authors thank two referees for their feedback. Furthermore, they thank Jon Leefmann for his critique and support.

References

Allen, Judy/McNamara, Beverley (2011): "Reconsidering the Value of Consent in Biobank Research." In: Bioethics 25/3, pp. 155–166.

Almassi, Ben (2014): "Trust and the Duty of Organ Donation." In: Bioethics 28/6, pp. 275–283.

Baier, Annette (1986): "Trust and Antitrust." In: Ethics 96/2, pp. 231–260.

Beard, T. Randolph/Kaserman, David L./Osterkamp, Rigmar (2013): The Global Organ Shortage: Economic Causes, Human Consequences, Policy Responses, Stanford: Stanford University Press.

Beier, Katharina/Frebel, Lisa (2018): "Brain Banking für die Forschung – eine empirisch-ethische Analyse praktischer Herausforderungen." In: Ethik in der Medizin 30/2, pp. 123–139.

Beier, Katharina (2019): "Biobanking at the Baltic Sea. An Analysis of the Swedish, Estonian and German Approaches." In: Nils Hansson/Jonatan Wistrand (eds.), Explorations in Baltic Medical History 1850–2015, Rochester: University of Rochester Press, pp. 203–228.

Bochud, Murielle/Currat, Christine/Chapette, Lawrence/Roth, Cindy/Mooser, Vincent (2017): "High Participation Rate among 25721 Patients with Broad Age Range in a hospital-based Research Project Involving Whole-Genome Sequencing – the Lausanne Institutional Biobank." In: Swiss Medical Weekly 147. DOI: 10.4414/smw.2017.14528

Boniolo, Giovanni/Di Fiore, Pier Paolo/Pece, Salvatore (2012): "Trusted Consent and Research Biobanks: Towards a 'New Alliance' between Researchers and Donors." In: Bioethics 26/2, pp. 93–100.

Brown, Sarah-Jane (2018): "Autonomy, Trust and Ante-Mortem Interventions to Facilitate Organ Donation." In: Clinical Ethics 13/3, pp. 143–150.

Caille-Brillet, Anne-Laure/Zimmering, Rebecca/Thaiss, Heidrun M. (2019): Bericht zur Repräsentativstudie 2018 "Wissen, Einstellung und Verhalten der Allgemeinbevölkerung zur Organ- und Gewebespende". Köln.

Caulfield, Timothy/Burningham, Sarah/Joly, Yann/Master, Zubin/Shabani, Masha/Borry, Pascal/Becker, Allan/Burgess, Michael/Calder, Kathryn/Critchley, Christine/Edwards, Kelly/ Fullerton, Stephanie M./ Gottweis, Herbert/Hyde-Lay, Robyn/ Illes, Judy/Isasi, Rosario/ Kato, Kazuto/Kaye, Jane/Knoppers, Bartha/Lynch, John/McGuire, Amy/Meslin, Eric/Nicol, Dianne/O'Doherty, Kieran/Ogbogu, Ubaka/Otlowski, Margaret/Pullman, Daryl/Ries, Nola/ Scott, Chris/Sears, Malcolm/Wallace, Helen/Zawati, Ma'n H. (2014): "A Review of the Key Issues associated with the Commercialization of Biobanks." In: Journal of Law and the Biosciences 1/1, pp. 94–110.

Critchley, Christine/Nicol, Dianne/Otlowski, Margaret (2015): "The Impact of Commercialisation and Genetic Data Sharing Arrangements on Public Trust and the Intention to Participate in Biobank Research." In: Public Health Genomics 18/3, pp. 160–172.

Dabrock, Peter/Taupitz, Jochen/Ried, Jens (2012): Trust in Biobanking, Berlin: Springer.

De Vries, Raymond G./Tomlinson, Tom/Kim, Hyungjin Myra/Krenz, Chris D./Haggerty, Diana/ Ryan, Kerry A./Kim, Scott Y.H. (2016): "Understanding the Public's Reservations about Broad Consent and Study-By-Study Consent for Donations to a Biobank: Results of a National Survey." In: PloS One 11/7. DOI: 10.1371/journal.pone.0159113

De Vries, Raymond G./Ryan, Kerry A./Gordon, Linda/Krenz, Chris D./Tomlinson, Tom/ Jewell, Scott/Kim, Scott Y.H. (2018): "Biobanks and the Moral Concerns of Donors: A Democratic Deliberation." In: Qualitative Health Research 29/13, pp. 1942–1953.

Dicks, Sean Glenton/Northam, Holly/Van Haaren, Fank M.P./Boer, Douglas P. (2018): "An Exploration of the Relationship between Families of Deceased Organ Donors and Transplant Recipients: A Systematic Review and Qualitative Synthesis." In: Health Psychology Open 5/1, pp. 1–25.

Dijker, Anton J.M./De Bakker, Erica/Bensen, Stanneke C./De Vries, Nanne K. (2019): "What Determines Support for Donor Registration Systems? The Influence of Sociopolitical Viewpoint, Attitudes toward Organ Donation, and Patients' Need." In: International Journal of Behavioral Medicine 26/2, pp. 195–206.

Ducournau, Pascal/Strand, Roger (2009): "Trust, Distrust and Co-Production: The Relationship between Research biobanks and Donors." In: Jan Helge Solbakk/ Soren Holm/Bjorn Hofmann (eds.), The Ethics of Research Biobanking, Boston: Springer US, pp. 115–130.

Falomir-Pichastor, Juan M./Berent, Jacques, & Pereira, Andrea (2013): "Social Psychological Factors of Post-Mortem Organ Donation: A Theoretical Review of Determinants and Promotion Strategies." In: Health Psychology Review 7/2, pp. 202–247.

Gambetta, Diego (1988): "Can We Trust Trust?" In: Diego Gambetta (ed.), Trust. Making and Breaking Cooperative Relations, Oxford: Basil Blackwell, pp. 213–237.

Gaskell, George/Stares, Sally/Allansdottir, Agnes/Allum, Nick/Castro, Paula/Esmer, Yilmaz/Fischler, Claude/Jackson, Jonathan/Kronberger, Nicole/Hampel, Jürgen/ Mejlgaard, Niels/Quintanilha, Alex/Rammer, Andu/Revuelta, Gemma/Stoneman, Paul/Torgersen, Helge/ Wagner, Wolfgang (2010): Europeans and Biotechnology in 2010: Winds of Change, Luxembourg: Publications of the European Union.

Gassner, Ulrich M/Kersten, Jens/Lindemann, Michael/Lindner, Josef Franz/Rosenau, Henning/ Schmidt am Busch, Birgit et al. (2015): Biobankgesetz: Augsburg-Münchner-Entwurf (AME-BiobankG). Tübingen: Mohr Siebeck.

German Ethics Council (2010): Human Biobanks for Research, Berlin: German Ethics Council.

Giddens, Anthony (1990): The Consequences of Modernity, Cambridge: Cambridge Polity Press.

Goddard, Katharina A.B./Smith, Sabina/Chen, Chuhe/McMullen, Carmit/Johnson, Cheryl (2009): "Biobank Recruitment: Motivations for Nonparticipation." In: Biopreservation and Biobanking 7/2, pp. 119–121.

Habermas, Jürgen (1984): Theory of Communicative Action, Volume One: Reason and the Rationalization of Society, Boston: Beacon Press.

Hansen, Solveig L/Pfaller, Larissa/Schicktanz, Silke (2020): Critical Analysis of Communication Strategies in Public Health Promotion: An Empirical-Ethical Study on Organ Donation in Germany. In: Bioethics, http://dx.doi.org/10.1111/bioe.12774.

Hansen, Solveig L./Eisner, Marthe I./Pfaller, Larissa/Schicktanz, Silke (2017): "'Are you in or are you out?!' Moral Appeals to the Public in Organ Donation Poster Campaigns – a Multimodal and Ethical Analysis." In: Health Communication 33/8, pp. 1020–1034.

Hansson, Mats G. (2005): "Building on Relationships of Trust in Biobank Research." In: Journal of Medical Ethics 31/7, pp. 415–418.

Hartmann, Martin (2011): The Practice of Trust, Frankfurt: Suhrkamp/Insel.

Hawkins, Alice K./O'Doherty, Kieran (2010): "Biobank Governance: a Lesson in Trust." In: New Genetics and Society 29/3, pp. 311–327.

Hawley, Katherine (2014): "Trust, Distrust and Commitment." In: Nous 48/1: pp. 1–20.

Hieronymi, Pamela (2008): "The Reasons of Trust." In: Australasian Journal of Philosophy 86/2, pp. 213–236.

Hoeyer, Klaus (2012): "Trading in Cold Blood?" In: Peter Dabrock/Jochen Taupitz/Jens Ried (eds.), Trust in Biobanking, Berlin: Springer, pp. 21–41.

Irving, Michelle J./Tong, Alisson/Jan, Stephen/Cass, Alan/Rose, John/Chadban, Steven/Allen, Richard D. et al. (2012): "Factors that Influence the Decision to Be an Organ Donor: a Systematic Review of the Qualitative Literature." In: Nephrology Dialysis Transplantation 27/6, pp. 2526–2533.

Jawoniyi, Oluwafunmilayo/Gormley, Kevin/McGleenan, Emma/Noble, Helen Rose (2017): "Organ Donation and Transplantation: Awareness and Roles of Healthcare Professionals – A Systematic Literature Review." In: Journal of Clinical Nursing 27/5–6, pp. e726–e738.

Johannsen, Richard L./Valde, Kathleen S./Whedbee, Karen E. (2008): Ethics in Human Communication, Long Grove: Waveland Press.

Johnsson, Linus (2013): Trust in Biobank Research. Meaning and Moral Significance, Uppsala: Uppsala University Publications.

Johnsson, Linus/Helgesson, Gert/Hansson, Mats G./Erikson, Stefan (2013): "Adequate Trust Avails, Mistaken Trust Matters: On the Moral Responsibility of Doctors as Proxies for Patient's Trust in Biobank Research." In: Bioethics 27/9, pp. 485–492.

Jones, Karen (1996): "Trust as an Affective Attitude." In: Ethics 107/1, pp. 4–25.

Kerasidou, Angeliki (2017): "Trust Me, I'm a Researcher!: The Role of Trust in Biomedical Research." In: Medicine, Health Care and Philosophy 20/1, pp. 43–50.

Kettis-Lindblad, Åsa/Ring, Lena/Viberth, Eva/Hansson, Mats G. (2006): "Genetic Research and Donation of Tissue Samples to Biobanks. What do Potential Sample Donors in the Swedish General Public Think?" In: European Journal of Public Health 16/4, pp. 433–440.

Lahno, Bernd (2001): "On the Emotional Character of Trust." In: Ethical Theory and Moral Practice 4, pp. 171–189.

Lipworth, Wendy/Morrel, Brownen M./Irvine, Rob Becky/Kerridge, Ian (2009): "An Empirical Reappraisal of Public Trust in Biobanking Research: Rethinking Restrictive Consent Requirements." In: Journal of Law and Medicine 17/1, pp. 119–132.

Luhmann, Niklas (1979): Trust and Power, Chichester: Wiley.

Master, Zubin/Nelson, Erin/Murdoch, Blake/Caulfield, Timothy (2012): "Biobanks, Consent and Claims of Consensus." In: Nature Methods 9/9, pp. 885–888.

Masui, Tohru (2009): "Trust and the Creation of Biobanks: Biobanking in Japan and the UK." In: Margaret Sleeboom-Faulkner (ed.), Human Genetic Biobanks in Asia: Politics of Trust and Scientific Advancemen, London: Routledge, pp. 66–91.

Melas, Philippe A./Sjöholm, Louise K./Forsner, Tord/Edhborg, Maigun/Juth, Niklas/Forsell, Yvonne/Lavebratt, Catharina (2010): "Examining the Public Refusal to Consent to DNA Biobanking: Empirical Data from a Swedish Population-Based Study." In: Journal of Medical Ethics 36, pp. 93–98.

McLeod, Carolyn (2000): "Our Attitude Towards the Motivation of Those we Trust." In: Southern Journal of Philosophy 38, pp. 465–480.

Molina-Pérez, Alberto/Rodríguez-Arias, David/Delgado-Rodríguez, Janet/Morgan, Myfanwy/Frunza, Mihaela/Randhawa, Gurch/Reiger-Van de Wijdeven, Jeantine et al./Schiks, Eline/Wöhlke, Sabine/Schicktanz, Silke (2018): "Public Knowledge and Attitudes towards Consent Policies for Organ Donation in Europe. A Systematic Review." In: Transplantation Reviews 33/1, pp. 1–8.

Möllering, Guido (2006): Trust. Reason, Routine and Reflexivity, Oxford: Elsevier.

Morgan, Susan E./Harrison, Tyler R./Afifi, Walid A./Long, Shawn D./Stephenson Michael T. (2008): "In Their Own Words: The Reasons Why People Will (Not) Sign an Organ Donor Card." In: Health Commuciation 23/1, pp. 23–33.

Morgan, Susan E. (2009): "The Intersection of Conversation, Cognitions, and Campaigns: The Social Representation of Organ Donation." In: Communication Theory 19/1, pp. 29–48.

Mühlfried, Florian (2018): Mistrust. Ethnographic Approximations, Bielefeld: transcript Verlag.

Mullin, Amy (2005). "Trust, Social Norms, and Motherhood." In: Journal of Social Philosophy 36/3, pp. 316–330.

Newton, Joshua D. (2011): "How Does the General Public View Posthumous Organ Donation? A Meta-Synthesis of the Qualitative Literature." In: BMC Public Health 11, pp. 791– 801.

Nobile, Hélène/Bergmann, Manuela M./Moldenhauer, Jennifer/Borry, Pascal (2016): "Participants' Accounts on their Decision to Join a Cohort Study with an Attached Biobank: A Qualitative Content Analysis Study within two German Studies." In: Journal of Empirical Research on Human Research Ethics 11/3, pp. 237–249.

O'Neill, Onora (2002): Autonomy and Trust in Bioethics, Cambridge: Cambridge University Press.

Pfaller, Larissa/Hansen, Solveig L./Adloff, Frank/Schicktanz, Silke (2018): "'Saying No to Organ Donation': an Empirical Typology of Reluctance and Rejection." In: Sociology of Health and Illness 40/8, pp. 1327–1346.

Pondrom, Sue (2013): "Trust is Everything." In: American Journal of Transplantation 13/5, pp. 1115–1116.

Porteri, Corinna/Pasqualetti, Patrizio/Togni, Elena/Parker, Michael (2014): "Public's Attitudes on Participation in a Biobank for Research: an Italian Survey." In: BMC Medical Ethics 15, pp. 81–90.

Prainsack, Barbara/Buyx, Alena (2013): "A Solidarity-Based Approach to the Governance of Research Biobanks." In: Medical Law Review 21/1, pp. 71–91.

Resnik, David B. (2018): The Ethics of Research with Human Subjects. Protecting People, Advancing Science, Promoting Trust, Cham: Springer.

Schicktanz, Silke/Pfaller, Larissa/Hansen, Solveig L./Boos, Moritz (2017): "A Comparison of Attitudes towards Brain Death and Body Concepts in Relation to Willingness or Reluctance to Donate: Results of a Students' Survey before and after the German Transplantation Scandals." In: Journal of Public Health 25, pp. 249–256.

Shaw, David (2013): "Lessons from the German Organ Donation Scandal." In: The Intensive Care Society 14, p. 3.

Sheach Leith, Valerie M. (2008): "Restoring Trust? Trust and Informed Consent in the Aftermath of the Organ Retention Scandal." In: Julie Brownlie/Alexandra Greene/Alexandra Howson (eds.), Researching Trust and Health, New York: Routledge, pp. 72–90.

Sheikh, Zeinab/Hoeyer, Klaus (2018): "'That is Why I Have Trust': Unpacking What 'Trust' Means to Participants in International Genetic Research in Pakistan and Denmark." In: Medicine, Health Care and Philosophy 21/2, pp. 169–179.

Simpson, Thomas W. (2012): "What is Trust?" In: Pacific Philosophical Quarterly 93, pp. 550–569.

Snell, Karoliina/Tarkkala, Heta (2019): "Questioning the Rhetoric of a 'Willing Population' in Finnish Biobanking." In: Life Sciences, Society and Policy 15/4. DOI: 10.1186/s40504-019-0094-5

Sprecher, Franziska (2017): "Biobanken sind im geltenden Recht nur unvollständig erfasst." In: Neue Züricher Zeitung, May 12, p. 9.

Steinsbekk, Kristin Solum/Ursin, Lars Øystein/Skolbekken, John-Arne/Solberg, Berge (2013a): "We're not in it for the Money – Lay People's Moral Intuitions on Commercial Use of 'their' Biobank." In: Medicine, Health Care and Philosophy 16/2, pp. 151–162.

Steinsbekk, Kristin Solum/Kåre Myskja, Bjørn/Solberg, Berge (2013b): "Broad Consent versus Dynamic Consent in Biobank Research: is Passive Participation an Ethical Problem?" In: European Journal of Human Genetics 21/9, pp. 897–902.

Urban Walker, Margaret (2006): Moral Repair. Reconstructing Moral Relations after Wrongdoing, Cambridge, New York: Cambridge University Press.

Ursin, Lars Øystein/Solberg, Berge (2008): "When is Normative Recruitment Legitimate?" In: Etikk i Praksis. Nordic Journal of Applied Ethics 2/2, pp. 93–113.

Van Zon, Sander K.R./Scholtens, Salome/Reijneveld, Sijmen A/Smidt, Nynke/Bültmann, Ute (2016): "Active Recruitment and Limited Participant-Load Related to High Participation in Large Population-Based Biobank Studies." In: Journal of Clinical Epidemiology 78, pp. 52–62.

Wiesemann, Claudia (2016): "Vertrauen als moralische Praxis – Bedeutung für Ethik und Medizin." In: Holmer Steinfath/Claudia Wiesemann (eds.), Autonomie und Vertrauen. Schlüsselbegriffe der modernen Medizin, Wiesbaden: Springer VS, pp. 69–99.

Zawati, Ma'n H. (2014): "There Will Be Sharing: Population Biobanks, the Duty to Inform and the Limitations of the Individualistic Conception of Autonomy." In: Health Law Review 21, pp. 97–140.

Zika, Eleni/Paci, Daniele/Braun, Anette/Rijkers-Defrasne, Sylvie/Deschênes, Myléne/Fortier, Isabel/Laage-Hellman, Jens/Scerri, Christian/Ibarreta, Dolores (2011): "A European Survey on Biobanks: Trends and Issues." In: Public Health Genomics 14/2, pp. 96–103.

II. HUMAN ORGAN SOURCES

5. Determining Brain Death
Controversies and Pragmatic Solutions

Dieter Birnbacher

1. Introduction

Part of the explanation of why questions of medical ethics in the field of transplantation are of enduring interest as well as enduring tenacity is that they arise from fundamental conflicts between ethics and anthropology. This is very much the case in the question of brain death. What sustains the debate on the ethical side are two convictions shared by most people engaged in the field: First, that transplantation of human organs from dead patients is a highly beneficial practice which should be extended rather than restricted. It saves a great number if lives and, in innumerable cases, raises the quality of life of otherwise severely ill patients. This practice should not be jeopardized by the seemingly never-ending debate about the validity of the brain death criterion as a criterion of death. Second, the conviction that organs for transplantation, with the exception of live donation of paired organs such as kidneys, should be retrieved only from patients that are truly dead. For the majority of transplantation surgeons, the appropriately named 'dead donor rule' is a central condition of the ethical legitimacy of their practice. Conversely, considerable uncertainties remain about the anthropology underlying the brain-death criterion, especially among the general public (see the recent survey of more than 1,400 students of the University of Göttingen, Schicktanz et al. 2017, 254). Among the brain death sceptics, as they might be called, there is a lingering uneasiness about whether brain death is a satisfactory and legitimate criterion of death. This divergence of perspectives is mirrored in an analogous gap between the views expressed in legal and professional documents on the one hand and popular ways of thinking about life and death on the other. While there is a high degree of consensus in legislatures and the official positions of international and national medical organizations that brain death is, or should be, regarded as identical with human death, both the general public and part of academia continue to hold reservations about the acceptability of the identification.

Doubts about the validity and legitimacy of the brain death criterion come from many quarters. Remarkably, however, some of these doubts continue to come from bioethicists. One of the early dissenters was philosopher Hans Jonas. In 1968, when the Harvard Ad hoc Committee published its proposal to identify human death with brain death, Jonas immediately attacked the proposal as a 'pragmatic re-definition of death', designed to legitimize postmortem organ transplantation but at odds with the traditional understanding of death as the irreversible cessation of bodily functioning (Jonas 1980). Jonas implied that the proposal was manipulative; it was, without saying so, created to safeguard the practice of explanting vasculated organs by securing its compatibility with the dead donor rule. Indeed, this was one of the aims of the proposal (Harvard Ad Hoc Committee 1968). Another one was to define a point in the development of a patient's disease at which treatment, curative or palliative, should be withdrawn. There can be no doubt, however, that this was only a secondary motive. The coincidence of the publication of the proposal with the emergence of transplantation medicine was in no way accidental. Even today, the ethical controversy regarding the validity of the brain death criterion is far from settled, as was recently demonstrated by a split vote in the *Ethikrat*, the German national advisory committee on bioethics, on this question. Remarkably, only a minority of the physicians on the committee voted with the majority that brain death should be identified with death.

It is useful to distinguish between the questions of whether brain death is a valid *definition* of death and whether it is a valid *criterion* of death. Even if many proposals make brain death the definition as well as a (or *the*) criterion of death, the two are conceptually distinct. The first question asks how 'death' should be understood in the relevant context. The second question seeks to specify the signs that indicate that the relevant definition of death has been met (Veatch 1989, 34ff.; Bernat et al. 1981). A criterion necessarily refers to something beyond itself; if observed, it allows us to draw the conclusion that the conditions of the thing or event for which it is a criterion have been fulfilled. For example, one criterion for the intensity of pain is the value given to it by a patient on a ten-point scale, from very weak to unbearably strong. Unlike the thing or event it indicates, a criterion must be publicly observable or measurable. Furthermore, the relation between the criterion and what it indicates is, as a rule, empirically verifiable. It is an empirical matter whether the ten-point scale of pain intensity is a good, bad, exact, or inexact criterion of pain intensity. By contrast, the definition referenced by any given criterion is an a priori matter for which empirical evidence is not directly relevant. A definition identifies the conditions that have to be met for a thing or event to answer a certain description, and these conditions must be clear before one is able to decide which criterion is most appropriate to indicate their being fulfilled. Furthermore, for a given concept, there can be more than one criterion, and more than one valid criterion.

2.   Good and Less Good Reasons for Doubt

Among the reasons for doubting the identification of death with brain death – understood as the complete and irreversible cessation of brain function – some deserve closer attention than others. One such argument by Hans Jonas in his seminal article belongs to the weaker sort: the argument that defining death the complete and irreversible cessation of brain functioning is too "uncertain" to serve as a basis for the practice of explanting organs (Jonas 1980). This objection seems to be based on the misunderstanding of the function of a definition; a definition seeks to explain what is, or should be, meant by a certain expression. As such, it cannot be right or wrong, precise or imprecise, reliable or unreliable in the way an empirical indicator can be. As an a priori matter, a definition does not depend on how the world is – at most it can be judged as adequate or inadequate, intelligible or intelligible, fruitful or sterile, or the like. The standard by which its validity is measured is a semantic or pragmatic standard, such as its agreement with common usage, with traditional conceptions, or with certain specified purposes. Given that it is now possible to maintain the biological functions of an organism with its brain functions completely and irreversibly lost, it is necessary to adapt the definition to the new options. There may be good reasons to doubt the wisdom of the Harvard Committee's choice, but these reasons cannot find any direct support in issues of veracity or conformity to fact.

There are, however, more compelling reasons to cast doubt on the identification of death with brain death. For example, one could argue that the definition of death used to assess the merits and demerits of a proposed criterion of death should be essentially *biological*. It is evident that life and death are primarily biological concepts. Therefore, their application to humans and non-human animals should follow the same criteria, at least as far as they do not essentially differ in their biological functioning. Because life and death in a non-human animal do not depend on the presence of consciousness or self-consciousness, it follows that mental aspects, and the brain functions on which they depend, cannot be crucial for deciding whether a human being is alive or dead. It is perfectly sufficient that central life functions such as circulation, breathing and metabolism are intact. This, at least at first sight, seems a strong reason to attribute life even to a brain dead human patient whose life functions are maintained by a ventilator, regardless of the fact that the patient has lost the capacity of consciousness and self-consciousness (DeGrazia 2005: 11ff.).

This argument gains support from further considerations that make the role of consciousness, and mental life in general, accidental rather than essential in the attribution of life and death. One is that the human organism is without consciousness over long stretches of time without thereby losing its property of being alive, for example in dreamless sleep or in deep narcosis. The life of consciousness is temporally embedded in biological life, which suggests that its emergence and continued existence is dependent on the life of the organism. One does not have to be an epiphenomenalist to assume that mental phenomena are causally dependent on a physical substrate. Another consideration is the observation that, ontologically, mental life is a phenomenon, not a substance. For one, the Cartesian thesis that 'l'âme pense toujours' is not borne out by experience, and the existence of consciousness without some physical substrate, though logically possible, does not seem compatible with the fundamental laws of the universe. Men are not, as has been said by dedicated dualists, "embodied minds" (McMahan 2002: 66f.) who accidentally happen to be provided with a physical body; rather, they are physical bodies that happen to be provided with minds and whose basic mechanisms are not essentially different from those of lower animals that lack mental life. Indeed, one striking phenomenon that convinces many observers that it is absurd to view the brain dead as 'really' dead is the range of complex bodily functions that are maintained, or can be maintained, in this state with relatively little outside stimulus, among them digestion, excretion, sweating, temperature regulation, wound healing, and, with the help of the fetal brain, prolonged pregnancy up to the birth of a healthy child.

Another reason to define life and death in purely biological terms, independently of the presence or absence of brain functioning, is the logical asymmetry that results from classifying a brain dead patient as dead while maintaining the common view that human embryos are alive, irrespective of whether their brain is functioning or whether the embryonic or fetal brain has developed to a stage in which it can be legitimately be said to function as a system of its own (Sass 1989). Both states, however, are structurally analogous. Given that life is defined as self-organization supported by external resources (Quante 2002: 69ff.), the processes in the early embryo and fetus and in brain death both satisfy the conditions for being alive. Self-organization means that the individual components of the organism interact in a systematic and coordinated way – a condition met in both cases – and depends for its maintenance on an external resource: the embryo and fetus on the resources provided by the uterus and the maternal organism, the brain dead patient on the stimuli coming from the ventilator. If the life of the embryo is 'real' life, so, it seems, is the life of the brain dead.

In response, it is sometimes objected that these two states are not really comparable because of two crucial differences: their very different temporal position in the course of a human life and the differences in potential. Of course, embryonic life comes before, and brain death after, the biographical life of the person, and there could be no greater difference in potential for further development. It is doubtful, however, that these features are relevant to the issue at hand. The differences in temporal position and potential do not affect the basic structural similarity between the two states (McMahan 2002: 436).

Due to its purely formal character, this argument on the side of the sceptics is particularly robust. It is independent of the question of which definition of life and death is most adequate. It does no more than to require consistency in the attribution of the concept of life to structurally similar states.

3.   Good and Less Good Reasons for the Identification of Brain Death with Death

On the side of the defenders of brain death as a valid criterion of death we also find arguments of different persuasiveness. A particularly strong case for identification maintained by some medical committees is the holistic integration argument, which states that with the complete and irreversible loss of brain function the organism has lost its central control organ – the control room as it were, from which all different parts and functions of the complex mechanism of the body are monitored and controlled (see, for example, SAMW 2011: 5). Furthermore, the body needs this central control to function as an integrated whole instead of being fragmented into a number of separate systems, which may work simultaneously but are not coordinated by a functioning brain as a central organ of regulation. This argument has played a prominent role in the justification of the brain death criterion by the German Medical Association, from the beginnings of brain death diagnostics (Birnbacher et al. 1993) through to its most recent relevant statement (Brandt/Angstwurm 2018). It is worth noting that this argument, again, is purely biological and does not refer to anything that might be distinctive for animals endowed with a mental life or for humans with a mental life including self-awareness and rationality. Its strength, however, essentially depends on the premise that the integration of bodily functions into a whole by a central regulative agency is a necessary condition of being alive, so that the irreversible cessation of the functioning of this agency becomes a sufficient condition of not being alive. This premise is doubtful, and it has been challenged.

Critics of this argument maintain either that it ascribes the brain a more exclusive position in the regulation of bodily functions than it really deserves, or that the brain's regulatory function is itself dependent on the autonomous functioning of integrative circuits outside the brain. In both arguments, the brain does not have the dominating position in the control of the organism as a whole ascribed to it by the holistic integration argument. Both theses were forcefully developed, among others, by the American neurologist Alan Shewmon in essays he published from 1998 onwards. These essays had considerable impact in the United States, challenging the President's Council on Bioethics to think anew about the definition of death. The majority of its members signed a White Paper designed to strengthen the criterion and to provide it with a less vulnerable foundation (President's Council on Bioethics 2008). Against the thesis that the brain holds an exclusive position in the regulation of bodily functions, Shewmon argued that the majority of somatic integrative processes are not, or not necessarily, mediated by the brain but are instead autonomous (Shewmon 2002: 311), which explains why so many them remain intact when brain-stem functions, such as the stimulation of the breathing reflex, are replaced by a ventilator. Shewmon further argued that most of the regulatory functions of the brain are in turn dependent on integrative mechanisms outside the brain. Indeed, the complex bodily functions that are maintained in the brain dead, such as blood circulation, digestion and wound healing, require the goal-directed coordination of a great variety of bodily mechanisms. They are not just isolated happenings, like the decay of a single cell, but holistic functions presupposing a system of interacting causal mechanisms. How else should it be possible, for example, that a brain dead patient manifests the so-called 'Lazarus sign' – raising both upper body and hands in reaction to being touched by a nurse – something that requires the coordinated integration of unconscious perception, motor impulses and muscle innervation? What Shewmon could not show, but only asserted, was that the sum of these autonomous bodily circuits and networks constitute a unity or whole comparable to that provided by a functioning brain. The rather vague way in which he formulated this unity, "an implicitly existing, intrinsically mediated somatic unity" (Shewmon 1998: 141), betrays some uncertainty on this point. It is, however, an open question how far this undermines his counterarguments, since the meaning of "somatic unity" is itself far from clear and is open to multiple interpretation. If it is taken to mean that the brain is strictly necessary for the control of every bodily function, this is obviously incompatible with the demonstrated capacity of the bodily functions of brain dead patients to remain intact with the support of a ventilator for days, weeks, and even months. If it is taken to mean that the body deprived of a functioning brain is no longer a complete whole, this is trivial because it is a truism that a human organism without a functioning brain can hardly be said to be complete. So far, it has not been made sufficiently clear what makes an organism governed by a functioning brain an 'integrated whole' in a sense that is illuminatingly distinct from when the same organism shows a number of autonomously working integrated circuits under stimulation from some artificial device (Truog/Robinson 2003: 2392).

A second argument put forward to bolster the brain death criterion was suggested by the President's Council in its abovementioned White Paper. In its majority vote it defined a living organism as consisting of three components, all of which must be absent for it to be legitimately classified as dead: "1. openness to the world – that is, receptivity to stimuli and signals from the surrounding environment; 2. the ability to act upon the world to obtain selectively what it needs; 3. the basic felt need that drives the organism to act as it must, to obtain what it needs and what its openness reveals to be available" (President Council on Bioethics 2008: 61). This definition, or rather re-definition, of death was a courageous step. It was one of the rare attempts to transcend the level of criteria and to confront the question of definition. However, addressing this question did not prevent the Council from pursuing a thoroughly pragmatic purpose: namely, to defend the legitimacy of the brain death criterion against the attacks of prominent critics such as Alan Shewmon, Franklin G. Miller, Robert D. Truog and others. This purpose was explicitly stated. The proposed definition should help "understand why an individual with total brain failure should be declared dead, even when ventilator-supported 'breathing' masks the presence of death" (ibid.: 61). It is doubtful, however, that this defense was as successful as the Council intended. One problem is condition one – openness to the world. If the definition is valid, the organism should have lost the capacity to receive anything from the outside world. But in fact it receives something from the outside world: the oxygen coming from the ventilator. Without this receptivity, it would be hard to explain why its lungs are taking in air and, in consequence, blood circulation and many other vital functions start working in roughly the same ways as in a living organism. Insofar as the organism is receptive to outside stimuli such as the oxygen, it does not meet all of the three components of the Council's definition and should not be classified as dead (Miller/Truog 2009: 189). In this case, consequently, the brain death criterion would become invalid. It would not show that the patient fulfils the requirements inherent in the concept of death.

A more promising defense of the brain death criterion that emerged from the discussion of the White Paper focused on the second condition, the capacity to act on the world. According to this argument, the brain dead patient is dead not because its organism is unreceptive (or insufficiently integrated) but because it is no longer able to breathe, or to show any other sign of vitality, on its own. In other words, any vital function it may exhibit is dependent on external impulses. This argument has been used in the recent defense of the brain death criterion by a working group of the German Medical Association. What is crucial, according to this argument, is that the brain dead organism is no longer able to initiate any "goal-oriented and purposefully directed activity" (Brandt/Angstwurm 2018: 678). It has lost, in short, the ability to do anything on its own. If the organism of the brain dead patient is still receptive, it is in a completely passive way, reacting to external impulses but in no way actively exerting any influence on the world except insofar as it is itself prompted by external impulses. If the organism reacts to a haptic stimulus with the "Lazarus sign", this may well be taken to constitute something the organism *does*, and such physical movements necessarily have an effect on the outside world. But they are not movements initiated by the organism itself. The crucial feature of life, according to this argument, is the autonomy of the organism in sustaining its own life by an autonomous integration of vital functions (Condic 2016: 257ff.). Accepting this argument leads to a full legitimization of the brain death criterion.

This conclusion is, however, bought at a price. Even if the autonomy-based definition of being alive or dead seems plausible for the standard situation of the brain dead patient on a ventilator, it inevitably has implications for non-standard situations.

Think, for example, of a situation, probably in the not-too-distant future, in which the ventilator of today is replaced by a device implanted into the brain. There can be no doubt that even such a device would have to be classified as 'external' to the organism, so any organic functioning enabled by this device in the absence of any capacity for autonomous functioning would not preclude classifying the organism as dead. The reason is that it does not seem to make a difference whether the device is outside or inside the organism as long as it is not part of the organism. In theory, it would not even make a difference whether this device is 'artificial' in the sense that it is a product of human engineering, mechanical or otherwise. Even a special kind of medicine might be suited to the task. It might even be a substance or mechanism that is completely 'natural'. The only property that it would have to possess in order to count as 'external' is that it is not part of the organism itself but an add-on deliberately used to maintain biological functioning which the organism itself cannot sustain on its own.

This suggestion invites the criticism that if followed to its logical conclusion, even a device like a pacemaker implanted to maintain the heart function of an indubitably living patient would have to be counted as an "external" condition of the maintenance of organ function, with the paradoxical result that a patient whose life depends on the functioning of this device would have to be counted as dead because he or she has irreversibly lost the capacity to maintain these functions autonomously (Deutscher Ethikrat 2015: 92f.). This is, no doubt, an objection of considerable weight. It shows that even if this argument is accepted in principle, it has to be qualified in order to avoid counterintuitive consequences, which means it cannot be valid in its most simple form. How might we qualify this argument? One suggestion is to add the proviso that it is only applicable when the patient concerned does not show any further sign of being alive, such as possessing the capacity for conscious experience. While it is possible to be alive without the capacity for conscious experience, this capacity seems categorically incompatible with death. That is, whether a patient is alive or dead cannot be determined by the presence or absence of consciousness or the capacity to be conscious. But it seems logically impossible for somebody to be simultaneously conscious and dead. It cannot be denied that any qualification of the argument along these lines amounts to a considerable weakening of its force. For one, the succinctness of the argument is dissolved. The definitions of being alive and being dead prove to be no less complicated than the brain death criterion and the neurological tests by which it is operationalized for practical purposes. An even weightier objection is that (re)introducing consciousness, or other mentalistic criteria, even as an additional component of the definition, falls back on a line of argument that most participants in the debate thought had been excluded once for all.

4.   How to Decide?

We have come to an impasse. There are, on both sides of the controversy, good and less good arguments, raising the question of who should have the last word. Even after mustering the most relevant arguments for and against, plenty of room remains for reasonable dissent regarding both the plausibility of the individual arguments and their relative weight. Again, it is worth stressing that this dissent does not concern the adequacy of the brain death criterion as such nor the tests into which it is translated for practical purposes; it concerns the underlying conception of what it means to be, or not to be, alive – the depth dimension, as it were, which is often left unmentioned but which constitutes the undissolved knot that explains the controversy's persistence and intensity.

In this situation there are various options we might choose to follow, some of them more obvious than others. Unfortunately, as will be shown, most of them have serious drawbacks, so that the help offered by passing the options in review is limited.

One proposal often heard in public discussion is to leave the accepted concepts of being and not being alive unchanged and to instead practice what has been called *definitional tutiorism* (Walton 1980: 22). This strategy promises to minimize irritation and controversy, which are inevitable when dealing with innovations that touch upon deep existential concerns. However, the problem with this proposal is that it is far from clear what the accepted view is. Public opinion is not unanimous on the matter, and even though the formal representative bodies of physicians generally favor a definition that legitimizes the brain death criterion, there is, even among them, a dissenting minority. Traditional views of life and death were suited to dealing with traditional cases and cannot resolve doubts about cases that have been made possible only by the rapid progress of medical technology in the 20th century. Traditionally, the signs of death occurred more or less simultaneously. Only modern medical technology has enabled the temporal separation of the cessations of brain activity and vital functions like respiration and circulation, respectively. The result is that the boundary between life and death has become ambiguous and drawing it requires a deliberate decision.

A second strategy favored by a great number of physicians is *naturalism*: basing the definition of death as far as possible on scientific fact. Again, this approach seems unlikely to be successful with regard to fundamentals such as the definition of life and death. Certainly, scientific medicine and especially neurology play a crucial role in formulating and spelling out the criterion of death as well as conducting the tests that make this criterion applicable in practice. Furthermore, medical science is essential for assessing the reliability of criteria and tests and, in the public sphere, correcting unjustified fears about their validity. Scientific expertise alone, however, cannot answer the central controversial question of how to define being and not being alive. Although any discussion of the adequacy and legitimacy of a certain definition must take into account the scientific evidence, the decision to accept or reject this definition cannot be based on this evidence alone. That is, scientific competence is a necessary, but not sufficient, condition for a decision of this kind.

A third methodological strategy is *pluralism*, which splits the concepts of being alive and being dead in two or more concepts, each adapted to certain contexts and not to others. There is more than one proposal in the literature to make such a split. Some propose concepts that refer to different points in the process of dying, for example 'passing away' versus 'deanimation' (Shewmon 2010). Ralf Stoecker proposed to add a third category to the dichotomy of being alive and dead in order to denote the 'hovering' of the brain dead patient between life and death (Stoecker 2010: XLVff.). The most prominent theory of this kind is the conceptual dualism proposed by the Oxford ethicist Jeff McMahan (2002). According to McMahan, there are two concepts of death with distinctly different ethical implications. According to the primary concept, a human being is dead when its capacity for conscious awareness is irreversibly lost – an openly mentalistic concept. The secondary concept is biological, according to which a human being is dead when its organism has irreversibly ceased to function. Both concepts have as their counterparts corresponding concepts of life. Life in the mentalistic sense begins and ends with the beginning and end of the capacity to have conscious experience. Life in the biological sense begins with conception and ends with the irreversible end of biological functioning. One of the consequences of this dichotomy is that there can be considerable differences between the respective – mental or biological – lifespans of a person. Sometimes they differ drastically, as in the case of the coma patient Nancy Cruzan, on whose tomb two dates of death are recorded: the end of her conscious life and the end of her biological life seven years later (ibid.: 423).

Obviously, duplicating the concepts of life and death along these lines is not merely strategic; it is rooted in a view of human life that goes beyond the issue at hand and has far-reaching metaphysical ramifications. McMahan's view is based on a spiritualist conception of human existence in which the mind is embodied but could, in principle, exist without embodiment, or at least the kind of embodiment we find in nature. Hence the priority given to the mentalistic concept of life. By contrast, materialists and evolutionists, who view the human being as a particularly gifted animal, would, if they were to adopt conceptual dualism, presumably reverse the equation and give priority to biology. Apart from that, any strangeness that this theory may have at first sight dissolves as soon as we interpret it as phenomenological account of the factual division of how we view our own life compared to the lives of others. From the first-person perspective, the central object of concern is the period of conscious experience. From this perspective, our life begins with the first "awakening" to consciousness at some unknown point in fetal development and comes to an end when we irretrievably lose the capacity for conscious experiences. From the third-person perspective, from which we view the lives of others, we tend to think in biological categories and take it for granted that their lives begin at the early embryo stage and end when their organisms have irreversibly ceased functioning.

The duplication of concepts of life and death only safeguards the dead donor rule if the mentalistic concept is given priority. Only then is it possible to say that the brain dead person is 'sufficiently' dead to allow the explantation of organs without infringing the rule. However, if this strategy were used to decide all cases in which it is applicable, it could lead to any patient who has irreversibly lost the capacity for consciousness to be declared dead, going far beyond the line drawn by the brain death criterion, which is commonly understood to require the irreversible cessation of *all* brain functions. This consequence is accepted by only a minority of medical ethicists (see, for example, Veatch 2004).

There are pragmatic reasons to avoid a duplication or multiplication of the concepts of life and death. The first is that these concepts function as fundamental orientations in thinking about ourselves and others and serve as reference points of communication about existential topics. Dissolving these concepts into a plurality of concepts risks confusion and irritation, such as those already provoked by the widespread use of the term 'clinical death', which misleadingly suggests that a patient who survives 'clinical death' has benefitted from some kind of miracle. Another reason is the requirement to provide a unitary concept for legal purposes; a multiplication of concepts would severely complicate the legal rules applying to life and death. A further reason to maintain a unitary concept of death is that multiple concepts can solve the conflict between the ethics and the anthropology of organ transplantation only when combined with the priority thesis. This thesis, however, will be acceptable to only very few of those involved in the practice of organ transplantation. Only few ethicists accept that organs can be explanted from irreversibly comatose patients or from anencephalics. And physicians tend to share the naturalistic worldview and to favor the evolutionary picture – according to which the mind phylogenetically emerged, and ontogenetically emerges, from living matter – in contrast to the Platonic view that a pre-existent soul is provided, at conception, with a body in which it then spends a lifetime.

The reservations expressed against the multiplication of concepts of life and death similarly apply to a fourth strategy to dissolve the definitional dilemma, *cultural pluralism*. It is a fact that although the brain death criterion is incorporated in all legal systems in countries where postmortem organ transplantation is practiced, acceptance of it in the general population differs greatly between cultures (Laurels 2005). For a long time, it was outright rejected by the populations of many East Asian countries, with the consequence that transplantation surgeons were charged with murder or manslaughter (Lock 2001). Often, religion plays a role in these cultural traditions, such as in orthodox Judaism and Christian fundamentalism, though most religious communities are no less divided on the issue than broader populations worldwide. Though cultural pluralism is a debatable option and was even indirectly defended with the proposal to leave the decision on the definition of death to individual choice (Veatch 1989: 30, 54ff.; Veatch/Ross 2016: 152), it meets with the criticism that, in a world increasingly characterized by more intensive communication, interaction, co-operation and international exchange, it seems misguided to leave central concepts like life and death to cultural particularism. Apart from that, the clear international convergence of legal criteria (which unfortunately co-exists with a great deal of divergence in required test procedures and quality safeguards) can be expected to lead, in the long run, to a similar convergence in opinion and attitude.

5.   A 'Pragmatic' Justification of the Brain Death Criterion

Instead of proposing a solution that heavily depends on uncertain *metaphysical* reasons, one might argue for a compromise between ethics and anthropology for more directly *pragmatic* reasons, with 'pragmatic' understood in a positive and constructive sense (Wiesemann 1995). After all, the concepts of life and death are not Platonic ideas, existing independently of language and convention. They are open concepts, leaving room for interpretation and specification. And how they are interpreted and specified can legitimately be made according to pragmatic, not least on ethical, reasons. Concepts are *man-made*, and the standard on which they have to be judged is not whether they are true or false but whether they are meaningful or not, adequate or not, and whether they serve their purposes.

Another methodological consideration is that, given the background of great differences between cultures, traditions and individuals in the interpretation of these concepts, it seems more appropriate to regard the quest for the *definition* underlying the brain death criterion as the quest for what in the philosophy of science has been called *explication* (Birnbacher 2018). An explication is an interpretation of an unclear or controversial concept that does not purport to mirror any common understandings but instead proposes a convention that, on the one hand, preserves the core of the various meanings given to the concept, and, on the other, is adapted to the purposes it is designed to serve in theoretical or practical contexts. Because there can be more than one context in which a concept needs explication, there can be more than one explication to a concept – as was explicitly conceded by Rudolf Carnap, who introduced the concept of explication in the context of probability. According to Carnap, explications can be introduced to meet more than one requirement, and these can have different weights in different contexts. One of Carnap's examples is the pre-scientific explicandum "fish" (1963: 6) for which there might be more than one scientific *explicatum* (the result of the explication), depending on the ends this explicatum is designed to serve and what amount of semantic agreement with common usage seems desirable.

The four requirements explications should meet, according to Carnap, are *similarity* with the explicandum, *exactness*, *simplicity* and *fruitfulness*. In the context of the concepts of life and death, similarity of meaning means that the conventionally fixed meaning of the explicatum should not deviate too heavily from the meaning or meanings traditionally associated with the *explicandum*. The criterion of exactness can be taken to mean that the explication should be consonant with well-confirmed anthropological theories and should not bring in speculative elements. As a matter of course, not all explications of life and death one may think of satisfy this condition, e.g. theological or esoteric conceptions of a substantial immaterial soul or an astral body governing bodily functioning. A further component of the exactness requirement is that the explicatum is sufficiently amenable to operationalization to be detected or measured by empirical methods. In the case of the concept of death, this implies that scientifically sound criteria and tests are available to determine whether the concept applies. Operational criteria are especially indispensable in the legal domain.

The third requirement, simplicity, is an obvious desideratum, especially in the case of everyday concepts such as life and death. The explication should make the concept easier to understand than in its original form. Furthermore, if we think of the necessity, in an increasingly integrated world, to communicate about life and death between individuals of different cultural backgrounds and different world views, the explicatum should ideally be acceptable even to people holding world views distinctly different from the scientific one.

The fourth requirement, fruitfulness, can be interpreted, for practical contexts, as the maxim to explicate a concept so that it is consonant with all or a substantial portion of the ethical principles and intuitions applying in the relevant domain. In analogy to fruitfulness in the theoretical field, where it means, among other things, the capacity to be introduced in and related to scientific laws, fruitfulness in the practical field can be understood as the capacity to become part of an ethically justified practice.

On this background, it may be argued that these requirements are in fact best served by an explicatum of the concept of death that corresponds to the brain death criterion, i.e. the irreversible and complete cessation of brain function. An explication along this line does not fully meet the first and the third requirement, but it meets the others better than its alternatives.

As to the first requirement, it cannot be denied that an explicatum of this kind deviates to a significant degree from both the traditional meaning of death and the meaning given to it by a great number of people today. These meanings, however, are profoundly inexact. For example, the proposed explication "death is the permanent cessation of the critical functions of the organism as a whole" (Laureys 2005: 900) leaves open exactly which functions count as 'critical'. By contrast, the explication of death as the irreversible cessation of the functioning of the whole brain is less ambiguous and enables physicians to unequivocally test the presence or absence of life in a patient. If done professionally and in accordance with the rules, no brain death diagnosis has ever been put in doubt by the "awakening" of a patient. Furthermore, these rules have been progressively differentiated on the basis of clinical experience and fine-tuned for special situations.

As far as simplicity and intelligibility are concerned, the definition of death as irreversible and complete cessation of brain activity is, admittedly, unsatisfactory. For many people, the definition is hard to accept because of its remoteness from the concrete experience of dying. In the situation of the intensive care unit, death has ceded its place in the *lebenswelt* to something purely cognitive and abstract, no longer accompanied by signs accessible to direct experience.

This defect is, however, more than offset by the important practical advantage that this explication enables the practice of postmortem organ transplantation without infringing the dead donor rule. Abandoning the brain death explication of death would either seriously limit the highly beneficial practice of organ transplantation or infringe a rule that is held by most physicians to be indispensable. Furthermore, abandoning it would require legislations that would greatly complicate the legal rules pertaining to life and death.

The question arises which normative status can be claimed for a pragmatically motivated explication that is, at least in part, motivated by 'pragmatic', in this case: ethical and praxeological considerations. Authors who tend to reject the identification of brain death and death have spoken of the brain death definition as a 'legal fiction' (Shah/Miller 2010). This manner of speaking can be interpreted as pejorative – a way of saying that brain death is only so-called death. Alternatively, it can be interpreted more neutrally, as a pragmatic manner of speaking aimed, in the first instance, at relieving the transplant surgeon from the risk of being held responsible for manslaughter. However, there is a crucial difference between this 'legal fiction' and others such as the fiction of a 'legal person'. In the case of 'legal persons' such as institutions and companies, it is clear to everyone that the term does not refer to a real person. The identification of brain death with death is different. By now, it has gained so much social acceptance that the conflict it is designed to solve is only rarely brought to attention. If acceptance increases in the future, the conflict between ethics and anthropology from which the debate started will largely be a matter of the past.

References

Bernat, James L./Culver, Charles M./Gert, Bernard (1981): "On the Definition and Criterion of Death." In: Annals of Internal Medicine 94, pp. 389–394.

Birnbacher, Dieter (2018): "Wie ‚pragmatisch' dürfen Explikationen des Begriffs ‚Tod des Menschen' sein? Überlegungen anlässlich der Vierten Fortschreibung der Richtlinien für die Todesfeststellung." In: Angewandte Philosophie 1, pp. 91–107.

Birnbacher, Dieter/Angstwurm, Hans/Eigler, Friedrich W./Wuermeling, Hans B. (1993): "Der vollständige und endgültige Ausfall der Hirntätigkeit als Todeszeichen des Menschen. Anthropologischer Hintergrund." In: Deutsches Ärzteblatt 90/44, pp. 2926–2929.

Brandt, Stephan A./Angsturm, Heinz (2018): "The Relevance of Irreversible Loss of Brain Function as a Reliable Sign of Death." In: Deutsches Ärzteblatt International 115, pp. 675–681.

Carnap, Rudolf (1963): The Logical Foundations of Probability. 2nd edition, Chicago: Chicago University Press.

Condic, Maureen L. (2016): "Determination of Death: a Scientific Perspective on Biological Integration." In: Journal of Medicine and Philosophy 41, pp. 257–278.

DeGrazia, David (2005): Human Identity and Bioethics, Cambridge: Cambridge University Press.

Deutscher Ethikrat (2015): Hirntod und Entscheidung zur Organspende. Stellungnahme. Berlin.

Harvard Ad Hoc Committee (1968): "A Definition of Irreversible Coma." In: Journal of the American Medical Association 205, pp. 85–88.

Jonas, Hans (1980): "Against the Stream. Comments on the Definition and Redefinition of Death." In: Hans Jonas (ed.). Philosophical Essays. From Ancient Creed to Technological Man, New York: Atropos Press, pp. 134–142.

Laureys, Steven (2005): "Death, Unconsciousness and the Brain." In: Nature Reviews Neuroscience 6, pp. 899–909.

Lock, Margaret (2001): "On Dying Twice: Culture, Technology and the Determination of Death." In: Margaret Lock/Alan Young/Alberto Cambrosio (eds.): Living and Working with the New Medical Technologies, Cambridge: Cambridge University Press, pp. 233–262.

McMahan, Jeff (2002): The Ethics of Killing. Problems at the Margins of Life, Oxford: Oxford University Press.

Miller, Franklin G./Truog, Robert D. (2009): "The Incoherence of Determining Death by Neurological Criteria: A Commentary on 'Controversies in the Determination of Death, A White Paper by the President's Council on Bioethics'." In: Kennedy Institute of Ethics Journal 19, pp. 185–193.

President's Council on Bioethics (2008): Controversies on the Determination of Death. A White Paper. Washington D. C.

Quante, Michael (2002): Personales Leben und menschlicher Tod. Personale Identität als Prinzip der biomedizinischen Ethik, Frankfurt: Suhrkamp.

Sass, Hans-Martin (1989): "Brain Life and Brain Death: a Proposal for a Normative Agreement." In: Journal of Medicine and Philosophy 14, pp. 45–59.

Schicktanz, Silke/Pfaller, Larissa/Hansen, Solveig Lena/Boos, Moritz (2017): "Attitudes Towards Brain Death and Conceptions of the Body in Relation to Willingness or Reluctance to Donate: Results of a Student Survey before and after the German Transplantation Scandals and Legal Changes." In: Journal of Public Health 25, pp. 249–256.

Shah, Seema K./Miller, Franklin G. (2010): "Can we Handle the Truth? Legal Fictions in the Determination of Death." In: American Journal of Law and Medicine 36, pp. 1–56.

Shewmon, D. Alan (2010): "Constructing the Death Elephant. A Synthetic Paradigm Shift for the Definition, Criteria, and Tests for Death." In: Journal of Medicine and Philosophy 35, pp. 256–298.

Shewmon, D. Alan (2001): "The Brain and Somatic Integration. Insights into the Standard Biological Rationale for Equating 'Brain Death' with Death." In: Journal of Medicine and Philosophy 26, pp. 457–478.

Shewmon, D. Alan (1998): "'Brainstem Death', 'Brain Death', and Death: A Critical Re-Evaluation of the Purported Equivalence." In: Issues in Law and Medicine 14, pp. 125–145.

Stoecker, Ralf (2010): Der Hirntod. Ein medizinethisches Problem und seine moralphilosophische Transformation, 2nd edition, Freiburg/München: Alber.

Swiss Academy of Medical Sciences (2011): Feststellung des Todes mit Bezug auf Organtransplantationen. Medizin-ethische Richtlinien und Empfehlungen. Basel.

Truog, Robert D./ Robinson, Walter M. (2003): "Role of Brain Death and the Dead-Donor Rule in the Ethics of Organ Transplantation." In: Critical Care Medicine 31, pp. 2391–2396.

Veatch, Robert M. (1989): Death, Dying and the Biological Revolution. Our Last Quest for Responsibility, rev. ed., New Haven/London: Yale University Press.

Veatch, Robert M. (2004): "Abandon the Dead Donor Rule or Change the Definition of Death?" In: Kennedy Institute of Ethics Journal 14, pp. 261–276.

Veatch, Robert M./Lainie F. Ross (2016): Defining Death. The Case for Choice, Washington: Georgetown University Press.

Walton, Douglas N. (1980): Brain Death. Ethical Considerations, West Lafayette: Purdue University Press.

Wiesemann, Claudia (1995): "Hirntod und Gesellschaft. Argumente für einen pragmatischen Skeptizismus." In: Ethik in der Medizin 6, pp. 16–28.

6. Defining Death in Donation after Circulatory Determination of Death
Medical Controversies

Anne Dalle Ave, David Shaw & James Bernat

1. Introduction

Over the past 50 years, the concept and the determination of death have been given increasing attention in the scientific literature. Death determination was not the prerogative of physicians until the 18th century, before which its determination was the responsibility of families or undertakers (Powner 1996). Mainly due to the fear of being buried alive and, later, due to the development of resuscitative technology, medicine has become the field of expertise for the determination of death. Beginning in the 18th and 19th centuries, death was determined by physicians based on the cessation of functions of the three vital organs: the heart, the lungs, and the brain. At that time, because the functions of these three vital organs were interdependent, death was a unitary phenomenon. When one vital organ ceased to function, the other two rapidly ceased to function as a result. The concept of death determination itself was straightforward and barely discussed in medical writings.

The development of mechanical ventilation in first half of the 20th century forever changed this paradigm (Rodríguez-Arias 2017). Advances in medical technologies now permitted physicians to sustain the functions of the heart and lungs despite the cessation of brain function resulting from severe brain damage. Medical technologies thus created a new human state, one in which the interdependency of functions among the three vital organs was lost. This new human state initiated the first serious discussions on the concept of death within the medical profession.

Since the 1960s, death determination has been conceptualized as either the cessation of functions of the whole brain (Mollaret 1959; Beecher 1968) or of circulatory and respiratory functions (President's Commission 1981). Throughout this time, as scholars have debated whether brain death was a coherent concept of death (Veatch 1993; Bernat 1981; Giacomini 1997), the acceptance of brain death as a criterion for death has grown worldwide (Capron 2001). The determination of brain death is now accepted by the international medical profession (Wijdicks 2010). When a patient is determined dead based on the brain criterion of death, his respiratory and circulatory functions are maintained by artificial means, such as the use of mechanical ventilation. Brain tests are used to prove the absence of any brain functions, particularly the absence of consciousness, brain stem functions, and spontaneous respiration.

Donation after circulatory determination of death (DCDD) programs were developed in the 1980s in order to address the scarcity of organs; they have since been developed in many countries around the world to increase the organ pool for transplantation. However, DCDD programs also challenge the concept and determination of death, and certain countries have chosen not to develop such programs, for moral, cultural, historical and also legal reasons. For example, DCDD remains illegal in Germany, possibly because of historical sensitivity around euthanasia.

The United States, Canada, the United Kingdom, and the Netherlands, among other countries, have mainly developed controlled DCDD programs (Magliocca 2005; Bos 2005; Summers 2015; Shemie 2006). Here, organ donation occurs after the cessation of the donor's circulation, following the withdrawal of life-sustaining therapies. The decision to withdraw life-sustaining therapies is made independently of the question of organ donation (Dalle Ave 2017a); it is made when the patient or family no longer desire the prolongation of life, and when doctors judge further medical treatment to be inappropriate or futile (Bosslet 2015).

France and Spain have pioneered the development of programs of uncontrolled DCDD (Burnod 2007; Antoine 2007; Mateos-Rodriguez 2010; Mateos-Rodriguez 2012). This system applies in cases of unexpected sudden cardiac arrest. Once it has been established that resuscitative efforts are futile, the patient is transferred to an uncontrolled DCDD medical center. Donation occurs once death has been determined at the hospital.

In DCDD programs (controlled and uncontrolled), death occurs after a cardiac arrest, which leads to the cessation of the circulatory and respiratory functions. Death is determined after a purposely short period of cardiac arrest and circulatory cessation, usually five minutes, to allow a sufficient quality of organs suitable for transplantation. The way death is determined in DCDD varies among countries.

In this chapter, we focus on the ethical issues raised by the determination of death in DCDD. Our purpose is to offer a conceptual justification for death determination in this context and to highlight practical pitfalls, but not to offer a normative analysis of the concept of death in general. We first describe and analyze the determination of death in DCDD by discussing the concepts of irreversible and permanent cessation of functions. Second, we discuss the issues raised by the use of extracorporeal membrane oxygenation (ECMO) in DCDD. Third, we analyze the unique issues raised by heart DCDD, and fourth, the issues raised by uncontrolled DCDD. Finally, we propose a new way to determine death in DCDD: the brain circulation determination of death.

2.   Description and Analysis of the Determination of Death in DCDD

In both uncontrolled and controlled DCDD programs, death is determined after a short stand-off (no-touch) period, defined as the time between complete circulatory cessation and the determination of death. Although the stand-off period varies among countries, five minutes has become the norm. A short stand-off period is desirable to minimize the warm ischemia time and thereby optimize graft outcome.

The criteria to determine death vary among countries. In the US and many other countries, death is determined by fulfilling one of two criteria: the irreversible cessation of circulatory and respiratory functions, or the irreversible cessation of all functions of the entire brain, including the brain stem (Uniform Determination of Death Act 1997).

Laws and codes of practice in other countries, including France, Canada (The Law Reform commission of Canada 1970), the United Kingdom (Academy of Medical Royal Colleges 2008), and Switzerland (Swiss Federal Act 2004), unify death determination under a single brain criterion. In Switzerland, for instance, "a person is dead when all cerebral functions, including the brain stem, have irreversibly ceased" (Swiss Federal Act 2004).

Several critics have argued, however, that DCDD donors are not dead at the time of the determination of death (Rady 2013; Joffe 2011; Potts 2007; Marquis 2010; Miller 2008). Death is, by definition, an irreversible state, and after only five minutes of circulatory cessation, the cessation of respiratory and circulatory functions might be potentially reversible. Thus, the five-minute stand-off period is obviously not sufficient to achieve the irreversible cessation of circulatory, respiratory, or brain functions. Several studies, unrelated to DCDD protocols, showed good neurological outcomes for some patients who suffered an out-of-hospital cardiac arrest with a no-flow period of 20 to 30 minutes (Hara 2015).[1] These studies reveal a fact known widely by physicians: after only five minutes of cardiac arrest, it may be possible to medically restore circulatory, respiratory and some brain functions. Furthermore, the use of advance resuscitative technique, such as extra-corporeal membrane oxygenation (ECMO), may also restore circulation after intractable cardiac arrest (Megarbane 2011). Additionally, animal studies have demonstrated evidence that circulatory, respiratory and some brain functions could be restored after cardio-circulatory cessation for as long as 30–60 minutes (Hossmann 1987; Hossmann 1973). Thus, it is clear that circulatory function may be restorable, even after a cessation of five minutes.

These facts have led some critics to conclude that DCDD protocols breach the dead donor rule, an ethical and legal guideline that requires that "donors must not be killed in order to obtain their organs" and that "organ retrieval cannot cause death" (Robertson 1999: 6).

One of us (James Bernat) has addressed the question of whether DCDD programs breached the dead donor rule by highlighting the distinction between the irreversible and permanent cessation of circulatory and respiratory functions). Bernat states that: "whereas, irreversibility is a requirement for the definition and criterion of death, [...] a circulatory-respiratory death determination requires demonstrating only that circulatory and respiratory functions have ceased permanently" (2010: 249).

Thus, an individual who has permanently lost his circulatory and respiratory functions is determined dead and the dead donor rule is not breached.

Bernat further points out that a function is said to be irreversibly lost when no available intervention or technology can restore that function. Irreversibility is thus an unequivocal state, which implies a technical impossibility, independent of our intention or action (Bernat 2006). By contrast, a function is said to be permanently lost when that function cannot restart spontaneously (autoresuscitation) and will not

---

1 No-flow is the time interval between collapse and the initiation of cardiopulmonary resuscitation.

be restored by medical intervention. Permanent cessation is thus an equivocal state, which implies a technical possibility, and one that is dependent on our intention and action (ibid.). After a cardiac arrest, a patient will have the permanent cessation of circulation after five minutes of observation, and this state will become irreversible with time if no actions to restore circulation are performed.

In practice, physicians typically determine death (particularly in the acute setting) once the cessation of respiratory and circulatory functions is permanent. For instance, in the intensive care unit after withdrawal of life-sustaining therapies, cardiac and respiratory functions progressively decrease until they cease completely. Once the heartbeat has stopped, physicians may determine death within as little as a few minutes.

To confirm permanent cessation, the physician must ensure that the period during which auto-resuscitation could occur has elapsed. From the point of death determination, the patient will evolve from a permanent to an irreversible cessation of circulation and respiration. Because no action will interfere with this process, permanency is a valid surrogate on which to base the determination of death, and in practice there is no need to wait longer.

Bernat argues that death could be determined in DCDD protocols based on the permanent cessation of respiratory and circulatory functions if two conditions are satisfied. First, spontaneous resumption of ceased functions (auto-resuscitation) cannot occur; and second, medical interventions will not be attempted to restart the ceased functions (Bernat 2010).

These necessary conditions in DCDD protocols raise two issues. First, how long must a physician wait to ensure the impossibility of auto-resuscitation? Second, how do resuscitative techniques (such as ECMO, Cardiopulmonary resuscitation (CPR), and mechanical ventilation) that are instituted after the determination of death interfere with the determination of death? Ethically, these questions are extremely important: if the patient is not truly dead when organs are retrieved, the dead donor rule would be breached and organ removal by physicians could actually cause death. This would be a grave violation of professional duties and the principle of non-maleficence.

To answer the first question regarding waiting time, we can cite studies that assess how many minutes of circulatory cessation confidently exclude the possibility of auto-resuscitation (Hornby 2010). Importantly, the answer differs between controlled and uncontrolled DCDD protocols. In controlled DCDD, no patients have demonstrated auto-resuscitation after one minute of circulatory cessation, whereas in uncontrolled DCDD after a primary cardiac arrest, no patients demonstrated auto-resuscitation after seven minutes of circulatory cessation. Because the number of patients studied has been relatively small, more studies are necessary to determine more accurately exactly how long it is necessary to wait after circulatory cessation to ensure the impossibility of auto-resuscitation, and thus to permit DCDD programs to determine an appropriate stand-off period. At present, it appears that a five-minute stand-off period in controlled DCDD is long enough to exclude the possibility of auto-resuscitation, but this is not long enough to confidently exclude the possibility of auto-resuscitation in uncontrolled DCDD, which requires ten minutes.

In the next two sections we address the second question: how the use of resuscitative techniques after the determination of death can interfere with the determination of death. We analyze the use of ECMO in DCDD and the unique case of DCDD heart transplantation.

3.   The Use of ECMO in DCDD

An ethical imperative of organ donation is to procure organs in good condition. Some controlled DCDD protocols use ECMO to resume bodily circulation following the determination of death, only to benefit the organs' condition (Magliocca 2005; Farney 2011; Lee 2005; Rojas-Pena 2014, Oniscu 2014). After a stand-off period, ECMO is initiated to decrease warm ischemia time before organ procurement begins.[2] ECMO can improve future graft outcome by maintaining organ perfusion until procurement. Some uncontrolled DCDD protocols in France and Spain (Burnod 2007; Mateos-Rodriguez 2010) also use ECMO as a method of organ preservation, after death has been determined.

The use of ECMO may be ethically justified from a utilitarian perspective because it may improve the organs that are donated. However, it raises ethical issues such as (temporarily) reversing the determination of death and thus potentially harming the patient. If it is used during a state of permanent cessation, before the cessation becomes irreversible, ECMO could restore brain, heart and circulatory functions. This situation creates a risk of harm to the donor. To avoid such risk, a supra-diaphragmatic aortic occlusion balloon is usually inserted to block ECMO blood flow to the brain and thorax and thereby to prevent the restoration of brain and heart circulation.

The risk of restoring brain and heart functions is not a fantasy or theoretical risk and was acknowledged in the initial controlled DCDD protocols using ECMO. In these protocols, instead of inserting an aortic occlusion balloon, intravenous lidocaine was administered to prevent the restoration of heartbeat, and/or phenobarbital was administered to prevent the restoration of brain functions. What effect on death determination would ECMO produce if circulation was resumed after death was determined? Even if upper body circulation was prevented through the use of the aortic occlusion balloon, lower body circulation would be resumed through the use of ECMO. Technology again forces us to reconsider our criteria for death, and whether they remain ethically appropriate. Is the patient dead under those conditions? The answer depends on which criterion of death one uses. If one determines death based on the circulatory criterion, it may be difficult to say whether the patient is dead or alive: above the aortic balloon there is no circulation, but below the aortic balloon circulation remains. Here, the brain criterion is more applicable, by which the donor is dead when his brain functions have ceased irreversibly, irrespective of what happens to his bodily circulation. In DCDD that means that brain death could occur under the condition that brain circulation is confidently prevented, even if bodily circulation persists. If brain circulation stops, brain function will cease, initially permanently, and then irreversibly. Later we discuss in greater detail the implication of the use of a brain criterion of death in DCDD.

Now, let us focus on the fact that to prevent harm, brain circulation must be confidently prevented despite the use of ECMO. Note that the balloon does not cause brain death; it prevents the brain being reoxygenated, which physicians must accomplish to maintain the pre-existing determination of death. But can one be certain that the aor-

---

2 The warm ischemia time is the interval between the moment donors develop severe ischemia (often at a systolic blood pressure threshold of 80 mmHg or from cardiac arrest) and the initiation of organ perfusion.

tic occlusion balloon is not misplaced when ECMO is started, or will not be displaced or malfunction during the use of ECMO? In the case of aortic occlusion balloon malfunction or displacement, because the brain tissue is sensitive to reperfusion for 30–60 minutes, there is a risk of restoring brain circulation, reviving the patient, and thus harming the donor. This risk is not theoretical; we have described such cases (Dalle Ave 2016a). We believe, as do others (Manara 2012), that no intervention should be used that may potentially restore brain functions after the determination of death (Dalle Ave 2016a; Bernat 2008).

4.   Heart DCDD

There are only a few heart DCDD programs currently operating around the world, probably because of the sensitivity of the heart to warm ischemia time and related technical difficulties. The first heart DCDD was performed in 1967 by Barnard in Cape Town (Barnard 1967). In 2008, Boucek et al. published three cases of heart DCDD transplanted in neonates (Boucek 2008). The stand-off period of this Denver DCDD protocol had been reduced from three minutes to 75 seconds, leading critics to question whether the neonatal heart donors were truly dead at the time of organ procurement. It is only since 2015 that heart DCDD programs have been developed elsewhere, principally in the United Kingdom (Ali 2009; Walsh 2015; Smail 2018; Messer 2017) and Australia (Dhital 2015; Chew 2019).

One of the two heart DCDD protocols of the United Kingdom is creative (Ali 2009; Walsh 2015). As in any controlled DCDD protocol, after withdrawal of life-sustaining therapies, circulatory cessation is followed by the determination of death. After a five-minute stand-off period, a thoracotomy is rapidly performed to clamp the aortic arch vessels and to insert ECMO catheters to resume bodily circulation. Instead of the aortic occlusion balloon, which excludes heart circulation, the UK heart DCDD protocol uses an aortic arch clamp. This heart DCDD protocol permits the resumption of full bodily circulation, including that of the heart, while excluding brain circulation. Once ECMO has resumed circulation, the UK heart DCDD protocol waits until the heart resumes normal function, after which ECMO is weaned. If the heart continues to demonstrate good function, it is deemed suitable for transplantation and is thus procured. The UK heart DCDD protocol thus essentially converts a DCDD organ donor into a brain-dead donor.

Like all DCDD protocols using ECMO, the UK heart DCDD protocol raises the issue of whether it retroactively interferes with the previous determination of death. Does the use of an aortic clamp confidently prevent the restoration of brain circulation during the use of ECMO? If not, the donor may incur harm. An aortic clamp may block blood circulation through the carotid and vertebral arteries, but it may "spare small collateral arteries from the segmental spinal arteries that arise from the thoracic aorta and anastomose the branches of the vertebral arteries. These collaterals conceivably could provide a small degree of perfusion to the brainstem" (Dalle Ave 2016b: 315).

Bedside assessment may provide some clues that the brain retains some brain perfusion with the use of ECMO. For instance, clinical signs of transtentorial brain herniation – such as sudden severe hypertension and bradycardia, followed by a rapid hypotension – after the determination of death and during the use of ECMO, may constitute evidence that the last brain functions are ceasing at that precise moment. This finding would imply that the brain had preserved some brain functions before the occurrence of this Cushing reflex, and thus that the donor was not dead, probably because ECMO permitted the preservation of a small degree of brain perfusion.

As we have explained elsewhere, to ensure that the aortic arch clamp completely blocks brain perfusion, brain circulation should be tested and proven absent. In particular, brain stem perfusion should be proven to have stopped because it can continue to function with a smaller blood flow than the cerebral hemispheres (Dalle Ave 2016b: 315).

The Australian heart DCDD protocol differs from that of the UK by not using ECMO (Dhital 2015; Chew 2019). In their protocol, a stand-off period of two or five minutes is used. To better preserve the future graft function, a "normothermic ex vivo cardiac perfusion device" is used to decrease the cold ischemia time, namely, the time from heart procurement to heart transplantation (Burnod 2007).

Controlled DCDD using a stand-off period as brief as two minutes (Boucek 2008; Dhital 2015) raises issues regarding the concept of permanent cessation. After circulatory cessation, the permanent cessation of circulation occurs once the possibility of auto-resuscitation has elapsed. A stand-off period as short as two minutes may put the donor at risk of auto-resuscitation, potentially breaching the DDR. That is why, until further studies of controlled DCDD programs have determined with greater accuracy the exact minimum duration of circulatory cessation that excludes the possibility of auto-resuscitation, we support a secure stand-off period of five minutes.

In addition to the previously described protocol using ECMO, the UK has developed a heart DCDD protocol similar to Australia's (Smail 2018; Messer 2017). After the stand-off period of five minutes, the heart is rapidly procured and reperfused in an *ex situ* normothermic platform using the Organ Care System. In this protocol, the donor's abdominal organs are perfused by the use of ECMO, but not the heart because the descending aorta is clamped.

5.   Uncontrolled DCDD

Uncontrolled DCDD programs raise several ethical issues. We focus here on those related to the determination of death. Uncontrolled DCDD programs (Burnod 2007; Mateos-Rodriguez 2010) concern donation after a sudden cardiac arrest, usually in an out-of-hospital setting. Once physicians deem them to be futile, resuscitations efforts are stopped. At that point, if the patient is suitable for an uncontrolled DCDD protocol, CPR efforts are resumed, and the patient is transferred to the uncontrolled DCDD medical center. The goal of CPR efforts at this stage is not to save the patient's life, which is no longer possible, but to preserve organ perfusion to ensure better future graft outcome. At the uncontrolled DCDD center, death is determined, followed by the initiation of ECMO or cold perfusion to preserve the organs for future transplantation. Organ procurement proceeds once consent to organ donation has been obtained. Four unresolved medical-ethical issues remain in the determination of death in uncontrolled DCDD programs, which we describe in the following.

5.1   The Use of CPR Once the Patient has been Considered Unsalvageable

As stated, when physicians judge that further resuscitation efforts are futile, CPR is stopped and the patient is considered to be dead (even though in some protocols, death is formally determined later at the hospital). The only justification for accepting the patient into an uncontrolled DCDD protocol – a decision that is made immediately after CPR has been stopped – is that the patient is unsalvageable and presumed dead. When CPR is resumed to preserve the organs, and despite no intent to save the patient's life, CPR produces a risk of restoring bodily circulation sufficient to restore brain circulation and thus brain function. This situation can harm the patient by temporarily returning him to life that will confer no benefit.

5.2   The Use of ECMO after the Determination of Death

The same considerations discussed in section III are relevant here. After the determination of death, no measure that could restore brain circulation and function should be used because it could revive the patient.

5.3   The Conflict of Interest between Uncontrolled DCDD Programs and ECMO-Assisted CPR (E-CPR)

E-CPR is a resuscitation technique using ECMO when conventional CPR cannot restore a patient's life (Stub 2015; Sakamoto 2014). There is evidence that advances in E-CPR may improve the outcome of patients suffering from an unexpected refractory cardiac arrest. E-CPR protocols and uncontrolled DCDD protocols are similar (Dalle Ave 2016c). The vexing question facing the resuscitative team is: given a patient with a refractory cardiac arrest, how should they decide between entering this patient into an E-CPR protocol to attempt to save his life, or into an uncontrolled DCDD protocol to convert him to an organ donor and save the life of a potential organ recipient? In some situations, there may be no hospital nearby that could save the patient's life, but there may be hospitals nearby with suitable organ donation programs (Dalle Ave 2016c). Attempting to save the patient's life with E-CPR may well be futile and might be judged inappropriate even if organ donation was not a possibility. The inherent conflict of interest has a major impact on the determination of death. If instead of attempting resuscitation by an E-CPR protocol, the patient was prematurely entered into an uncontrolled DCDD protocol, he would be declared dead, even though he might have been saved by a resuscitative technique.

To avoid a 'third world resuscitation-first world donation' situation (Dalle Ave 2016c), saving patients' lives in case of cardiac arrest should remain the highest priority. Countries should primarily focus on the development of resuscitation techniques, such as E-CPR, and donation should be considered only secondarily. One solution to avoid such a conflict of interest would be to have uncontrolled DCDD programs only in centers that use E-CPR. If E-CPR is not an option, and if no other lifesaving options are available, termination of resuscitation efforts could be considered. Only after the final step should death be determined following an adequate stand-off period, at which time organ procurement may be pursued.

5.4   The Optimal Duration of the Stand-Off Period

Usually, the stand-off period used in uncontrolled DCDD programs is five minutes. However, one survey showed that, in the context of an unexpected cardiac arrest, auto-resuscitation to restored circulation is possible for up to seven minutes (Hornby 2010). To ensure that a state of permanent cessation of circulation exists, death should be declared only after a stand-off period of at least ten minutes in the context of uncontrolled DCDD.

6.   The Brain Circulation Determination of Death

In DCDD, the permanent cessation of circulation as a criterion of death can be retro-actively negated using resuscitative technologies such as ECMO. Previously, we suggested that the permanent cessation of brain circulation is the essential underlying determinant of death in the context of DCDD. We therefore suggested a new acronym in place of DCDD: DBCDD – organ *donation after brain circulation determination of death* (Dalle Ave 2017b). We now analyze the role of the permanent cessation of brain circulation in determining death in DCDD.

After circulatory cessation, ischemia develops progressively in different organs. Because the brain is the organ most sensitive to ischemia, it is affected first and heart ischemia follows. After circulatory cessation, brain functions cease within minutes, first permanently, and after 30-60 minutes, irreversibly. If one accepts brain death as a valid criterion of death, one may apply this same criterion in the DCDD context. The concept of brain death holds that patients whose brain functions have ceased irreversibly, but who have their circulation sustained artificially, are considered dead (see also chapter 5 in this book). In the discussion that follows, we assume that the irreversible cessation of brain functions is a theoretically valid criterion of death. However, we will show that it is not how death is usually determined in practice, and it may also not be the best way to determine death at the bedside, including in DCDD programs.

If DCDD programs employed the standard brain death criterion to determine death, they would become impossible. Because proving the irreversible cessation of all brain functions would require at least 30–60 minutes of circulatory cessation, most organs would be unsuitable for transplantation.

Another option would be to require only the permanent cessation of all brain functions to determine death. This step would be a departure from the usual understanding of the brain death criterion, which requires irreversibility. The justification to switch from the irreversible to the permanent cessation of all brain functions is the same as the justification used to switch from the irreversible to the permanent cessation of circulatory functions. In practice, physicians often determine death during a state of permanent cessation, whether the functions which are permanently lost are those of the heart, the circulation, or the brain. Thus, in DCDD, one could use the same standard to determine death, ensuring the two conditions proposed by James Bernat, i.e. that brain circulation must not be restored after death, and there can no longer be a possibility of auto-resuscitation.

An additional necessary condition is that the permanent cessation of all brain functions must be complete. It is necessary to wait long enough after circulatory cessation that all brain functions have ceased. Death should never be determined (or organs procured) while the patient retains brain functions because it could create the potential of awareness and suffering. Only a few minutes of circulatory cessation are necessary to assure that all brain functions have ceased permanently. A stand-off period of five minutes would ensure that the possibility of auto-resuscitation has elapsed and that all brain functions are permanently lost.

The requirement that brain circulation not be restored after the determination of death demands that any technologies that could restore bodily circulation must be omitted after the determination of death. These technologies include ECMO, CPR, and even lung inflation, all of which may stimulate the heart to restart functioning and restore circulation. If those techniques are used after the determination of death, brain circulation must be excluded, and the absence of brain circulation proven with certainty. This requirement may be a challenge to achieve in practice.

To use the brain circulation criterion of death to determine death in DCDD, one should determine which tests will be used to confirm death. We argue that because circulatory cessation irremediably leads to the cessation of brain function, the confirmation of the cessation of systemic circulation is sufficient to confirm death. This can be done using an echocardiography, proving no opening of the aortic valve, or of an electrocardiogram, proving the absence of electrical cardiac activity. The use of specific brain death tests is unnecessary, despite claims to the contrary (Swiss Academy of Medical Sciences 2019).

The proposal of basing the determination of death in DCDD on the brain circulation criterion has the advantage of unifying death under a single criterion. Elsewhere, we have explained the proposal of proving the absence of brain circulation in the context of organ donation after brain death (DBD) (Dalle Ave 2018). There is evidence that some patients determined dead by the brain death criterion – i.e. patients who have no apparent brain functions but who have their circulation artificially sustained – may retain some brain functions despite having been declared dead. To reduce the inconsistency between the brain death criterion and the tests for brain death, we proposed the requirement of showing the absence of brain circulation by a validated neuroimaging test. We argue that showing absence of brain circulation could be a unique criterion to determine death in both DCDD and in DBD. Because currently no method completely excludes brain circulation, further research is necessary before this idea can be implemented.

7.   Conclusion and Future Perspectives

The controversy over whether the DCDD donor is dead after five minutes of complete circulatory cessation can be resolved by accepting the medical practice standard for death determination as the permanent cessation of circulation and respiration. Even though many death statutes employ the term 'irreversible cessation' of circulation and respiration, and the biological concept of death requires irreversibility, the medical practice standard for death determination has always been their permanent cessation (Bernat 2013). There is no compelling reason why death determination in the context of organ donation should require a change in medical practice from the standard that physicians widely use to declare death in non-donation circumstances.

All existing DCDD programs implicitly accept permanent cessation as death by requiring only two to five minutes of circulatory and respiratory cessation before death is declared, despite knowing that the loss of these functions may not be irreversible at that point. Only a few groups have explicitly accepted the permanent vs. irreversible distinction (American Academy of Pediatrics Committee on Bioethics 2013), but there is no justification for hospitals to sponsor DCDD programs other than endorsing this conceptual distinction. We are simply making the concept underlying prevailing DCDD practices explicit. Clear definitions of the underlying concepts of DCDD are essential for ethical decision-making, because without them patients might be harmed by unnecessary interventions, or organs removed when patients are not really dead. Clarity is also essential for transparency and trust.

For physicians to accurately declare death on the basis of permanent cessation of circulation and respiration, there must be no subsequent interventions that restore circulation because the cessation would then no longer be permanent. If cessation is not permanent, organ removal could in some cases constitute killing the patient. That is why there must be a complete proscription against the use of CPR, ECMO, and all other resuscitative technologies that restore or partially restore brain circulation. There also must be a reliable method to determine that circulatory cessation is complete, such as showing zero forward blood flow by an arterial catheter or Doppler, or by an echocardiogram showing no opening of the aortic valve. The third condition is that the no-touch interval after circulatory cessation must be of sufficient duration to exclude the possibility of auto-resuscitation. Auto-resuscitation to restoration of circulation is extremely unlikely after one minute in the controlled DCDD patient but may occur up to seven minutes after circulatory cessation in cases of uncontrolled DCDD because of the prior resuscitative treatments.

We believe that for their future success, all DCDD programs should use the determination of death that requires showing only the permanent cessation of brain circulation. Fulfilling this criterion also requires that any resuscitative efforts including ECMO and chest compressions must not restore any circulation to the brain. Ultimately, both circulatory and brain criteria of death depend on the permanent and total absence of brain circulation.

References

Academy of Medical Royal Colleges (2008): A Code of Practice for the Diagnosis and Confirmation of Death. London.

Ali, Ayyaz/White, Paul/Dhital, Kumud/Ryan, Marian/Tsui, Steven/Large, Stephen (2009): "Cardiac Recovery in a Human Non-Heart-Beating Donor after Extracorporeal Perfusion: Source for Human Heart Donation?" In: The Journal of Heart and Lung Transplantation 28/3, pp. 290–293.

American Academy of Pediatrics Committee on Bioethics (2013): "Policy Statement: Ethical Controversies in Organ Donation after Circulatory Death." In: Pediatrics 131/5, pp. 1021–1026.

Antoine, Corinne/Tenaillon, Alain (2007): "Conditions à respecter pour réaliser des prélèvements de reins sur des donneurs à Cœur arrêté dans un établissement de santé autorisé aux prélèvements d'organes." Agence de la biomédecine. Available at: http://www.urgences-serveur.fr/IMG/pdf/DVprotocole_V12_avril_2007.pdf (accessed June 28, 2020)

Bernard, Christian N. (1967): "A Human Cardiac Transplant: an Interim Report of a Successful Operation Performed at Groote Shuur Hospital, Cape Town." In: South African Medical Journal 41/48, pp. 1271–1274.

Beecher, Henry K. (1968): "A Definition of Irreversible Coma. Special Communication: Report of the Ad Hoc Committee of the Harvard Medical School to Examine the Definition of Brain Death." In: Journal of the American Medical Association 205/6, pp. 337–340.

Bernat, James L./Culver, C. M./Gert, B. (1981): "On the Definition and Criterion of Death." In: Annals of Internal Medicine 94/3: 389–394.

Bernat, James L. (2006): "Are Organ Donors after Cardiac Death Really Dead?" In: Journal of Clinical Ethics 17/2, pp. 122–132.

Bernat, James L. (2008): "The Boundaries of Organ Donation after Circulatory Death." In: New England Journal of Medicine 359/7, pp. 669–671.

Bernat, James L. (2010): "How the Distinction between 'Irreversible' and 'Permanent' Illuminates Circulatory-Respiratory Death Determination." In: Journal of Medicine and Philosophy 35/3, pp. 242–255.

Bernat, James L. (2013): "On Noncongruence between the Concept and Determination of Death." In: Hastings Center Report 43/6, pp. 25–33.

Bos, M. A. (2005): "Ethical and Legal Issues in Non-Heart-Beating Organ Donation." In: Transplantation 79/9: 1143–1147.

Bosslet, Gabriel T./Pope, Thaddeus M./ Rubenfeld, Gordon D./Lo, Bernard/Truog, Robert D./ Rushton, Cynda H./Curtis, J. Randall/Ford, Dee W./Osborne, Molly/Misak, Cheryl/Au, David H./Azoulay, Elie/Brody, Baruch/Fahy, Brenda G./Hall, Jesse B./ Kesecioglu, Jozef/ Kon, Alexander A./Lindell, Kathleen O./Lindell, Kathleen O./ White, Douglas B./ American Thoracic Society ad hoc Committee on Futile and Potentially Inappropriate Treatment; American Thoracic Society; American Association for Critical Care Nurses; American College of Chest Physicians; European Society for Intensive Care Medicine; Society of Critical Care (2015): "An Official ATS/AACN/ACCP/ESICM/SCCM Policy Statement: Responding to Requests for Potentially Inappropriate Treatments in Intensive Care Units." In: American Journal of Respiratory and Critical Care Medicine 191/11, pp. 1318–1330.

Boucek, Mark M./Mashburn, Christine/Dunn, Susan M./Frizell, Rebecca/Edwards, Leah/ Pietra, Biagio/Campbell, David/Denver Children's Pediatric Heart Transplant Team (2008): "Pediatric Heart Transplantation after Declaration of Cardio-circulatory Death." In: New England Journal of Medicine 359/7, pp. 709–714.

Burnod, A./Antoine C., et al. (2007): "Resuscitation of Non-Heart-Beating Donors in the Prehospital Setting." In: Réanimation 16/7–8, pp. 687–694.

Capron, Alexander M. (2001): "Brain Death – Well Settled yet Still Unresolved'. In: New England Journal of Medicine 344/16, pp. 1244–1246.

Chew, Hong Chee/Iyer, Arjun/Connellan, Mark/Scheuer, Sarah/Villanueva, Jeanette/ Gao, Ling/Hicks, Mark/Harkness, Michelle/Soto, Claudio/Dinale, Andrew/Nair, Priya/Watson, Alasdair/Granger, Emily/Jansz, Paul/Muthiah, Kavitha/Jabbour, Andrew/Kotlyar, Eugene/ Keogh, Anne/Hayward, Chris/Graham, Robert/Spratt, Phillip/Macdonald, Peter/Dhital, Kumud (2019): "Outcomes of Donation after Circulatory Death Heart Transplantation in Australia." In: Journal of the American College of Cardiology 73/12, pp. 1447–1459.

Code de la Santé Publique. Article R 1232-1 et R 1232-2

Dalle Ave, Anne L./Shaw, David M./Bernat, James L. (2016a): "Ethical Issues in the Use of Extracorporeal Membrane Oxygenation in Controlled Donation after Circulatory Determination of Death." In: American Journal of Transplantation 16/8: 2293–2299.

Dalle Ave, Anne L./Shaw, David /Bernat, James L. (2016b): "An Analysis of Heart Donation after Circulatory Determination of Death." In: Journal of Medical Ethics 42/5, pp. 312–317.

Dalle, Ave Anne L./Shaw, David M./Gardiner, Dale (2016c): "Extracorporeal Membrane Oxygenation (ECMO) Assisted Cardiopulmonary Resuscitation or Uncontrolled Donation after the Circulatory Determination of Death Following Out-of-Hospital Refractory Cardiac Arrest – an Ethical Analysis of an Unresolved Clinical Dilemma'. In: Resuscitation 108, pp. 87–94.

Dalle Ave, Anne L./Shaw, David M. (2017a): "Controlled Donation After Circulatory Determination of Death." In: Journal of Intensive Care Medicine 32/3, pp. 179–186.

Dalle Ave, Anne L./Bernat, James L. (2017b): "Donation after Brain Circulation Determination of Death." In: BMC Medical Ethics 18/1, 15. DOI: 10.1186/s12910-017-0173-1

Dalle Ave, Anne L./Bernat, James L. (2018): "Inconsistencies Between the Criterion and Tests for Brain Death." In: Journal of Intensive Care Medicine 1–9. DOI: 10.1177/0885066618784268

Dhital, Kumud K./Iyer, Arjun/Connellan, Mark/Chew, Hong C./Gao, Ling/Doyle, Aoife/ Hicks, Mark/Kumarasinghe, Gayathri/Soto, Claude/Dinale, Andrew/Cartwright, Bruce/Nair, Priya/Granger, Emily/Jansz, Paul/Jabbour, Andrew/Kotlyar, Eugene/ Keogh, Anne/Hayward, Christopher/Graham, Robert/Spratt, Phillip/Macdonald, Peter (2015): "Adult Heart Transplantation with Distant Procurement and Ex-Vivo Preservation of Donor Hearts after Circulatory Death: a Case Series." In: Lancet 385/9987, pp. 2585–2591.

Farney, Alan C./Hines, Michael H./al-Geizawi, Samer/Rogers, Jeffrey/Stratta, Robert J. (2011): "Lessons Learned from a Single Center's Experience with 134 Donation after Cardiac Death Donor Kidney Transplants." In: Journal of the American College of Surgeons 212/4, pp. 440–451.

Giacomini, M. (1997): "A Change of Heart and a Change of Mind? Technology and the Redefinition of Death in 1968." In: Social Science and Medicine 44/10, pp. 1465–1482.

Hara, Masahiko/Hayashi, Kenichi/Hikoso, Shungo/Sakata, Yasushi/Kitamura, Tetsuhisa (2015): "Different Impacts of Time from Collapse to first Cardiopulmonary Resuscitation on Outcomes after Witnessed Out-of-Hospital Cardiac Arrest in Adults." In: Circulation: Cardiovascular Quality and Outcomes 8/3, pp. 277–284.

Hornby, K./Hornby, L./Shemie, S. D. (2010): "A Systematic Review of Autoresuscitation after Cardiac Arrest." In: Critical Care Medicine 38/5, pp. 1246–1253.

Hossmann, Konstantin-A./Kleihues, Paul (1973): "Reversibility of Ischemic Brain Damage." In: Archives of Neurology 29/6, pp. 375–384.

Hossmann, Konstantin-A./Schmidt-Kastner, Rainald/Grosse Ophoff, B. (1987): "Recovery of Intergrative Central Nervous Function after One Hour Global Cerebro-Circulatory Arrest in Normothermic Cat." In: Journal of the Neurological Sciences 77/2–3, pp. 305–320.

Joffe, Ari R./Carcillo, Joe/Anton, Natalie/deCaen, Allan/Han, Yong Y./Bell, Michael J./Maffei, Frank A./Sullivan, John/Thomas, James/Garcia-Guerra, Gonzalo (2011): "Donation after Cardiocirculatory Death: a Call for a Moratorium Pending Full Public Disclosure and Fully Informed Consent." In: Philosophy, Ethics, and Humanities in Medicine 6: 17. DOI: 10.1186/1747-5341-6-17.

Lee, Chih-Yuan/Tsai, Meng-Kun/Ko, Wen-Je/Chang, Chee-Jen/Hu, Rey-Heng/Chueh, Shih-Chieh/Lai, Ming-Kuen/Lee, Po-Huang (2005): "Expanding the Donor Pool: Use of Renal Transplants from Non-Heart-Beating Donors Supported with Extracorporeal Membrane Oxygenation." In: Clinical Transplantation 19/3, pp. 383–390.

Magliocca, Joseph F./Magee, John C./Rowe, Stephen A./Gravel, Mark T./Chenault, Richard/ Merion, Robert M./Punch, Jeffrey D./Bartlett, Robert H./Hemmila, Mark R. (2005): "Extracorporeal Support for Organ Donation after Cardiac Death Effectively Expands the Donor Pool." In: The Journal of Trauma 58/6, pp. 1095–1102.

Manara, Alex R./Murphy, P. G./O'Callaghan, G. (2012): "Donation after Circulatory Death." In: British Journal of Anaesthesia 108/S1, pp. 108–21.

Marquis, Don (2010): "Are DCD Donors Dead?" In: Hastings Center Report 40/3, pp. 24–31.

Mateos-Rodríguez, Alonso A./Pardillos-Ferrer, Luis/Navalpotro-Pascual, José María/ Barba-Alonso, Carlos/Martin-Maldonado, María Eugenia/Andrés-Belmonte, Amado (2010): "Kidney Transplant Function Using Organs from Non-Heart-Beating Donors Maintained by Mechanical Chest Compressions." In: Resuscitation 81/7, pp. 904–907.

Mateos-Rodríguez, Alonso A./Navalpotro-Pascual, José Maria/Del Rio Gallegos, Francisco/ Andrés-Belmonte, Amado (2012): "Out-Hospital Donors after Cardiac Death in Madrid, Spain: A 5-Year Review." In: Australasian Emergency Nursing Journal 15/3, pp. 164–169.

Mégarbane, Bruno/Deye, Nicolas/Aout, Mounir/Malissin, Isabelle/Résière, Dabor/ Haouache, Hakim/Brun, Pierre/Haik, William/Leprince, Pascal/Vicaut, Eric/Baud, Frédéric J. (2011): "Usefulness of Routine Laboratory Parameters in the Decision to Treat Refractory Cardiac Arrest with Extracorporeal Life Support." In: Resuscitation 82/9, pp. 1154–1161.

Messer, Simon/Page, Aravinda/Axell, Richard/Berman, Marius/Hernández-Sánchez, Jules/ Colah, Simon/Parizkova, Barbora/Valchanov, Kamen/Dunning, John/ Pavlushkov, Evgeny/ Balasubramanian, Sendhil K./Parameshwar, Jayan/Omar, Yasir Abu/Goddard, Martin/Pettit, Stephen/Lewis, Clive/Kydd, Anna/Jenkins, David/Watson, Christopher J./Sudarshan, Catherine/Catarino, Pedro/Findlay, Marie/Ali, Ayyaz/Tsui, Steven/Large, Stephen R. (2017): "Outcome after Heart Transplantation from Donation after Circulatory-Determined Death Donors." In: The Journal of Heart and Lung Transplantation 36/12, pp. 1311–1318.

Miller, Franklin G./Truog, Robert. (2008): "Rethinking the Ethics of Vital Organ Donations." In: Hastings Center Report 38/6, pp. 38–46.

Mollaret, P./Goulon, M (1959): "Le coma dépassé." In: Revista de Neurología 101, pp 3–15.

Oniscu, G. C./Randle, L. V./Muiesan, A. P./Butler, J./Currie, I. S./Perera, M. T. P. R./ Forsythe, J. L./Watson, C. J. E. (2014): "In Situ Normothermic Regional Perfusion for Controlled Donation after Circulatory Death – the United Kingdom Experience." In: American Journal of Transplantation 14/12, pp. 2846–2854.

Potts, Michael (2007): "Truthfulness in Transplantation: Non-Heart-Beating Organ Donation. Commentary." In: Philosophy, Ethics, and Humanities in Medicine 24/2: 17. DOI: 10.1186/1747-5341-2-17

Powner, D. J./Ackerman, B. M./Grenvik, A. (1996): "Medical Diagnosis of Death in Adults: Historical Contributions to Current Controversies." In: Lancet 348/9036, pp. 1219–1223.

President's Commission for the Study of Ethical Problems in Medicine and Biomedical and Behavioral Research (1981): Defining Death: a Report on the Medical, Legal and Ethical Issues in the Determination of Death. Washington.

Rady, Mohamed Y./Verheijde, Joseph L. (2013): "No-Touch Time in Donors after Cardiac Death [Nonheart-Beating Organ Donation]." Current Opinion in Organ Transplantation 18/2, pp. 140–147.

Robertson, John (1999): "The Dead Donor Rule." In: Hastings Center Report 29/6, pp. 6–14.

Rodriguez-Arias, David (2017): "Together and Scrambled. Brain Death was Conceived in Order to Facilitate Organ Donation." In: Dilemata 23, pp. 57–87.

Rojas-Peña, Alvaro/Sall, Lauren E./Gravel, Mark T./Cooley, Elaine G./Pelletier, Shawn J./Bartlett, Robert H./Punchal, Jeffrey D. (2014): "Donation after Circulatory Determination of Death: the University of Michigan Experience with Extracorporeal Support." In: Transplantation 98/3, pp. 328–334.

Sakamoto, Tetsuya/Morimura, Naoto/Ken Nagao, Yasufumi/Asai, Hiroyuki/Yokota, Satoshi/ Nara, Mamoru/Hase, Yoshio/Tahara, Takahiro/Atsumi, SAVE-J Study Group (2014): "Extracorporeal Cardiopulmonary Resuscitation versus Conventional Cardiopulmonary Resuscitation in Adults with Out-of-Hospital Cardiac Arrest: a Prospective Observational study." In: Resuscitation 85/6, pp. 762–768.

Shemie, Sam D./Baker, Andrew J./Knoll, Greg/Wall, William/Rocker, Graeme/Howes, Daniel/Davidson, Janet/Pagliarello, Joe/Chambers-Evans, Jane/Cockfield, Sandra/ Farrell, Catherine/Glannon, Walter/Gourlay, William/Grant, David/Langevin, Stéphan/Wheelock, Brian/Young, Kimberly/Dossetor, John (2006): "National Recommendations for Donation after Cardiocirculatory Death in Canada: Donation after Cardiocirculatory Death in Canada." In: Canadian Medical Association Journal 175/8, pp. S1–S24.

Smail, Hassiba/Garcia-Saez, Diana/Stock, Ulrich/Ahmed-Hassan, Hesham/Bowles, Christopher/Zych, Barlomiej/Mohite, Prashant N./Maunz, Olaf/Simon, Andre R. (2018): "Direct Heart Procurement after Donation after Circulatory Death with Ex Situ Reperfusion." In: Annals of Thoracic Surgery 106/4, pp. e211–214.

Stub, Dion/Bernard, Stephen/Pellegrino, Vincent/Smith, Karen/Walker, Tony/Sheldrake, Jayne/Hockings, Lisen/Shaw, James/Duffy, Stephen J./Burrell, Aidan/Cameron, Peter/De Villiers Smit, David M Kaye (2015): "Refractory Cardiac Arrest Treated with Mechanical CPR, Hypothermia, ECMO and Early Reperfusion [the CHEER trial]." In: Resuscitation 86, pp. 88–94.

Summers, Dominic M./Watson, Christopher J. E./Pettigrew, Gavin J./Johnson, Rachel J./ Collett, David/ Neuberger, James M./Bradley, J. Andrew (2015): "Kidney Donation after Circulatory Death (DCD): State of the Art." In: Kidney International 88/2, pp. 241–249. Doi: 10.1038/ki.2015.88

Swiss Academy of Medical Sciences (2019): Ethical Guidelines on the Determination of Death in the Context of Organ Transplantation. Bern.

Swiss Federal Act on Transplantation of Organs, Tissues and Cells. 8th October 2004 (SR 810.21)

The law reform commission of Canada. Act, R.S.C. 1970, C. I-23: Section 28A – Criteria of Death

Uniform Determination of Death Act, 12 uniform laws annotated 589 (West 1993 and West suppl 1997)

Veatch, Robert M. (1993): "The Impending Collapse of the Whole-Brain Definition of Death." In: The Hastings Center Report 23/4, pp. 18–24.

Walsh, F. (2015): Europe's First Non-Beating Heart Transplant. BBC, 26th of March. Available at: http://www.bbc.com/news/health-32056350 (accessed June 28, 2020)

Wijdicks, Eelco F. M./Varelas, Panayiotis N./Gronseth, Gary S./Greer, David M./American Academy of Neurology (2010): "Evidence-Based Guideline Update: Determining Brain Death in Adults: Report of the Quality Standards Subcommittee of the American Academy of Neurology." In: Neurology 74/23, pp. 1911–1918.

7. Deciding about Living Organ Donation
Balancing Risk Management and Autonomy

Dominique E. Martin

1. Introduction

The maxim *primum non nocere* – first do no harm – is beloved by medical practitioners. It is also valued by the public, who must place their vulnerable bodies in the hands of physicians and surgeons, trusting that doing so will leave them at least no worse off, and hopefully, somewhat better. Nevertheless, it is the more nuanced interpretation of the principle of nonmaleficence that has guided medical practice. This principle adjures practitioners to avoid and prevent harm to patients, and to ensure that if some risk of harm related to a medical intervention is inevitable it will be proportionate to the expected benefits of the intervention. The use of potentially harmful medical therapies and procedures has historically been justified by the claim that unavoidable risks are necessary, in order to restore or enhance the health of a person who would likely be worse off in the absence of the intervention. Thus, more practical advice was offered, allegedly, by Hippocrates to physicians, "As to diseases, make a habit of two things – to help and not to harm." (Jonsen 2000: 2)

The principle of nonmaleficence accordingly entails a degree of caution, while permitting the experimentation and trial of innovations that have underpinned centuries of medical progress in the care of unwell or injured individuals. In 1954, this foundational norm of medical ethics was rocked by the first successful living donor kidney transplant (LDKT). (Mueller and Luyckx 2012: 1462) While the procedure posed risks for the transplant recipient, who otherwise faced an untimely death, it was the intervention in the living donor (LD) that established a paradigm shift in medical ethics: a fit young man underwent major surgery to remove a healthy organ for the purpose of improving his brother's health. Since that time, ongoing developments in living organ donation (henceforth "living donation") and transplantation have repeatedly challenged the established norms and frameworks of clinical ethics.

Ten years after the first successful LDKT, living kidney donation was still an infrequent and somewhat experimental procedure. At this time, Woodruff described necessary, but not perhaps sufficient, conditions for "volunteer kidney donation" (1964: 1458) to be ethically permissible. In essence he argued that the donation must be necessary; the intended transplant recipient must lack alternative treatment for their "gross and irreversible renal failure" (ibid.), that the donor must be healthy, such that they face little risk of harm from nephrectomy, and that the decision to donate must be voluntary and informed. Further, there must be reasonable certainty regarding the likely outcomes of individual procedures, in particular the probability of successful transplantation; "there must be no grounds for thinking that the chances of success are exceptionally poor in the case under discussion" (ibid.). These conditions reflect the ethical considerations that continue to guide living donation decision-making today, however the landscape in which they are applied has changed dramatically.

In this chapter, I explore a range of longstanding and emerging ethical considerations in directed living organ donation in the context of emerging clinical and scientific knowledge, changing clinical practices, and evolving norms.[1] I focus on the most common types of living donation, kidney and partial liver donation.[2] First, I consider the gradual change in attitudes towards the quality and proportionality of risks and benefits associated with living donation. I discuss the influence of emerging evidence and knowledge gaps relating to risks and benefits, and of the nature of prospective donor and recipient relationships on perceived ethical acceptability of donation. Second, I discuss ethical concerns about consent for donation with regards to decision-making capacity and voluntariness of prospective LDs. Third, I explore the issue of paternalism in donation decision-making, and tensions that arise between contemporary norms regarding respect for patient autonomy and the physician duty of nonmaleficence. In conclusion, I suggest that instead of considering the ethics of LDT as inherently challenging the norms of clinical ethics, we ought instead to consider what we have learned from the ethically complex relational context of LDTs, and how this understanding might be applied in the wider field of health care decision-making.

2.   Rethinking the Risks and Benefits of Living Donation

Overriding physicians' aversion to harming the healthy by surgically removing an organ was likely made possible by the fact there is an even more compelling professional intuition, namely that every effort must be made to save lives. When the likely benefits of donation include the sole opportunity to save the life of the intended transplant recipient, this heavily weights the scales of proportionality in favor of donation. For example, the imperative to save a life remains influential in the context of donations that may pose significant risks to donor health, such as liver donation which has

---

1   Broader ethical concerns regarding LD transplantation such as inequities in access to living donation and living donor transplants (LDTs), and inequities in the distribution of burdens of donation are explored only briefly in this Chapter. Factors that may influence decision-making about living donation are discussed primarily from the more individualistic perspective of clinical ethics. For example, financial status and gender of potential donors may contribute to systemic inequities in donation and transplantation and also represent important systemic socioeconomic inequities that are beyond the scope of this chapter. Instead such factors are considered with regards to their potential impact on the risks of donation. For instance, poverty may pose an additional risk to donor wellbeing if donation-related expenses are not covered. With regard to autonomy of donation decision-making, , a gender bias within some cultures may exert a coercive influence on female potential donors.

2   Living lung lobe donation is also possible, however this is uncommon except in Japan (Date 2017). Living donation of intestines and pancreas is also possible but rarely occurs (Barr et al. 2005). Living uterus donation will be explored in the context of Chapter 15 of this book.

a donor mortality as high as 1 in 200 (Dew et al 2017: 881). Furthermore, in countries where access to dialysis is limited or prohibitively costly for much of the population and deceased donation programs are virtually nonexistent, as is the case in most parts of Africa and Asia, LDKT remains a life-saving opportunity for those with end stage kidney disease (ESKD) who can afford transplantation (Liyanage et al. 2015; Reese et al. 2015: 2004). However, LDTs are now widely practiced in the absence of life-saving necessity.

Many people with ESKD now have access to alternative life sustaining interventions such as dialysis, if not deceased donor transplants, yet living kidney donation has increased over time. LDKTs represented approximately 40 per cent of all kidney transplants performed worldwide in 2016, with more than 36.000 LDKTs reported to the Global Observatory on Donation Transplantation (2018: 2). In the absence of immediate high stakes in the form of life-saving necessity, determining the balance of risks and benefits that will justify living donation requires careful consideration of a range of potential outcomes of donation decision-making. In particular, it requires consideration of the prospective donor's potential interests in donation in the context of their relationships. Individuals are socially embedded and make decisions about donation in the context of relationships with family, friends and broader social communities. They also have longstanding roles and responsibilities that are influenced by and often enacted through interpersonal relationships. Hence, individuals may have "other-regarding" interests in donation in addition to personal welfare interests that should be considered when estimating potential benefits and risks of donation and of non-donation (Williams 2018: 19; Reese et al. 2018).

2.1   Risks and Burdens

In the early days of LDKT, despite the fact that there were few alternative treatments for people with ESKD, concern for donor wellbeing and uncertainty regarding risks underpinned a cautious approach. However, over time, the number of LDTs increased dramatically. This growth was in part influenced by the widespread perception that living kidney donation was a minimal risk activity. Comparison of the physical risks of donation with those of dangerous employment or leisure activities was often used in arguments that financial incentives could be offered to donors without fear of harmful exploitation (Cherry 2000: 343). The introduction of laparoscopic nephrectomy in the mid 1990s led to a decrease in perioperative morbidity associated with kidney donation and hence the immediate risk of harm to kidney donors has diminished considerably (Kok et al. 2006). However, the commonly cited risks of perioperative mortality (1 in 3000) and perioperative complications (1 in 6 donors) are not necessarily reflective of risks in all populations (Lentine et al. 2016). Increasing acceptance of higher risk donors, such as older people with comorbidities and obese donors has led to higher rates of both short and long term complications of donation (ibid).

A more dramatic shift in the level of risk considered acceptable in living donation was evident in the emergence of living liver donation during the 1990s. Abecassis and colleagues reported an overall incidence of complications associated with liver donation in the United States of 40 per cent, and a "1% incidence of residual disability, liver failure or death" (2012: 1216). The absence of alternative treatment for patients with end stage liver failure means that receiving a transplant is often a time critical matter of life and death. Initially considered acceptable when required to save the life of a child (Singer et al. 1989), living liver donation is now widespread despite the rate of perioperative complications. In the South East Asian region, limited availability of deceased donors means that LDs now supply more than 90 per cent of liver transplants (Global Observatory on Donation Transplantation 2018: 12). The total liver transplants from LDs per annum is estimated at 6012, or 19.8 per cent of total liver transplants worldwide (ibid).

Despite greater acceptance of significant risks to LDs in some contexts, it is the magnitude of the donor risk that usually sets the limit of what may be ethically permitted in a prospective LDT case, rather than the magnitude of the benefit that the recipient may gain from transplantation. Duties of beneficence to those in need of transplantation are thus trumped by obligations of nonmaleficence to potential donors. Evidence suggests this is consistent with the attitudes of clinicians, in particular surgeons, who may struggle with the burdens of responsibility involved in facilitating a major intervention that may be perceived as harming the healthy for the sake of the sick (Tong et al. 2013).

Harm to the donor is thus not considered a justifiable trade-off in return for improvements to the health of the recipient *per se*; in contrast to the more utilitarian framework of public health ethics, the separateness of persons is not overlooked in LDT ethics. In keeping with the traditional approach to clinical ethics, protecting and promoting the individual donor's welfare and interests ("benefits") are considered the primary duties of clinicians *vis a vis* prospective donors. In calculating the proportionality of potential benefits and risks of living donation, the potential benefits of transplantation for the intended recipient are effectively considered only in so far as they may be instrumental in producing benefits for the donor. The nature of risks and benefits that may be considered pertinent when determining whether a proposed LDT is ethically justifiable has also changed over time, as well as the relative value accorded to particular risks and benefits. While the immediate physical risks to the donor remain a primary concern, and the potential to save a life through transplantation is often a key priority, the longer term risks to donors both physically and psychosocially have assumed a greater importance together with the potential long-term psychosocial benefits of enabling a transplant – whether life-saving or not.

Despite widespread emphasis on the need for confidence in the assessment of risks and benefits of donation, several gaps in knowledge of risks and benefits persist, in particular with regards to outcomes in donor populations resident outside North America and Europe (Reese et al. 2015), longer term (>1 year) outcomes for living liver donors (Dew et al. 2017), and psychosocial outcomes that may be of particular interest to donors (Hanson et al. 2018).

Increasing awareness of the longer term impact of uninephrectomy on the health of LDs has fostered a renewed wave of caution with regards to living kidney donation, particularly in the light of evidence indicating that donors are at a higher relative risk for renal failure (Maggiore et al. 2017). Risk stratification has revealed that some donors have a much higher risk than others (Lentine et al. 2016). Nephrologists and transplant surgeons commonly cite the risks of kidney donation as a primary concern, particularly when dealing with younger donors for whom risk evaluation is less certain (Tong et al. 2013; Steiner 2019).

Potential psychosocial burdens of living donation are also increasingly recognized as relevant considerations (Delmonico 2005; Barr et al. 2006), although there has been comparatively little research investigating the psychological and non-economic social impact of donation. Much of the research in this field has been conducted in America. Accordingly, there is little evidence-based guidance available to facilitate risk assessment of prospective donors in their local socioeconomic and cultural context, and psychosocial screening is neither standardized nor routinely performed even in high income countries (Anderson et al. 2007; Massey et al. 2018). Nevertheless, the results of American research provide valuable insights into ethical considerations of relevance around the world. For example, the impact of lost income experienced by American donors is likely to be exacerbated in the context of donors living in low income countries in which even the basic protections of social welfare available in the United States may be lacking.

LDs may suffer significant financial harms as a result of taking time off work to donate, and in some cases may be required to cover the costs of evaluation as a donor (Delmonico et al. 2015; Dew and Jacobs 2012; DiMartini et al. 2017). Their ability to access follow up care to protect against longer term health risks, particularly in the context of kidney donation, may be conditional upon their financial situation. Donors may also experience higher health insurance costs (Dew and Jacobs 2012; Dimartini et al 2017). In recent years efforts have been made to evaluate and address the financial risks of donation in several high income countries, including Australia, the United States, and several European countries, for example through governmental programs providing paid leave for donors and coverage of costs associated with donation (Hays et al. 2016).

Studies suggest that while donation generally has a positive psychosocial impact on donors, some donors may suffer from depression or anxiety, and donation may negatively impact on relationships with their recipient and/or family (Lentine et al. 2019; Timmerman et al. 2016). Concern for the psychosocial risks of donation has primarily focused on those of unrelated donors for whom guidelines have been developed and for whom psychosocial screening is routinely performed (Dew et al. 2007). This may reflect assumptions that such donors may be more likely to have a psychological disorder and perhaps the belief that the potential benefits of donation are diminished in the absence of a close relationship between donors and recipients, thus entailing greater concern to ensure that psychosocial risks are minimized.

2.2   Benefits and Interests

The multifaceted potential benefits of donation for the LD herself are now well recognized. These may include the emotional and psychological benefits of helping others such as improved self-esteem, as well as the positive impact of transplantation on a relationship and/or family by greatly improving an individual's health and/or preserving their life (Leventine et al. 2017, Schulz et al. 2009; Erim et al. 2007, Clemens et al. 2006). Although the immediate stakes of living kidney donation decision-making may be less compelling in so far as the ethical imperative to save a life is concerned, LKDTs may offer significant advantages for recipients (and hence indirectly to donors) compared with transplants from deceased donors or dialysis, particularly when considered in the longer term. The relative benefits of living compared with deceased donor kidney transplants may be somewhat overstated, as it is often those who are in better health and socioeconomically advantaged who are able to access a LDT and avoid time on dialysis that may undermine their health in the longer term (Schold et al. 2018). However compared with dialysis, LKDTs generally provide far better health and psychosocial outcomes for most people with ESKD. In addition to survival gains, quality of life is greater and costs of ongoing care are lower. LD liver transplants also presently offer health advantages for recipients when compared with deceased donor transplants (Montenovo et al. 2019). Improved health may enable recipients to assume roles within the family that are beneficial to the donor, for example by returning to work and/or being able to fulfill parenting duties and so on.

A key benefit of kidney or liver donation is also the avoidance of what may reasonably be assumed a significant harm to most prospective donors, namely the death of a loved one or their continued reliance on dialysis. Very little is known of the potential risks of declining a prospective LD candidate, although recent research suggests some declined donor candidates may suffer psychosocial harm (Jennings et al. 2013; Reese et al. 2018). It is conceivable that in some cases, the potential negative impact of missing the opportunity to preserve the life of a loved one may cause greater harm in the longer term than would have occurred if a higher risk donor had been permitted to proceed. Such risks may include guilt at failure to be approved, or anger or regret that they were denied the opportunity to donate (Allen et al. 2014; Jennings et al. 2013).

2.3   Risks and Benefits in the Context of Relationships

Many of the psychosocial risks and benefits described above are largely premised on the assumption of a close relationship between the LD and the transplant recipient. Early donors were usually identical twins, and then parents of children, due to the need for close genetic matching and the belief that for parents or twins the loss of a child or twin was a sufficiently great harm to balance the potential risks of donation. Spouses were soon accepted as donors, and over time, in addition to biologically related donors and spousal donors, acceptance of so-called "emotionally related" donation has emerged which includes more distant familial relationships, friends and even social acquaintances in some transplant programs (Spital 2000). The depth and nature of relationships between prospective donors and recipients have implications for the assessment of risks and benefits as well as the voluntariness of donation. Closer relationships may offer more benefits to the donor as the positive impact of transplantation on recipient health can improve the donor's own life and family wellbeing. The intimacy of a loving relationship between donor and recipient also means the harm avoided when transplantation prevents loss of life is proportionately greater (Van Pilsum Rasmussen et al. 2017). Closer relationships may also reduce concerns that the motivation for donation may be due to problematic factors such as a coercive influence, or desire for personal fame or emotional reward from the recipient as it is often discussed in unspecified living organ donation (see chapter 8 in this book). On the other hand, closer relationships may also be coercive with multiple ties binding the donor to a potential recipient such that they feel they have no option but to donate to preserve the breadwinner of a family or under pressure from other relatives (Wöhlke 2017).

3.   Consent for Donation Decision-Making

Considerable attention has been given to concerns regarding the validity of consent to become a LD. Several factors may be considered to undermine the quality of prospective donor decision-making and/or the validity of their consent, which requires the donor to be competent to make a decision, sufficiently informed, and able to make a voluntary decision free of coercion, deception or manipulation. As noted above, the limited availability of robust evidence regarding longer term risks and benefits of donation – as well as those associated with a decision not to donate – may undermine the ability of prospective donors to make a fully informed decision. Living kidney donation might ideally be deferred, for example, until prospective donors are middle aged, to enable a more accurate assessment of their lifetime risk of renal disease (Steiner 2019). Nevertheless, ethical concerns about consent for donation predominantly focus on questions of competency and voluntariness.

3.1   Competency to Consent

Arguably, many prospective donors might lack the ability to make a fully rational and considered decision about donation. Faced with a loved one's need for transplantation, many donors have reported making an impulsive decision to donate prior to receipt and processing of relevant information about donation (Papachristou et al. 2010). Concerns that internal or self-imposed pressures to donate are unduly influencing decision-making or undermining the quality of decision-making are in part addressed by strategies such as rigorous psychosocial evaluation, use of 'cooling off' periods for decision-making and of LD advocates (ibid.; Gordon et al. 2015).

Potential donors who may have limited decision-making capacity – as the term generally applies to medical decision-making – include children or adolescents below the legal age of majority and individuals with cognitive impairments or mental illness that may temporarily or permanently undermine their ability to weigh the relevant information and form an enduring decision about donation in accordance with their own values, beliefs and preferences. In some countries, legal minors or adults lacking legal competency to make their own decisions are excluded from living donation programs (Thys et al. 2013; Thys et al. 2016). In others, they may be permitted to donate if judged competent to consent to donation, or if they assent to a donation that has been authorised by their legal guardian (ibid). In its *Guiding Principles on Human Cell, Tissue and Organ Transplantation*, the World Health Organization (WHO) notes that where donation by a legally incompetent person is legally permitted, "Specific measures should be in place to protect" the donor (Sixty-Third World Health Assembly 2010: 8). The WHO suggests that such donations should only occur in exceptional circumstances (ibid.: 9).

3.2   Voluntariness in the Context of Donor Relationships

Concerns relating to the decision-making capacity of a prospective donor are often intertwined with concerns regarding voluntariness; understandably, those who may lack decision-making capacity are often at the greatest risk of exploitation or coercion (Van Assche et al. 2014). Biller-Andorno (2011) notes that a donor's autonomy may be under threat if there is coercion, or pressure intentionally exerted by others to compel a donation decision, but also by virtue of the fact that autonomy and decision-making are inherently relational. Family members or close friends, for example, may often influence and inform important decisions that individuals make, particularly when they have a shared interest in the decision being made (Verkerk et al. 2015) as is the case in living donation (Wöhlke 2017). In the context of related donation, concerns regarding potential conflicts of interest in decision-making may be difficult to address without isolating the prospective donor from the customary supports they would have when making important decisions in their lives. Baylis et al. observe that "rather than pretending that individuals can make decisions 'free' of outside influences, relational autonomy encourages us to pay close attention to the types of forces that may shape an individual's decisions" (2008: 202). Thus Biller-Andorno (2011) argues that understanding the many factors that may undermine donor autonomy and assessing these effectively during evaluation of prospective donors is essential, as is implementation of safeguards to protect the donor from undue influence and to ensure their freedom to refuse donation. Accordingly, independent donor advocates are recommended in the United States to help ensure that donors are making a competent and voluntary decision (Hays et al. 2015). Other strategies that may be implemented to protect the autonomy of prospective donors include provision of a medical "alibi" that may be used as a reason for donation to be declined instead of disclosing the prospective donor's refusal to donate (Thiessen et al. 2015b).

In some countries, concerns about external coercion of prospective donors rather than internal factors or impaired decision-making capacity may predominate. Familial or sociocultural hierarchies and values in some communities may directly or indirectly exert pressure on individuals to donate. For example, women may be expected to donate for the benefit of spouses, children or male siblings because of their perceived role as a caregiver or lower instrumental value to the family (Scheper-Hughes 2007). Gender disparities in rates of living kidney donation and transplantation are well described, although higher rates of female donation and lower rates of LKDTs in females in some countries are not wholly attributable to gender norms or bias influencing consent or even donor selection (Carrero et al 2018; Gill et al 2018). In other contexts, concerns about the voluntariness of donation may focus on risk factors for human trafficking, particularly in countries with large economically vulnerable populations such as India or Pakistan (see chapter 11). The socioeconomic status of prospective donors, and the comparative status of their intended recipient, for example, may indicate potentially coercive relationships, irrespective of potential familial or social relationships. Prospective donors and recipients who travel abroad for transplantation despite the existence of programs in their own country may also raise suspicion of human trafficking for the purpose of organ removal (Domínguez-Gil et al. 2018).

4.   Paternalism

While greater efforts to detect and prevent coercion and to optimize the quality of informed and voluntary decision-making by prospective donors are needed, concerns regarding the autonomy of donation decision-making are likely to persist. To some extent, these concerns reflect the habitual challenges of decision-making in health care more generally; often patients are required to select from a limited range of imperfect options for treatment of serious conditions, each with risks and potential benefits that may be difficult to assess. The ethical stakes of donation decision-making however, may be considered greater, given the greater potential for conflicts of interest that may influence decision-making and the fundamental problem that any donation imposes some degree of physical risk to the donor that cannot be offset by the usual justification that intervention of some kind may be therapeutically necessary, as is the case for an ordinary patient. Unsurprisingly, questions regarding the autonomy of a prospective donor's decision may therefore be used to justify a degree of paternalism that may be considered unacceptable in the normal setting of health care decision-making.

4.1   Acceptance of Risk is a Right of Competent Persons in Health Care

Respect for autonomy has widely assumed a primary position in ethical decision-making in clinical practice. When an adult is ill or injured, if she is deemed competent to make informed decisions for herself, then she is permitted to refuse even life-saving treatment, and to choose between available options in accordance with her own values, beliefs and preferences. When more than one treatment option is available, the competent patient herself is usually considered best placed to evaluate the potential risks and benefits in the context of their own life, particularly as these usually entail qualitative judgements and personal preferences regarding the assumption of risk. It is the place of health professionals to support such decision-making, and to identify the options that should be considered. For example, interventions that are deemed to have no evidence base for success in a particular case may be considered futile and are hence not offered – particularly if they have associated risks or costs. Although some procedures may offer uncertain benefits, have a relatively low probability of success, and/or carry significant risks, these are often still presented as options, particularly in the absence of alternatives with a better risk-benefit profile or when they offer a chance – however small - of restoring vital functions or prolonging life. Thus, people may undergo experimental cancer treatments or risky surgical procedures in life or death situations.

4.2   Clinician Involvement in the Setting of Risk Thresholds for Donation

While clinicians play a leading role in determining the range of therapeutic options that may reasonably be offered to a patient, there appears to be greater scope for clinicians to apply their own value judgements regarding proportionality of risks and benefits for a prospective LD. This is significant given research indicating that transplant professionals are more risk averse that prospective LDs (Young et al. 2008). Spital (2004: 107) observes that, "it is the potential donor herself who is best able to determine if the expected benefits are worth the risks. On the other hand, physicians must make their own assessments, and they should never be forced to perform a procedure that they think will do more harm than good."

Thus, whereas patients are routinely permitted to undergo invasive procedures with high risk of short and/or long term harms in the hope of achieving a therapeutic benefit, prospective donors may be declined with an equivalent or more favorable risk-benefit profile simply because the clinical benefit will accrue to the transplant recipient rather than the donor herself.

In defining the limits of acceptable risk for living donation, there is general consensus that donation should not be likely to cause the death of the donor. Further, the anticipated gain in health for the recipient should be greater than the anticipated loss of health for the donor. (Authors for the live organ donor consensus group 2000: 2924)

Despite such principles, and frequent references to the importance of benefits for the donor outweighing the risks, there is considerable scope for disagreement regarding the proportionality of risks and benefits that would fall within the "reasonable" range considered acceptable by clinicians. Donors who lack life time health insurance are frequently accepted in some countries, such as the Philippines or India, despite the risk they may be unable to access long term follow up care in the event of complications, whereas such coverage is a necessary condition for donation in others. In South Korea, adolescents are not infrequently accepted as living liver donors from the age of 16 (if donating to a parent), (Hwang et al 2006) whereas this is considered unacceptable in European countries (Thys et al. 2016). There is evidence of considerable variation in practice across transplant programs, even within countries, with regards to criteria used to evaluate donor risk and determine when to exclude prospective donors (Gabolde et al. 2001; Rodrigue et al. 2007; Thiessen et al. 2015a).

Variation in guidelines and practice around the world and within countries is to be expected, given risks and potential benefits of living donation will be influenced not only by factors specific to particular donor and recipient populations but also by factors specific to the local health care context. The level of experience and expertise within specific transplant programs may, for example, influence the risk of surgical complications for particular procedures. Nevertheless, clinician assessments of proportionality in risks and benefits may be subject to cognitive biases, personal values and beliefs, and/or conflicts of interest that may influence their acceptance or refusal of potential donors. Financial interests might, for example encourage the acceptance of higher risk donors in order to enable lucrative transplants to be performed, or alternatively encourage risk avoidance for fear of impairing quality indicators associated with clinician or institutional reputations.

4.3   Balancing Patient Autonomy and Moral Agency of Transplant Professionals

Thiessen and colleagues (2015a: 2315) advocate a donor-centered approach to risk assessment that would give greater weight to prospective donor values and preferences when dealing with "discretionary donors", that is, "medically complex" donors with a slightly higher level of risk who nevertheless wish to proceed with donation despite potential disagreement regarding the acceptability of risk from clinicians. While helpful in resolving some potential conflicts between respect for donor autonomy and the clinician's duty of nonmaleficence, this approach is unlikely to resolve all disagreements between prospective donors and clinicians regarding acceptable risk thresholds or proportionality of risks and benefits. In such cases, several authors have defended the clinician's right to decline a donor. (Authors for the live organ donor consensus group 2000: 2925) Ross and Thistlethwaite argue that to proceed otherwise would be unethical: "the members of the transplant team are moral agents who must concur that the risks and benefit: risk to both parties individually and jointly is reasonable or they should refuse to proceed with performing the living donor surgery" (2018: 844).

In such cases, however, how might the risks of undue paternalism or bias in clinical risk assessment for prospective donors – and their intended transplant recipients – be managed? Paternalistic decision-making is most likely to affect populations that already suffer from exclusion and poorer health outcomes in the setting of donation and transplantation. For example, African Americans and Indigenous prospective donors are more likely to have a higher risk profile, and their intended recipients are also more likely to miss out on deceased donor transplants (Reese et al. 2015). Reluctance to accept donors from these populations may have a significant impact on equity in transplantation.

One partial solution is to promote transparency in clinical decision-making and routine reporting of outcomes of prospective donor assessment, to enable evaluation of transplant center decision-making. Alternatively, one might treat such cases as a form of conscientious objection by health professionals. The right of conscientious objection allows clinicians to refuse to provide a clinical intervention that is legal and would be considered clinically appropriate by professional peers, on the grounds that providing such an intervention would violate the clinician's personal moral values and beliefs. At least some decisions to decline a prospective donor on the grounds that the expected risks of donation are disproportionate should be recognized as reflecting a clinician's personal judgment that to proceed with donation would be ethically unjustified, whereas another clinician may find the risk-benefit ratio within the range of reasonable options to be chosen at the discretion of prospective donors.

The controversial right to conscientious objection is often deemed conditional, in order to minimize inequities in access to care for patients and to prevent serious harm to patients. For example the right may not be exercised in an emergency setting when refusal of treatment would endanger the patient, and it may be associated with an obligation to inform the patient of alternative opportunities to receive the intervention in question, if not refer the patient to a clinician willing to provide the intervention. If disagreements regarding acceptable risk thresholds and proportionality of risks and benefits are regarded as a matter of conflicting ethical values rather than tension between the autonomy of prospective donors and that of clinicians, this may facilitate a more constructive response in the event of some decisions to decline prospective donors. Clinicians or transplant centers might be encouraged to refer donors to alternative care providers for a new assessment, for example, rather than treating an assessment as a conclusive judgment regarding donor suitability.

5.   Conclusion

The perennial issues of proportionality in risks and benefits of donation and limits of prospective donor autonomy are regularly invigorated by the emergence of novel procedures and policies, and experimentation by clinicians willing to test the boundaries of accepted practice. Various populations of 'marginal risk' donors and recipients, such as those of older age (see chapter 12 in this book), have gradually become established in some settings. Most recently, an HIV-positive woman donated part of her liver to her daughter, in a transplant justified on the grounds of life-saving necessity given that the child had no prospect of receiving a suitable organ from a deceased donor or from an HIV-negative LD (Botha et al. 2018). Specific types and novel forms of directed living donation, such as paired kidney exchanges, transorgan paired exchanges and advanced donation programs have also presented new ethical dilemmas, or significant variations on longstanding ethical concerns (Kranenburg et al. 2004; Fortin 2013; Samstein et al. 2018; Martin/Danovitch 2017).

The field of living organ donation situates familiar ethical dilemmas of clinical practice, namely tensions between physician duties of beneficence and nonmaleficence and respect for patient autonomy, in a particularly challenging context. The physician customarily has the comfort of therapeutic necessity when performing a potentially harmful procedure on a patient. In living donation, exposing the healthy donor to harm requires a significant shift in the framing and evaluation of risks and benefits of clinical interventions. In this context, the duty of beneficence is perhaps best understood not as an obligation to address a deficit in the patient-donor's health status, but rather to help them to address an actual or foreseeable deficit in their broader well-being, or simply to enhance their wellbeing by enabling them to fulfil a personal goal of donation. This approach is not, in theory, dissimilar from ethical decision-making in clinical practice in the non-transplant context. Determining whether an intervention is in the best interests of a patient requires careful attention not only to their physical or psychological health but also to their complex and varied life goals, values and preferences which are shaped by interpersonal relationships, experiences and broader interests.

As more information emerges regarding LD risks and potential benefits in particular populations and contexts, and new practices are introduced that challenge the values we place on specific types of risks and benefits and disrupt traditional frameworks for decision-making and consent, ethical analysis of LDT should provide ongoing opportunities for reflection on the ethical standards we apply in clinical practice more generally. As we question, for example, the limits of physician paternalism in LDT, we should be prompted to explore potential paternalism in other contexts. Is it possible that similar values and concerns influence – explicitly or not – the range of therapeutic options deemed 'reasonable' for patients in other contexts? Research investigating living organ donation sheds invaluable light on the relational nature of individual autonomy and of benefits and harms, and on the way that broader socioeconomic and cultural factors may shape – both positively and negatively - opportunities for health care and health outcomes. Rather than challenging the ethical values and principles that are espoused in health care policy and practice, LDTs should challenge us to think critically about the way these values and principles are applied in practice across our health care systems.

References

Abecassis, Michael M./Fisher, Robert A./Olthoff, Kim M./Freise, Chris E./Rodrigo, Del R./ Samstein, Benjamin/Kam, Igal/Merion, Robert M./A2ALL Study Group (2012): "Complications of Living Donor Hepatic Lobectomy – a comprehensive report." In: American Journal of Transplantation 12/5, pp. 1208–1217.

Allen, Matthew B./Abt, Peter L/Reese, Peter P. (2014): "What are the Harms of Refusing to Allow Living Kidney Donation? An Expanded View of Risks and Benefits." In: American Journal of Transplantation 14/3, pp. 531–537.

Anderson, Kate/Cass, Alan/Cunningham, Joan/Snelling, Paul/Devitt, Jeannie/Preece, Cilla (2007): "The Use of Psychosocial Criteria in Australian Patient Selection Guidelines for Kidney Transplantation." In: Social Science & Medicine 64/10, pp. 2107–2114.

Authors for the Live Organ Donor Consensus Group (2000): "Consensus Statement on the Live Organ Donor." In: Journal of the American Medical Association 284, pp. 2919–2926.

Barr, Mark L./Belghiti, Jacques/Villamil, Federico G./Pomfret, Elizabeth A./Sutherland, David S./Gruessner, Rainer W./Langnas, Alan N./Delmonico, Francis L. (2006): "A Report of the Vancouver Forum on the Care of the Live Organ Donor: Lung, Liver, Pancreas, and Intestine Data and Medical Guidelines. " In: Transplantation 81/10, pp. 1373–1385.

Baylis, Francoise/Kenny, Nuala P./Sherwin, Susan (2008): "A Relational Account of Public Health Ethics." In: Public Health Ethics 1/3, pp. 196–209.

Biller-Andorno, Nikola. (2011): "Voluntariness in Living-Related Organ Donation." In: Transplantation 92/6, pp. 617–619.

Botha, Jean/Conradie, Francesca/Etheredge, Harriet/Fabian, June/Duncan, Mary/Mazanderani, Ahmad Haeri/Paximadis, Maria/Maher, Heather/Britz, Russell/Loveland, Jerome/Strobele, Bernd/Rambarran, Sharan/Mahomed, Adam/Terblanche, Alta/Beretta, Marisa/Brannigan, Liam/Pienaar, Michael/Archibald-Durham, Lindsay/Lang, Allison/ Tiemessen, Caroline T. (2018): "Living Donor Liver Transplant from an HIV-positive Mother to her HIV-negative Child: Opening up New Therapeutic Options." In: AIDS 32/16, pp. F13–F19.

Carrero, Juan Jesu/Hecking, Manfred/Chesnaye, Nicholas C./Jager, Kitty J. (2018): "Sex and Gender Disparities in the Epidemiology and Outcomes of Chronic Kidney Disease." In: Nature Reviews Nephrology 14/3, pp. 151–164

Cherry, Mark J. (2000): "Is a Market in Human Organs Necessarily Exploitative." In: Public Affairs Quarterly 14/4, pp. 337–360.

Clemens, Kristin K./Thiessen-Philbrook, Heather/Parikh, Chirag R./Yang, Robert C./Karley, Mary Lou/Boudville, Neil/Ramesh Prasad, G. V./Garg, Amit X./Donor Nephrectomy Outcomes Research (DONOR) Network (2006): "Psychosocial Health of Living Kidney Donors: a Systematic Review." In: American Journal of Transplantation 6/12, pp. 2965–2977.

Date, Hiroshi (2017): "Living-Related Lung Transplantation." In: Journal of Thoracic Disease 9/9, pp. 3362–3371.

Delmonico, Francis L. (2005): "A Report of the Amsterdam Forum on the Care of the Live Kidney Donor: Data and Medical Guidelines." In: Transplantation 79/6, pp. S53–66.

Delmonico, Francis L./Martin, Dominique E./Domínguez-Gil, Beatriz/Muller, Elmi/Jha, Vivek/Levin, Adeera/Danovitch, Gabriel M./Capron, Alexander M (2015): "Living and Deceased Organ Donation Should be Financially Neutral Acts." In: American Journal of Transplantation 15/5, pp. 1187–1191.

Delmonico, Francis L. Harmon, William E. (2002): "The Use of a Minor as a Live Kidney Donor." In: American Journal of Transplantation 2/4, pp. 333–336.

Dew, Mary Amanda/Jacobs, Cheryl L./Jowsey, Sheila G./Hanto, Ruthanne/Miller, Charles/ Delmonico, Francis L. (2007): "Guidelines for the Psychosocial Evaluation of Living Unrelated Kidney Donors in the United States." In: American Journal of Transplantation 7/5, pp. 1047–1054.

Dew, Mary Amanda/Jacobs, Cheryl L. (2012): "Psychosocial and Socioeconomic Issues Facing the Living Kidney Donor." In: Advances in Chronic Kidney Disease 19/4, pp. 237–243.

Dew, Mary Amanda/Butt, Zeeshan/Humar, Abhinav/DiMartini, Andrea F. (2017): "Long-Term Medical and Psychosocial Outcomes in Living Liver Donors." In: American Journal of Transplantation 17/4, pp. 880–892.

DiMartini, Andrea/Dew, Mary Amanda/Liu, Qian/Simpson, Mary Ann/Ladner, Daniela P./ Smith, Abigail R./Zee, Jarcy/Abbey, Susan/Gillespie, Brenda W./Weinrieb, Robert/Mandell, Mercedes S./Fisher, Robert A./Edmond, Jean C./Freise, Chris E./ Sherker, Averell H./Butt, Zeeshan (2017): "Social and Financial Outcomes of Living Liver Donation: A Prospective Investigation Within the Adult-to-Adult Living Donor Liver Transplantation Cohort Study 2 (A2 ALL-2)." In: American Journal of Transplantation 17/4, pp. 1081–1096.

Domínguez-Gil, Beatriz/Danovitch, Gabriel/Martin, Dominique E./López-Fraga, Marta/Van Assche, Kristof/Morris, Michele L./Lavee, Jacob (2018): "Management of Patients Who Receive an Organ Transplant Abroad and Return Home for Follow-Up Care: Recommendations from the Declaration of Istanbul Custodian Group." In: Transplantation 102/1, pp. e2–e9.

Erim, Yesim/Beckmann, Mingo/Kroencke, Sylvia/Valentin-Gamazo, Camino/Malago, Massimo/Broering, Dieter/Rogiers, Xavier/Frilling, Andrea/Broelsch, Christoph E./Schulz, Karl-Heinz (2007): "Psychological Strain in Urgent Indications for Living Donor Liver Transplantation." In: Liver transplantation 13/6, pp. 886–895.

Fortin, Marie Chantal (2013): "Is it Ethical to Invite Compatible Pairs to Participate in Exchange Programmes?" In: Journal of Medical Ethics 39/12, pp. 743–747.

Gabolde, Martine/Hervé, Christian/Moulin, Anne-Marie (2001): "Evaluation, Selection, and Follow-Up of Live Kidney Donors: a Review of Current Practice in French Renal Transplant Centres." In: Nephrology Dialysis Transplantation 16/10, pp. 2048–2052.

Gill, Jagbir/Joffres, Yayuk/Rose, Caren/Lesage, Julie/Landsberg, David/Kadatz, Matthew/ Gill, John (2018): "The Change in Living Kidney Donation in Women and Men in the United States (2005–2015): a Population-Based Analysis." In: Journal of the American Society of Nephrology 29/4, pp. 1301–1308.

Global Observatory on Donation and Transplantation (2018): "Organ Donation and Transplantation activities 2016." Available at: http://www.transplant-observatory. org/download/2016-activity-data-report/ (accessed June 1, 2019)

Gordon, Elisa J./Rodde, Jillian/Skaro, Anton/Baker, Talia (2015): "Informed Consent for Live Liver Donors: a Qualitative, Prospective Study." In: Journal of Hepatology 63/4, pp. 838–847.

Hanson, Camilla S./Chapman, Jeremy R./Gill, John S./Kanellis, John/Wong, Germaine/Craig, Jonathan C./Teixeira-Pinto, Armando/Chadban, Steve J./Garg, Amit X./ Ralph, Angelique F./Pinter, Jule/Lewis, Joshua R./Tong, Allison (2018): "Identifying Outcomes that are Important to Living Kidney Donors: A Nominal Group Technique Study." In: Clinical Journal of the American Society of Nephrology 13/6, pp. 916–926.

Hays, Rebecca E./LaPointe Rudow, Diane/Dew, Mary Amanda/Taler, S. J./Spicer, H./Mandelbrot, Didier (2015): "The Independent Living Donor Advocate: a Guidance Document from the American Society of Transplantation's Living Donor Community of Practice (AST LDCOP)." In: American Journal of Transplantation 15/2, pp. 518–525.

Hays, Rebecca/Rodrigue, James R./Cohen, David/Danovitch, Gabriel/Matas, Arthur/Schold, Jesse/LaPointe Rudow, Diane (2016): "Financial Neutrality for Living Organ Donors: Reasoning, Rationale, Definitions, and Implementation Strategies." In: American Journal of Transplantation 16/7, pp. 1973–1981.

Hwang, Shin/Lee, Sung-Gyu/Lee, Young-Joo/Sung, Kyu-Bo/Park, Kwang-Min/Kim, Ki-Hun/Ahn, Chul-Soo/Moon, Deok Bog/Hwang, Gyu Sam/Kim, Kyung Mo/Ha, Tae Yong/ Kim, Dong-Sik/Jung, Jae Pil/Song, Gi Won (2006): "Lessons Learned from 1,000 Living Donor Liver Transplantations in a Single Center: how to Make Living Donations Safe." In: Liver Transplantation 12/6, pp. 920–927.

Jennings, Tiane/Grauer, Danielle/LaPointe Rudow, Dianne (2013): "The Role of the Independent Donor Advocacy Team in the Case of a Declined Living Donor Candidate." In: Progress in Transplantation 23/2, pp. 132–136.

Jonsen, Albert R. (2000): A Short History of Medical Ethics, New York: Oxford University Press.

Kok, Niels F. M./Lind, May Y./Hansson, Birgitta M. E./Pilzecker, Desiree/RAM Mertens zur Borg, Ingrid/Knipscheer, Ben C./Hazebroek, Eric J./Dooper, Ine M./Weimar, Willem/Hop, Wi C. J./Adang, Eddy M. M./van der Wilt, Gert J./Bonjer, Hendrik J./van der Vliet, Jordanus A./IJzermans, Jan N.M. (2006): "Comparison of Laparoscopic and Mini Incision Open Donor Nephrectomy: Single Blind, Randomised Controlled Clinical Trial." In: British Medical Journal 333/7561, pp. 221. DOI: 10.1136/bmj.38886.618947.7C

Kranenburg, Leonieke W./Visak, Tatjana/Weimar, Willem/Zuidema, Willij/de Klerk, Marry/ Hilhorst, Medard/Passchier, Jan/IJzermans, Jan N. M./Busschbach, Jan J. V. (2004): "Starting a Crossover Kidney Transplantation Program in the Netherlands: Ethical and Psychological Considerations." In: Transplantation 78/2, pp. 194–197.

Lentine, Krista L./Lam, Ngan N./Axelrod, David/Schnitzler, Mark A./Garg, Amit X./Xiao, Huiling/Dzebisashvili, Nino/Schold, Jesse D./Brennan, Daniel C./Randall, Henry/King, Elizabeth A./Segev, Dorry L. (2016): "Perioperative Complications after Living Kidney Donation: a National Study." In: American Journal of Transplantation 16/6, pp. 1848–1857.

Lentine, Krista L/Lam, Ngan N./Segev, Dorry L. (2019): "Risks of Living Kidney Donation: Current State of Knowledge on Outcomes Important to Donors." In: Clinical Journal of the American Society of Nephrology 14/4, pp. 597–608.

Liyanage, Thaminda/Ninomiya, Toshiharu/Jha, Vivekanand/Neal, Bruce/Patrice, Halle Marie/Okpechi, Ikechi/Zhao, Ming-hui/Lv, Jicheng/Garg, Amit X./Knight, John/Rodgers, Anthony/Gallagher, Martin/Kotwal, Sradha/Cass, Alan/Perkovic, Vlado (2015): "Worldwide Access to Treatment for End-Stage Kidney Disease: a Systematic Review." In: The Lancet 385/9981, pp. 1975–1982.

Maggiore, Umberto/Budde, Klemens/Heemann, Uwe/Hilbrands, Luuk/Oberbauer, Rainer/ Oniscu, Gabriel C./Pascual, Julio/Schwartz Sorensen, Soren/Viklicky, Ondrej/Abramowicz, Daniel (2017): "Long-Term Risks of Kidney Living Donation:

Review and Position Paper by the ERA-EDTA DESCARTES working group." In: Nephrology Dialysis Transplantation 32/2, pp. 216–223.

Martin, Dominique E./Danovitch, Gabriel M. (2017): "Banking on Living Kidney Donors – a New Way to Facilitate Donation without Compromising on Ethical Values." In: Journal of Medicine and Philosophy 42/5 pp. 537–558.

Massey, Emma K./Timmerman, Lotte/Ismail, Sohal Y./Duerinckx, Nathalie/Lopes, Alice/ Maple, Hannah/Mega, Inês/Papachristou, Christina/Dobbels, Fabienne/ ELPAT Psychosocial Care for Living Donors and Recipients Working Group (2018): "The ELPAT Living Organ Donor Psychosocial Assessment Tool (EPAT): from 'What' to 'How' of Psychosocial Screening – a Pilot Study." In: Transplant International 31/1, pp. 56–70.

Montenovo, Martin I./Bambha, Kiran/Reyes, Jorge/Dick, Andre/Perkins, James/ Healey, Patrick (2019): "Living Liver Donation Improves Patient and Graft Survival in the Pediatric Population." In: Pediatric Transplantation 23/1, e13318. DOI: 10.1111/petr.13318

Mueller, Thomas F./Luyckx, Valerie A. (2012): "The Natural History of Residual Renal Function in Transplant Donors." In: Journal of the American Society of Nephrology 23/9, pp. 1462–1466.

Murray, Joseph E./Hartwell Harrison, J. (1963): "Surgical Management of Fifty Patients with Kidney Transplants Including Eighteen Pairs of Twins." In: American Journal of Surgery 105/2, pp. 205–218.

Papachristou, Christina/Marc, Walter/Frommer, Jeorg/Klapp, Burghard F. (2010): "Decision-Making and Risk-Assessment in Living Liver Donation: how Informed is the Informed Consent of Donors? A Qualitative Study." In: Psychosomatics, 51/4, pp. 312–319.

Reese, Peter P./Boudville, Neil/Garg, Amit X. (2015): "Living Kidney Donation: Outcomes, Ethics, and Uncertainty." In: The Lancet 385/9981, pp. 2003–2013.

Reese, Peter P./Allen, Matthew B./Carney, Caroline/Leidy, Daniel/Levsky, Simona/ Pendse, Ruchita/Mussell, Adam S./Bermudez, Francisca/Keddem, Shimrit/Thiessen, Carrie/Rodrigue, James R./Emanuel, Ezekiel J. (2018): "Outcomes for individuals turned down for living kidney donation." In: Clinical transplantation 32/12, e13408.

Rodrigue, James R./Pavlakis, Martha/Danovitch, Gabriel M./Johnson, S. R./Karp, S. J./ Khwaja, K./Hanto, Douglas W./Mandelbrot, Didier A. (2007): "Evaluating Living Kidney Donors: Relationship Types, Psychosocial Criteria, and Consent Processes at US transplant Programs." In: American Journal of Transplantation 7/10, pp. 2326–2332.

Ross, Lainie F./Thistlethwaite, J. Richard (2018): "Developing an Ethics Framework for Living Donor Transplantation." In: Journal of Medical Ethics 44/12, pp. 843–850.

Samstein, Benjamin/de Melo-Martin, Inmaculada/Kapur, Sandip/Ratner, Lloyd/ Emond, Jean (2018): "A Liver for a Kidney: Ethics of Trans-Organ Paired Exchange." In: American Journal of Transplantation 18/5, pp. 1077–1082.

Scheper-Hughes, Nancy (2007): "The Tyranny of the Gift: Sacrificial Violence in Living Donor Transplants." In: American Journal of Transplantation 7/3, pp. 507–511.

Schold, Jesse D./Poggio, Emilio D./Augustine, Joshua J. (2018): "Gathering Clues to Explain the Stagnation in Living Donor Kidney Transplantation in the United States." In: American Journal of Kidney Disease 71/5, pp. 608–610.

Schulz, Karl-Heinz/Kroencke, Sylvia/Beckmann, Mingo/Nadalin, Silvio/Paul, Andreas/ Fischer, Lutz/Nashan, Björn/Senf, Wolfgang/Erim, Yesim (2009): "Mental and physical quality of life in actual living liver donors versus potential living liver donors: a prospective, controlled, multicenter study." In: Liver Transplantation 15/12, pp. 1676–1687.

Singer, Peter A./Siegler, Mark/Whitington, Peter F./Lantos, John D./Emond, Jean C./Thistlethwaite, J. Richard/Broelsch, Christoph E. (1989): "Ethics of Liver Transplantation with Living Donors." In: New England Journal of Medicine 321/9, pp. 620–622.

Spital, Aaron (2000): "Evolution of Attitudes at US Transplant Centers toward Kidney Donation by Friends and Altruistic Strangers." In: Transplantation 69/8, pp. 1728–1731.

Spital, Aaron (2004): "Donor Benefit is the Key to Justified Living Organ Donation." In: Cambridge Quarterly of Healthcare Ethics 13/1, pp. 105–109.

Steiner, Robert W. (2019): ""You can't get there from here": Critical Obstacles to Current Estimates of the ESRD Risks of Young Living Kidney Donors." In: American Journal of Transplantation 19/1, pp. 32–36.

Thiessen, Carrie/Gordon, Elisa J./Reese, Peter P./Kulkarni, Sanjay (2015a): "Development of a Donor-Centered Approach to Risk Assessment: Rebalancing Nonmaleficence and Autonomy." In: American Journal of Transplantation 15/9, pp. 2314–2323.

Thiessen, Carrie/Kim, Yunsoo A. Kim/Formica, Richard/Bia, Margaret/Kulkarni, Sanjay (2015): "Opting Out: Confidentiality and Availability of an 'Alibi' for Potential Living Kidney Donors in the USA." In: Journal of Medical Ethics 41/7, pp. 506–510.

Thys, Kristof/Van Assche, Kristof/Nobile, Hélène/Siebelink, Marion/Aujoulat, Isabelle Aujoulat/Schotsmans, Paul/Dobbels, Fabienne/Borry, Pascal (2013): "Could Minors be Living Kidney Donors? A Systematic Review of Guidelines, Position Papers and Reports." In: Transplant International 26/10, pp. 949–960.

Thys, Kristof/Van Assche, Kristof/Nys, Herman/Sterckx, Sigrid/Borry, Pascal (2016): "Living Organ Donation by Minors: An Analysis of the Regulations in European Union Member States." In: American Journal of Transplantation 16/12, pp. 3554–3561.

Timmerman, Lotte/Laging, Mirjam/Timann, Reinier/Zuidema, Willij C./Beck, Denise K./IJzermans, Jan N. M./Bezjes, Michiel G. H./Busschbach, Jan J. V./Weimar, Willem/Massey, Emma K. (2016): "The Impact of the Donors' and Recipients' Medical Complications on Living Kidney Donors' Mental Health." In: Transplant International 29/5, pp. 589–602.

Tong, Allison/Chapman, Jeremy R./Wong, Germaine/Craig, Jonathan C. Craig (2013): "Living Kidney Donor Assessment: Challenges, Uncertainties and Controversies among Transplant Nephrologists and Surgeons." In: American Journal of Transplantation 13/11, pp. 2912–2923.

Van Assche, Kristof/Genicot, Gilles/Sterckx, Sigrid Sterckx (2014): "Living Organ Procurement from the Mentally Incompetent: the Need for More Appropriate Guidelines." In: Bioethics 28/3, pp. 101–109.

Van Pilsum Rasmussen, Sarah E./Henderson, Macey L. Henderson/Kahn, Jeffrey/Segev, Dorry (2017): "Considering Tangible Benefit for Interdependent Donors: Extending a Risk–Benefit Framework in Donor Selection." In: American Journal of Transplantation 17/10: pp. 2567–2571. Sixty-Third World Health Assembly (2010):

"WHO Guiding Principles on Human Cell, Tissue and Organ Transplantation." In: Cell Tissue and Banking 11/4, pp. 413–419.

Verkerk, Marian A./Lindemann, Hilde/McLaughlin, Janice/Sculla, Jackie Leach/Kihlbom, Ulrik/Nelson, Jamie/Chin, Jacqueline (2015): "Where Families and Healthcare Meet." In: Journal of Medical Ethics 41/2, pp. 183–185.

Williams, Nicola Jane (2018): "On Harm Thresholds and Living Organ Donation: Must the Living Donor Benefit, on Balance, from his Donation?" In: Medicine, Health Care and Philosophy 21/1, pp.11–22.

Wöhlke, Sabine (2017): "Self-Determination in Living Organ Donation: an Empirically Informed Contribution to Ethical Issues in Decision Making." In: Dilemata 23, pp. 1–8.

Woodruff, Michael F. A. (1964): "Ethical Problems in Organ Transplantation." In: British Medical Journal 1/5396, pp. 1457–1460.

Young, Ann/Karpinski, Martin E./Treleaven, Darin J./Waterman, Amy/Parikh, Chirag R./ Thiessen-Philbrook, Heather/Yang, Robert C./Garg, Amit X./Donor Nephrectomy Outcomes Research (DONOR) Network (2008): "Differences in Tolerance for Health Risk to the Living Donor among Potential Donors, Recipients, and Transplant Professionals." In: Kidney international 73/10, pp. 1159–1166.

8. Unspecified Living Organ Donation
A Challenge to the Duty to 'First Do No Harm'

Heather Draper & Greg Moorlock

1. Introduction

In this chapter, we will discuss ethical issues associated with unspecified living organ donation. We start by providing some background information about the practice, and explaining how it differs from other forms of donation. We then focus in detail on how the medical ethical principle of 'first do no harm' operates within this context, and consider whether unspecified living organ donation falls foul of this principle. In the final section, we explore whether, given the preceding discussion, facilitating unspecified living organ donation is broadly consistent with the aims and values of the medical profession.

2. Background

Most living organ donations occur within the context of existing relationships, normally between family members or close friends (see also chapter 7 in this book). In the early days of transplantation, there was little option but to use family members, as close genetic relatedness was required in order for transplants to be successful. Subsequent developments have, however, reduced the need for this, thereby expanding the pool of potential donors for any recipient. In the majority of living donations, the recipient is specified by the donor: the whole point of the donation is that the organ goes to this specific recipient, who the donor particularly wants to help. In recent years, however, there has been a significant number of *un*specified living donors. These are people who are motivated to help someone in need of the organ[1] they are willing to donate, but they do not choose or specify who this is. For this reason, this type of donation has also been known variously as 'altruistic', 'Samaritan' or 'stranger' donation but can be referred to more precisely as non-directed altruistic or unspecified living donation. We will use the term 'unspecified donation' going forward, as this appears to be the current preferred terminology (Dor et al. 2011). In principle, living donation

---

1 We refer to 'organ' throughout, but this should be taken to include 'partial organ', as living donors can also donate part of their liver or lung.

– and therefore unspecified donation – could include the survivable donation of any organ: single kidney, liver lobe, lung lobe, uterus and even a testicle or ovary. The latter two options raise particular ethical and legal issues with respect to genetic relatedness and procreation and are still experimental so we will not discuss them further in this chapter. We will also not discuss blood, skin and other tissue donation.

2.1   What Can Be Donated?

The most common living donation is donation of a single kidney. This is perhaps because it is regarded as a relatively low risk procedure and a near normal level of renal function can be achieved for the donor with their single remaining kidney. Additionally, kidney patients make up the majority of transplant waiting lists so demand is high. Although donating a kidney is considered to be low risk in medical terms, the process does involve some negative effects for the donor. The risk of death as a consequence of donating a kidney is approximately 3 in 10.000 (Lentine/Patel 2012), and around three per cent of donors experience major perioperative complications (Lentine et al. 2019). Although it used to be thought that donating a kidney did not increase a donor's risk of developing end stage kidney disease themselves, recent and more nuanced analysis has suggested that donating a kidney is linked to a small but significant increase in risk of developing end stage kidney disease later in life (Mjøen et al. 2014; Muzaale et al. 2014). Although all of these risks are relatively low and broadly considered to be within the realms of acceptability according to the transplant community, they are nonetheless risks that the person would not have faced but for their donation.

Numbers of unspecified donors are much lower than other types of living donor. In the United Kingdom in 2018–2019, there were 62 unspecified kidney donations (compared to 872 specified living donations) (NHS Blood and Transplant 2019: 2). Although kidneys are the most common organ donated via living donation, other organs can potentially be donated. Living liver donation is rarer than kidney donation, and entails the complete removal of one of the liver lobes – usually the smaller, left lobe. Although the liver is a remarkable organ, capable of significant regeneration, living donation of a liver lobe is a much more serious and risky procedure than kidney donation. Risk of donor mortality following liver donation ranges from 1 in 250 to 1 in 500 (Winder/Fontana 2019), and there is a 15–25 per cent risk of complications, which is even higher if the donation is adult-to-adult (approximately 40 per cent) (Dew et al. 2016). Donors can expect significant postoperative pain (Winder/Fontana 2019), and around a third of living liver donors report "lingering physical symptoms" (Dew et al. 2016: 881): despite this, few donors regret donating. Donation of a liver lobe can therefore come at a higher cost than kidney donation, but is still permitted via unspecified donation. Costlier still is the donation of a lung lobe, which occurs only very rarely and requires two donors, one giving the lower right lobe and the other the lower left lobe. No deaths have occurred in recent studies examining the risks of these donations, although risk of complications was fairly high. 19.8 per cent of donors in one study experienced complications (Bowdish et al. 2004), while another study found the risk of serious complications to be around 18 per cent (Yusen et al. 2014). Because lungs are not regenerative organs, lung capacity is permanently lost: one study suggests that the loss may not be as great as anticipated, with donors recovering around 90 per cent of their pre-donation lung function (Chen et al. 2011). We are not aware of any unspecified lung donors. Living uterus donation forms the backbone of the uterus transplant research programme in Sweden (Brännström 2015; see also chapter 15 in this book). This arguably represents a significant extension of living donation practice, as the main aim of uterus donation is not to extend life or restore health as such, but rather to enable the recipient to experience pregnancy. Here, although the surgery is more complex and takes longer, the risks to the donor are similar to those associated with a radical hysterectomy, which include haemorrhage, infections of the wound site, pelvis and urinary tract, as well as potential for bladder or intestinal injury (Kisu et al. 2013).

2.2 Legal and Regulatory Context

The practice of living donation is widely considered to be acceptable, and norms such as the requirement of freely given informed consent, screening for physical or psychosocial contraindications, and availability of long-term medical follow-up are well established parts of the ethical and regulatory framework (Ethics Committee of the Transplantation Society 2004: 491; Council of Europe Committee of Ministers 2008). Despite widespread acceptance of living donation, unspecified donation appears to be less well accommodated. Although many European countries (including Spain, Italy, and Austria, for examples) do not place restrictions on the types of relationships between donor/recipient that render living donation permissible, thereby potentially permitting unspecified donation, such donations are performed rarely (Lopp 2013). The United Kingdom and The Netherlands, along with the United States of America, are responsible for the majority of unspecified living donations world-wide (if trade in living-donor organs (legal and illegal) is excluded.[2] In this chapter, we will refer to unspecified donation within the context of the system we understand best, namely that operating in England within the *National Health Service* (NHS). The UK is comprised of several devolved and partly autonomous governments. Legislation, particularly in relation to organ donation and transplantation differs slightly between these regions. Organ donation and transplantation in England is governed by the *Human Tissue Act 2004*. These practices are regulated by the *Human Tissue Authority* with services run by *NHS Blood and Transplant* (NHSBT) and delivered in local NHS Trusts (one or more hospitals under a single administration).

Living organ donation is legal in England if the conditions imposed by the Human Tissue Act are met, otherwise it is an offense (which covers both the removal and use of organs) that is punishable by imprisonment and fines. These legal requirements are that the donor must give written and signed consent (witnessed by one person) and thus must have capacity to consent, and must not receive/solicit any reward. The regulator requires all living donors to be independently counselled prior to donation, by personnel it trains, in order to be satisfied that these conditions have been met, and that the donor has capacity, properly understands the procedure and its associated risks and consequences, and is not being coerced or otherwise pressured into donating. Until fairly recently, the regulator also required unspecified living donors to receive an independent mental health assessment. Although this formal requirement has been dropped, the British Transplantation Society and NHSBT both recommend that psychological testing continues (British Transplantation Society 2018: 43). These

---

2 Iran is the only country that permits organ sales, and has a centrally organised system to facilitate this.

'screening' processes are in addition to careful medical screening, the aim of which is to ensure that the donor is able to withstand surgery and is at an acceptably low risk of both short and longer term negative outcomes of donation.

Not only is unspecified living donation legal in the UK, one of the goals of NHSBT is to increase the numbers of those donating kidneys in this way (NHSBT 2014: 3). This has been echoed by recommendations from the *Ethical, Legal and Psychosocial Aspects of Transplantation* (ELPAT) group of the European Society of Transplantation (Burnapp et al. 2019). The benefits of unspecified donations go beyond just the number of organs from unspecified donors. Such donations can also be used to commence chains of donations and transplants via paired/pooled donations, and this is now the preferred use for unspecified living kidney donation in the UK. Chains occur when someone needing a transplant has identified someone who would be willing to donate to them, but their chosen donor is not a suitable match for them. If other donor/recipient pairs are in similar positions, it can be possible to organise things so that the donor from Pair one donates to a recipient in Pair two, and the donor in Pair two donates to a recipient in Pair three and so on. Long chains of donors and recipients can be created, but they sometimes require the introduction of a single unspecified donation to kick-start this process. A single unspecified donation can therefore make many more transplants possible. Despite this, those involved in the delivery of transplant services seem to have mixed views about the ethical acceptability of unspecified donation, which clearly remains controversial as far as much of Europe is concerned. We will now explore some of the ethical challenges presented by unspecified living donation and consider why the practice has not been universally embraced.

3.   Ethical Challenges Raised by Unspecified Living Donation

3.1   First Do No Harm

It is often said that the first principle of medical ethics is *'primum non nocere'* – first do no harm (see also chapter 7 in this book). Although the precise interpretation of this principle is open to debate, it is clearly reasonable to think that doctors should try to avoid harming their patients. All forms of living donation superficially appear to contravene this principle, since donation entails invasive surgery and the loss of a healthy body part. Obviously, many forms of surgery entail similar harms and the risk of further harm: at the very least, invasive surgery involves the risks associated with anaesthetic, and recovery is likely to entail pain, however well managed, and analgesics also have side-effects. 'First do no harm' is, however, not regarded as an absolute principle, rather it is a *prima facie* obligation that must be weighed against other relevant considerations. Ordinarily, the harms of surgery are thought to be outweighed by the anticipated benefits of surgery when it is performed in response to disease or other abnormality. Removing a tumour, for example, can present complex risks and harms for a patient, but by the end of the surgery the tumour will hopefully have been successfully removed thereby alleviating risks of other harms. The harms of surgery are therefore regarded as unavoidable side-effects that are necessary to achieve the intended benefit for the patient. In normal practice, potential side-effects are balanced against anticipated benefits and provided the benefits outweigh the harms, 'first do no harm' is not regarded as compromised because it would be more harmful for the patient if no action were taken.

3.2   First Do No Harm and Specified Living Donation

In the case of living donation, a similar approach to justifying the process has been applied, but is made more complex in light of a fundamental but uncomfortable truth: there is no clinical reason to operate on a healthy living person and remove a healthy organ from their body (see also chapter 7 in this book). In order to justify living donation, the outweighing benefits to the donor therefore must be defined somewhat differently, and more broadly, to include benefits that could arguably be considered non-medical (where 'medical' is defined in a fairly narrow sense). In the case of living-related donation, some benefits to the *recipient* (e.g. extended life or quality of life) are thought to also accrue to the donor by virtue of their relationship with the recipient: the donor's life is improved by having their family member or friend return to better health. The closer the relationship, the greater these benefits are thought to be, particularly if the recipient is in peril. In a more formal sense, the interests of the recipient are entangled with the interests of the donor, so furthering the former also serves to further the latter. 'First do no harm' is satisfied if we assume that the donor arguably faces a *greater* harm if the donation does not proceed (e.g. the significant distress caused by bereavement or the shared distress of the intended recipient's highly constrained life). Insisting on a favourable balance of harms and benefits sets some limits on what is acceptable: for instance, no matter the pain resulting from the death of a child, a parent would not be permitted to donate their heart to save that child's life. Equally, and perhaps more realistically, a parent is unlikely to be accepted as a living kidney donor more than once (although some have argued that this should be accepted (Bailey/Huxtable 2016), though a parent has in the past donated both a kidney and a liver lobe. Medical screening of potential donors is used to assess the potential risks/harms, and where more than one person volunteers the least risky donor may be preferred, other things being equal.

Although it seems entirely reasonable to think that donors obtain benefit from donating to relatives or friends, quantitative evidence for nonmedical benefits that outweigh known harms and projected risks is somewhat elusive. Maple et al. (2017) found no improvement in psychosocial outcomes post donation, leading them to acknowledge that they were not able to demonstrate measurable benefit (twelve months post-surgery), even though the majority of respondents still felt positively about their donation. Maple et al. conclude, that although there was no measurable benefit, the unchanged outcome scores suggested that respondents were, at least, not harmed; 10.7 per cent are, however reported as regretting the decision. Other research has suggested that quality of life decreased following living kidney donation (Chien et al. 2010), and another study highlights the emotional cost of donation (Smith et al. 2004). Evidence of this nature could suggest that the benefits to donors from living donation are overstated, or alternatively perhaps that the qualitative benefits that are frequently described by donors are just difficult to capture quantitatively using existing survey tools.

It is worth noting that the factoring of psychosocial benefits into risk/benefit calculations has occurred somewhat inconsistently over the history of transplantation.

For instance, Van Pilsum Rasmussen et al. state that "[f]rom its outset, the transplant community has dismissed any potential benefits to the donor in live donor transplantation" (2017: 2567), and altruism (understood broadly as being motivated to act by a selfless desire to help others) has always played a central role in justifying donation practice. There are now, however, increasing moves to expand consideration of richer accounts of benefits (ibid) (and the avoidance of other harms (Allen et al. 2014)). Although precisely specifying and measuring these broader benefits (and avoidance of counterfactual harms) may be challenging, for our purposes here, we need only posit that in some cases where donor and recipient are in a close relationship, the donor is likely to accrue some meaningful benefit from their donation, and that this can outweigh the downsides of donation and thereby justify the process.[3]

3.3   First Do No Harm and Unspecified Living Donation

Unspecified living donation poses a greater challenge to 'first do no harm' because the donor and recipient have no existing relationship through which the recipient benefits may be shared. Given the ordinarily anonymous nature of unspecified donation, no future relationship is anticipated. Even if the harms to the donor are outweighed by the benefits to the recipient, the donor is physically harmed without deriving any obvious physical or recipient-originating benefit themselves. In the early days of unspecified donation, the lack of obvious benefit prompted speculation about the motivations or mental health of those who wanted to become unspecified donors. Given that donating an organ comes at a physical cost involving discomfort, pain and risk, some people thought that a willingness to go through this process for little or no benefit to oneself was more likely to indicate personality disorders or more worrying motivations than a purely altruistic disposition. Research on the motivations of unspecified donors has made clear that these concerns were largely misplaced, however, and that some people do simply want to help others who are in dire need (Clarke et al. 2013).

There are two ways that the issue of 'first do no harm' could be addressed in the context of unspecified donation:

i.   Include consideration of other benefits into the calculations of risks/benefit, to produce a favourable balance.
ii. Accept that unspecified donation does cause some harm to the donor, but that this is normally an acceptable level of harm that an autonomous person can voluntarily consent to, and that frustrating a person's autonomous wishes can itself cause harm.

3.4   Including Other Considerations in Risk/Benefit Calculations

In order to justify unspecified donation, the notion of benefit could perhaps be extended to include some kind of specific but abstract moral benefit that accrues to the donor for, at some personal cost, doing a good deed for the recipient. Although it

---

3 There is further debate about whether donors must themselves receive overall benefit in order to living donation to be justified, or whether it is sufficient for donor and recipient benefit to outweigh harms when combined (Williams 2018: 11).

is no longer the preferred terminology, unspecified donation was for a long period of time also known as 'altruistic donation'. Altruism is an elusive concept to pin down with precision philosophically and is used inconsistently in relation to organ donation (Moorlock et al. 2014), but within this context can be understood to broadly mean being motivated by the interests of others to act selflessly. Performing altruistic acts is generally considered to be a good and praiseworthy thing to do, and this seems especially true when that act is potentially life-saving. We normally laud altruistic life-saving acts as heroic, especially when there is a cost to the agent or significant risks involved, and living organ donation would seem to fall into this category. The argument here must go that acting heroically, or more generally altruistically, is either intrinsically beneficial to the agent (it is intrinsically good *for* that agent to do good things), and/or that it results in some psychological 'warm glow' that is instrumentally good for the agent. An obvious issue arises here though: if acting altruistically is considered to be of benefit to an agent, especially if the permissibility or possibility of the action hinges upon the existence of this benefit, then one may wonder whether the action is really correctly characterised as altruistic since the agent stands to foreseeably benefit from it. It is also difficult to see how evidence for this type of benefit can be collected because it is challenging to imagine how it can be isolated and measured or a reliable proxy measure identified. Moreover, it is very difficult to see how abstract 'moral benefit' could be weighed against physical harm. In terms of less abstract benefits, one study found similar post-operative psychosocial measures for specified and unspecified living kidney donors, and that both groups felt good about themselves, though neither reported any increase in their sense of self-esteem, and levels of regret were also similar (Maple et al. 2014). Given that there is actually little evidence to suggest measurable benefit to specified donors, the lack of difference in post-operative psychosocial measures between specified and unspecified donors could merely suggest that measurable benefit for unspecified donors is also questionable. On a theoretical level, moreover, to outweigh the harms incurred, account also needs to be taken of other ways of doing good (deriving similar benefit) that would not generate these harms. In normal medical treatment, if one treatment option offered a more favourable balance of risks and benefits than another, other things being equal, the option with the more favourable balance should be preferred. And just as there may be more than one way to treat a medical condition, there are other ways to be altruistic. Relatively small donations to carefully selected charities can accrue significant benefit to others, which might allow a person to achieve the 'warm glow' of acting altruistically without having to undergo significant surgery. The harms, in this respect, are not unavoidable side-effects of virtuous behaviour in general, but rather just of this virtuous act of kidney donation in particular. It has been suggested elsewhere that excessive altruism should not necessarily be considered virtuous, and that it may be better characterised as intrinsically bad in some situations of organ donation (Saunders 2018). A further issue with reliance on altruism to do work in justifying the acceptability of unspecified donation is that people's motivations for wishing to donate may be multi-faceted and complex. Determining with confidence whether someone is truly motivated by altruism or, for example, narcissism is likely to be extremely difficult, even with the latest approaches to screening of potential donors.

3.5   Adding in Autonomy

Although abstract moral benefit, and the notion of related psychosocial benefit, are sometimes cited as reasons to permit unspecified donation, the real justificatory force increasingly appears to be grounded in respect for autonomy: it has been noted that unspecified donation is very much a 'donor-driven' process (Burnapp et al. 2019), and that if someone comes forward wanting to donate, it could be wrong to stand in their way. Ross states the autonomy argument clearly: "[i]f a competent adult seeks to act altruistically and offers to donate a solid organ unconditionally, and the adult understands the risk and benefits of the procedure, and voluntarily consents to the procurement, then his or her wishes should be respected" (2002: 441). The challenge to 'first do no harm' tends to be met by including donor autonomy in the balance of harms and benefits. According to this justification, the decision as to whether the harms incurred are outweighed by the benefits is one for the donor to make, and blocking an autonomous person's wishes is *itself* harmful, insofar as it prevents them from living their life in the way that they determine to be best for them. Liberal societies generally accept and respect different conceptions of the good life, and donating a kidney does not seem objectionable in this respect. Autonomy is engaged by claiming that placing obstacles in the way of the donor – like adhering too closely to 'first do no harm' – is excessively paternalistic and assumes that the doctor is in a better position than the autonomous donor to judge what is best for that donor. This kind of argument includes within the understanding of 'first do no harm' the harm of frustrating autonomy. The implication of this assumption is that something *prima facie* harmful can be, on balance, good for somebody, by virtue of them wanting it, if this is compared with the counterfactual and allegedly harmful scenario of ignoring their wishes. This is not, however, taken to be true for all actions that a person may conceivably want to take. If someone simply wished to have a kidney removed but had no desire to donate it to anyone, it seems extremely unlikely that any doctor would consider it to be acceptable to remove their kidney (absent any medical indication for doing so). In the case of unspecified organ donation, it is the autonomous wish to do a good thing (hence terminology focussed on altruism as an indicator of their goodness) that makes it an autonomous wish deserving of respect. It also assumes, although this is rarely articulated in the transplant literature, an understanding of respect for autonomy that includes promoting or even maximising opportunities for autonomous action. This is, perhaps, a broader understanding of autonomy than that which underpins the concerns of the *Human Tissue Authority* that the donor has capacity, is fully informed and understands the information. Here respect for the bodily integrity of an autonomous agent is perhaps the driving concern. Moreover, it is clear that the many countries that do not permit unspecified donation either have concerns about the psychological wellbeing and motives of those wishing to donate in this manner (although evidence suggests that these concerns would be incorrect), or do not consider either the 'abstract benefit' or 'autonomy' arguments to be sufficient to permit a healthy person to undergo surgery for another's benefit.

Hilhorst et al. (2011) point out that the determination of acceptable risk is not always left to autonomous individuals: seatbelt legislation, safe speed limits on roads and risks in relation to research are broadly determined by wider society, although these decisions may also be justified with reference to harm to other people. In both the Netherlands and the UK, a wider social decision was taken to permit unspecified living donation where it was previously unlawful. As we have seen, in the UK, the regulator itself imposes some safeguards in relation to consent and motivation but the process of regulation cuts across whether the harms and benefits can be balanced, and accepts that valid consent to be physically harmed in these circumstances legitimises what would otherwise be wrong-doing. This change was brought about in part as a result of pressure from medical professionals and has not been resisted by the *General Medical Council*. Donors are routinely medically screened using standardised processes, which incorporate mental health assessment even though this is no longer required by the regulator. Standardised screening, and the clearly stated possibility of not being accepted as a donor as a result of screening, denotes a general view that there is a threshold for acceptable risk that must be met prior to any processes that may result in a legal consent being sought and given. Individual clinicians may feel more or less comfortable with this threshold, and this may explain why some clinicians are reluctant to actively promote unspecified living donation (Burnapp et al. 2019), and some are unwilling to participate in some forms of living donation. Although our discussion has focussed primarily on kidney donation, as kidneys are by far the most common unspecified donation, the additional risks and harms posed by the prospect of unspecified living liver donation may explain why this is much less common. Nonetheless, rather than engaging increasingly tenuous justifications in relation to 'first do no harm', its advocates could simply accept that unspecified living donation is a licenced medical procedure where, despite the *complete* absence of medical need, any patient meeting this threshold is legally permitted to consent to be harmed and the doctor performing the intervention is not behaving unlawfully. This suggests that unspecified living donation may occupy a similar legal and ethical space as e.g. cosmetic enhancement, where similar difficulties arise in relation to 'first do no harm', nonmedical reasons and the balance of harm/benefit.

To recap, 'first do no harm' is thought to be consistent with specified living donation to the extent that the donor may be regarded as being, overall, more harmed by the failure to proceed, then by proceeding. It is also used to limit the harms by e.g. limiting the number and type of organs that can be donated to a close friend or relative. Likewise, donors are screened and the healthiest donor/the donor most able to withstand surgery may be preferred when more than one donor is available. In the case of unspecified living donation, where there is unlikely to be tangible benefit to the donor, other more abstract benefits have to be considered, or the harm of frustrating autonomy (by deciding for the donor what harms are worth what benefits) is incorporated into the notion of 'first do no harm'. Nonetheless, it remains the case that there are no medical grounds on which the surgical procedure on the donor can be justified, and patient autonomy does not usually extend to insisting on being given an intervention. The question remains, then, of whether unspecified donation is something that the medical profession should facilitate or even promote, or whether a more paternalistic approach may be justified.

4.   Considerations beyond First Do No Harm

Moving on from here, and given the potential challenges in terms of 'first do no harm', it is important to consider in more detail whether facilitating unspecified donation is something that the medical profession should be doing, given the values, aims and responsibilities that doctors should have.

4.1   A Reason to Permit Unspecified Donation

Doctors' involvement in the procurement of organs from the living is presumably not primarily motivated by a desire to promote the autonomy of potential donors, but rather an awareness of the need to acquire the resources necessary to extend or improve recipients' lives. The underlying question of whether it is ethical for medical professionals to expose healthy people to the risks of living donation, whether specified or unspecified, cannot be answered in theoretical isolation, and depends upon whether there is a sufficient need for this to occur.

It would be difficult, for example, to justify living donation and its associated risks in a country with a surplus of good quality organs from deceased donors. Although no country is in this situation, the operation of parallel living and deceased donation systems does raise the question of where each donation system should stand relative to the other (see also chapter 9 in this book). We would suggest that, all other things being equal, a source of organs that involves risks to healthy people should not be preferred over a source of organs that involves no risks to healthy people. Of course, all other things are not equal, and factors such as decreased waiting time, increased control over the circumstances of donation/transplantation, and potentially better post-transplant outcomes for the recipient all add something to the case in favour of living donation.

A further claim can also be made then, that living donors should not be used unless serious attempts to maximise rates of deceased donation have been made (Moorlock/ Draper 2018). Although the medical risks of living donation are the same regardless of whether a donation is specified or unspecified, it seems reasonable to think that benefits to donors are likely at their thinnest or most minimal in cases of unspecified donation, and so these should be of particular last resort. It is unfortunately the case that people die on a daily basis as a consequence of not receiving a transplant in time, so it is true to say that there is a need for more donors. It is also true to say that significant efforts are being made to increase the number of deceased donors (see England's move to an opt-out donation system, for example), but that this will still not meet demand. Specified living donors go a significant additional way to meeting demand, but there remains a shortfall. There is a need for more donors, and unspecified donors, particularly when used to start chains of living donors, do help to ensure that more lives are extended and/or improved.

4.2   Resource Acquisition and the Roles of Doctors

Given that there is a need, albeit a qualified one, for unspecified living donors, the question still remains of whether it is ethically permissible for doctors to obtain organs from this source. Transplantation itself is regarded as a relatively uncontroversial and legitimate medical procedure when looked at from the point of view of the *recipient* (for this perspective, see also chapter 13 in this book). It is a procedure performed on a patient, intended to provide clear medical benefit. Arguably one of the main ethical difficulties has been associated with ensuring that the organs used in transplantation have been obtained in an ethical way.

Explantation, the surgical process of donation, is a medical procedure, requiring medical skills, but is not performed for the usual medical reason of trying to make a patient better, as far as the donor is concerned. The donor *becomes* a patient by virtue of donating. Justification is therefore required for using medical skills to make someone a patient, rather than *stopping* them from being a patient. This is not such a concern in the case of deceased donors because they are dead, although an argument could also be made that acting on wishes made during life about what happens after death is part of respect for autonomy. We have seen that some living donors, particularly those in a close relationship with the imperilled recipient – may reasonably be assumed to benefit from the procedure. Since becoming a donor may prevent some harms that may themselves lead to health problems, at a stretch some people have argued that these benefits are potentially health benefits (Freeman/Whiteman 2018). In the case of unspecified living donors this is much less obviously the case and, from the donor perspective, the procedure is being done for purely non-medical reasons. There is a question, therefore, of whether doctors could permissibly, or even should, invoke a paternalistic approach towards unspecified donation.

It is clear that a desire to increase the numbers of organs available for transplantation is driving doctors' involvement with unspecified living donors: it is a matter of resource acquisition. Absent the need for transplantable organs, there would clearly be no justification for unspecified living donation, regardless of donor autonomy. In this respect the principle 'first do no harm' seems to be being applied across the donation/transplantation procedure as a whole – balancing the harm to the donor against the benefits to the recipient. From a purely utilitarian perspective, this does not pose a problem, particularly if the harms to the donor are indeed minimal. But traditionally 'first do no harm' applies to the individual patient, and not interpersonally or across populations. Moreover, in the case of individual patients, transplant practitioners have traditionally scrupulously avoided allowing the benefits to the recipient to cloud their professional judgement: this is why the person treating the recipient is not supposed to play any part in the screening, consenting or operation on the donor, deceased or living (British Transplantation Society 2018: 31). Nonetheless, it seems clear that it is the potential benefit to recipients of having timely access to good quality grafts that is driving the increase in the number of living donors in general, and unspecified donors in particular. Even those many doctors who do support unspecified donation can conceive of circumstances under which the practice is unacceptable. Donors are carefully screened to minimise risk, which suggests that there is a risk threshold beyond which the practice would not be considered acceptable, regardless of a willing autonomous donor. This seems to be a decision for the profession as a whole, and can be considered to be part of the determination of the circumstances under which the practice is permissible.

We should be cautious too of both placing too much weight on the harm of frustrating potential donor autonomy and tying medical decision-making too closely to utilitarianism. Suppose for hypothetical example, someone was willing to have a kidney removed to raise money for charity, and suppose that they had managed to gain several million pounds in sponsorship money that they proposed to donate to a cause that would directly result in life-saving treatment being given to several young adults. Let's also suppose that although they had two functioning kidneys, a pre-surgical assessment shows that neither kidney was suitable for transplantation. Would it be acceptable for this person to have a kidney removed, even though the kidney removed could not be transplanted into a recipient? The harms experienced would be no greater than for any other donor, and although no single recipient would benefit, several other people would. Presumably, having expended such effort in raising money the potential donor would feel frustrated if the surgery was refused. The onus remains on the medical professionals in those countries that have legalised unspecified donation to justify their support for legalising the practice in such a way that adheres to the legitimate ends of medicine and its values, such as 'first do no harm', without using arguments that could also permit, if applied consistently the facilitation of other – even charitable – surgical procedures that they would be unlikely to consider acceptable. Retaining a perspective on the fact that unspecified donation is performed with the justifiable aim of acquiring a particular life-saving resource that is consistent with the aims of medicine, and that the autonomous consent of the donor is a legitimacy requirement, would appear to be one way of achieving this without centring donor autonomy as the *justification* for the practice.

4.3   Case-by-Case Considerations

Against a backdrop of clear reasoning for the permissibility of living donation as a whole, and agreement on where the limits of acceptability lie, the acceptability of proceeding with particular unspecified donations must then be determined by individual clinicians, albeit guided by the considered views of the profession. If a clinician makes a clinical judgment that the risks of donation for a particular potential donor are above the acceptable levels agreed by the profession, then respect for donor autonomy cannot require the clinician to proceed with the donation. This may be considered paternalistic, but this does not seem problematic in this type of scenario: it has been argued that when offering procedures to patients, physicians have the right to impose their own sense of acceptable risk (Reese et al. 2006).

Assuming that levels of risk for a potential donor do fall within the agreed bounds of acceptability, and that a doctor is therefore willing to proceed with the donation, the final judgment rests with the potential donor. Given that unspecified donation is legal in England, the regulator has chosen to concentrate their efforts on ensuring that sufficiently informed and capacitous consent is gained. A formal mental health assessment is no longer required but it is regarded as good practice. This perhaps addresses the concerns that have been raised about the motivations of unspecified living donors, particularly when compared to specified living donors. The benefits for the latter by virtue of their connection to the recipient appear to provide a motivation that is at least accessible or comprehensible to those who are more sceptical about the motivations of unspecified donors. Even though the law in England does not automatically assume that those with mental health problems lack the capacity to consent or refuse consent to treatment, mental illness may cast doubt on capacity so it is essential to be certain that potential living donors have capacity before they embark on a surgical process that is, in part, permitted and sometimes even seemingly justified by respect for a capacitous person's autonomous wishes. Guidelines (Lentine et al. 2017) and psychosocial assessment tools (Massey et al. 2018) have been developed to ensure appropriate assessment and screening of potential living donors. There is a difficult balance to be struck between the doctors' adherence to 'first do no harm' and respectful treatment of well-motivated individuals wishing to donate organs to strangers. For example, the screening process should not feel stigmatising and should not create an unnecessarily large obstacle for donors to overcome. Nonetheless, on balance, when it comes to the doctor's duty to the donor, we would err on the side of caution over causing offence or even deterring donation. Unspecified donation should not proceed unless the donor is really sure it is the right decision. A few additional hurdles (as opposed to barriers), including taking time over the assessment, are one way of ensuring that the donor will not later regret their generosity.

5.   Conclusions

We have outlined the commonly cited ethical justifications for living donation in general, and have highlighted how unspecified donation poses some particular challenges to these. The particular issue of 'first do no harm' requires careful consideration in this context. It has conventionally been addressed by expanding the notion of 'benefit' within organ donation to include abstract moral benefit derived from doing something good, or to weigh in the harms of frustrating the wishes of an autonomous potential donor. We have then considered issues beyond 'first do no harm', specifically whether there is a sufficient need for unspecified donors and whether the practice is compatible with the roles of doctors. We remain somewhat sceptical about elaborate manoeuvres intended to fit unspecified donation within a traditional risk/benefit model of medical justification. The emphasis on risks/benefits for donors and respect for the autonomy of potential donors risks losing sight of the primary reason for permitting unspecified donation, which is that it helps to meet a significant need that would otherwise remain unmet via deceased or specified donation. We would welcome more transparency and openness around the fact that unspecified donation *does*, from a medical perspective, cause harm to donors. The level of harm is, in most cases, relatively low but it is nonetheless harm that the donor would not experience but for their donation. It is precisely the willingness to undergo this harm, however, that makes unspecified donation a remarkably generous and courageous thing for people to do.

References

Allen, Matthew B./Abt, Peter L./Reese, Peter P. (2014): "What are the Harms of Refusing to Allow Living Kidney Donation? An Expanded View of Risks and Benefits." In: American Journal of Transplantation 14/3, pp. 531–537.

Bailey, Phillippa/Huxtable, Richard (2016): "When Opportunity Knocks Twice: Dual Living Kidney Donation, Autonomy and the Public Interest." In: Bioethics 30/2, pp. 119–128.

Bowdish, Michael E./Barr, Mark L./Schenkel, Felicia A./Woo, Marlyn S./Bremner, Ross M./Horn, Monica V./Baker, Craig J./ Barbers, Richard G./Wells, Winfield J./Starnes, Vaughn A. (2004): "A Decade of Living Lobar Lung Transplantation: Perioperative Complications after 253 Donor Lobectomies." In: American Journal of Transplantation 4/8, pp. 1283–1288.

Brännström, Mats (2015): "The Swedish Uterus Transplantation Project: the Story Behind the Swedish Uterus Transplantation Project." In: Acta Obstetricia et Gynecologica Scandinavica 94/7, pp. 675–679.

British Transplantation Society (2018): "Guidelines for Living Donor Kidney Transplantation". Available at: https://bts.org.uk/wp-content/uploads/2018/07/FINAL_LDKT-guidelines_June-2018.pdf (accessed April 01, 2021)

Burnapp, Lisa/Van Assche, Kristof/Lennerling, Annette/Slaats, Dorthe/Van Dellen, David/Mamode, Nizam/Citterio, Franco/Zuidema, Willij/Weimar, Willem/Dor, Frank J. M. F. (2019): "Raising Awareness of Unspecified Living Kidney Donation: an ELPAT* view." In: Clinical Kidney Journal 13/2, pp. 159–165.

Chien, Ching-Hui/Wang, Hsu-Han/Chiang,Yang-Jen/Chu, Shenghsien/Liu Hsueh-Erh/Liu, Kuanlin (2010): "Quality of Life after Laparoscopic Donor Nephrectomy." In: Transplantation Proceedings 42/3, pp. 696–698.

Chen, Fengshi/Fujinaga, Takuji/Shoji, Tsuyoshi/Sonobe, Makoto/Sato, Toshihiko/ Sakai, Hiroaki/ Bando, Toru/Date, Hiroshi (2012): "Outcomes and Pulmonary Function in Living Lobar Lung Transplant Donors." In: Transplant International 25/2, pp. 153–157.

Clarke, Alexis/Mitchell, Anne/Abraham, Charles (2014): "Understanding Donation Experiences of Unspecified (Altruistic) Kidney Donors." In: British Journal of Health Psychology 19/2, pp. 393–408.

Council of Europe Committee of Ministers (2008): "Resolution CM/Res(2008)6 on Transplantation of Kidneys from Living Donors Who Are Not Genetically Related to the Recipient."

Dew, Mary Amanda/Butt, Zeeshan/Humar, Abhinav/DiMartini, Andrea F (2017): "Long-Term Medical and Psychosocial Outcomes in Living Liver Donors." In: American Journal of Transplantation 17/4, pp. 880–892.

Dor, Frank J. M. F./Massey, Emma K/Frunza, Mihaela/Johnson, Rachel/Lennerling, Annette/Loven, Charlotte/Mamode, Nizam/Pascalev, Assya/Sterckx, Sigrid/Van Assche, Kirstof/Zuideme, Willij C./Weimar, Willem (2011): "New Classification of ELPAT for Living Organ Donation." In: Transplantation 91/9, pp. 935–938.

Ethics Committee of the Transplantation Society (2004): "The Consensus Statement of the Amsterdam Forum on the Care of the Live Kidney Donor." In: Transplantation 78/4, pp. 491–492.

Freeman, Michael A/Wightman, Aaron G (2018): "Did Parents Have it Right all Along? Parents, Risk, and Living Kidney Donation: Revisiting the Arguments for and against Parental Living Donation of Kidneys." In: Pediatric Transplantation 22/3, pp. 1–6.

Hilhorst, Medard/Wijsbek, Henri/Erdman, Ruud/Metselaar, Herold/van Dijk, Gert/ Zuidema, Willij/Weimar, Willem (2011): "Can We Turn Down Autonomous Wishes to Donate Anonymously?" In: Transplant International 24/12, pp. 1164–1169.

Kisu, Iori/Mihara, Makoto/Bannom, Kouji/Umene, Kiyoko/Araki, Jun/Hara, Hisako/ Suganuma, Nobuhiko/Aoki, Daisuke (2013): "Risks for Donors in Uterus Transplantation." In: Reproductive Sciences 20/12, pp. 1406–1415.

Lentine, Krista L./Patel, Anita (2012): "Risks and Outcomes of Living Donation." In: Advances in Chronic Kidney Disease 19/4, pp. 220–228.

Lentine, Krista L./Kasiske, Bertram L./Levey, Andrew S./Adams, Patricia L./Alberú, Josefina/Bakr, Mohamed A./Gallon, Lorenzo/Garvey, Catherine A./Guleria, Sandeep/Li Philip Kam-Tao/Segev, Dorry (2017): "KDIGO Clinical Practice Guideline on the Evaluation and Care of Living Kidney Donors." In: Transplantation 101/8, pp. S1–S109

Lentine, Krista L./Lam, Ngan N./Segev, Dorry L. (2019): "Risks of Living Kidney Donation: Current State of Knowledge on Outcomes Important to Donors." In: Clinical Journal of the American Society of Nephrology 14/4, pp. 597–608.

Lopp, Leonie (2013): Regulations Regarding Living Organ Donation in Europe: Possibilities of Harmonisation, Berlin: Springer.

Maple, Hannah/Chilcot, Joseph/Burnapp, Lisa/Gibbs, Paul/Santhouse, Alastair/Norton, Sam/ Weinman, John/Mamode, Nizam (2014): "Motivations, Outcomes, and Characteristics of Unspecified (Nondirected Altruistic) Kidney Donors in the United Kingdom." In: Transplantation 98/11, pp. 1182–1189.

Maple, Hannah/Chilcot, Joseph/Weinman, John/Mamode, Nizam (2017): "Psychosocial Wellbeing after Living Kidney Donation – a Longitudinal, Prospective Study." In: Transplant International 30/10, pp. 987–1001.

Massey, Emma K./Timmerman, Lotte/Ismail, Sohal Y./Duerinckx, Nathalie/Lopes, Alice/ Maple, Hannah/Mega, Inês/Papachristou, Christina/Dobbels, Fabienne/ ELPAT Psychosocial Care for Living Donors and Recipients Working Group (2018): "The ELPAT Living Organ Donor Psychosocial Assessment Tool (EPAT): from 'What' to 'How' of Psychosocial Screening – a Pilot Study." In: Transplant International 31/1, pp. 56–70.

Mjøen, Geir/Hallan, Stein/Hartmann, Anders/Foss, Aksel/Midtvedt, Karsten/Øyen, Ole/Reisæter, Anna/Pfeffer, Per/Jenssen, Trond/Leivestad, Torbjorn/Line Pal-Dag/ Øvrehus, Magnus/Dale, Dag Olav/Pihlstrom, Hege/Holme, Ingar/Dekker, Freido/ Holdaas, Hallvard (2014): "Long-Term Risks for Kidney Donors." In: Kidney International 86/1, pp. 162–167.

Moorlock, Greg/Ives, Jonathan/Draper, Heather (2014): "Altruism in Organ Donation: an Unnecessary Requirement?" In: Journal of Medical Ethics 40/2, pp. 134–138.

Moorlock, Greg/Draper, Heather (2018): "Empathy, Social Media, and Directed Altruistic Living Organ Donation." In: Bioethics 32/5, pp. 289–297.

Muzaale, Abimereki D./Massie, Allan B./Wang, Mei-Cheng/Montgomery, Robert A./ McBride, Maureen A./Wainright, Jennifer L./Segev, Dorry L. (2014): "Risk of End-Stage Renal Disease Following Live Kidney Donation." In: Journal of the American Medical Association 311/6, pp. 579–586.

NHS Blood and Transplant (2019): "Annual Report on Living Donor Kidney Transplantation". Available at: https://nhsbtdbe.blob.core.windows.net/umbraco-assets-corp/16883/annual-report-on-living-donor-kidney-transplantation-2018_19. pdf (accessed June 28, 2020)

NHS Blood and Transplant (2014): "Living Donor Kidney Transplantation 2020: A UK Strategy Available at: https://nhsbtdbe.blob.core.windows.net/umbraco-assets-corp/1434/ldkt_2020_strategy.pdf (accessed June 28, 2020)

Reese, Peter P./Caplan, Arthur L./Kesselheim, Aaron S./Bloom, Roy D. (2006): "Creating a Medical, Ethical and Legal Framework for Complex Living Kidney Donors." In: Clinical Journal of American Society of Nephrology 1, pp. 1148–1153.

Ross, Lainie F. (2002): "Solid Organ Donation between Strangers." In: The Journal of Law, Medicine & Ethics 30/3, pp. 440–445.

Saunders, Ben (2018): "How Altruistic Organ Donation May Be (Intrinsically) Bad." In: Journal of Medical Ethics 44/10, pp. 681–684.

Smith, Graeme C./Trauer, Thomas/Kerr, Peter G./Chadban, Steven J. (2004): "Prospective Psychosocial Monitoring of Living Kidney Donors Using the Short Form-36 Health Survey: Results at 12 Months." In: Transplantation 78/9, pp. 1384–1389.

Van Pilsum Rasmussen, Sarah E./Henderson, Macey L./Kahn, Jeffrey/Segev, Dorry (2017): "Considering Tangible Benefit for Interdependent Donors: Extending a Risk–Benefit Framework in Donor Selection." In: American Journal of Transplantation 17/10, pp. 2567–2571.

Williams, Nicola J. (2018): "On Harm Thresholds and Living Organ Donation: Must the Living Donor Benefit, on Balance, from his Donation?" In: Medicine, Health Care and Philosophy 21/1, pp. 11–22.

Winder, Gerald Scott/Fontana, Robert J. (2019): "Outcomes in Living Liver Donor 'Heroes' After the Spotlight Fades." In: Liver Transplantation 25/5, pp. 685–687.

Yusen, R D./Hong, B. A./Messersmith, E. E./Gillespie, B. W./Lopez, B. M./Brown, K. L./Odim, J./Merion, R. M./Barr, M. L. and RELIVE Study Group (2014): "Morbidity and Mortality of Live Lung Donation: Results from the RELIVE Study." In: American Journal of Transplantation 14/8, pp. 1846–1852.

III. ORGAN ALLOCATION AND TRANSPLANTATION SYSTEMS

9. Allocating Organs
Fairness, Transparency, and Responsibility

Søren Holm

1. Introduction

Since organ transplantation was first developed as a treatment option for organ failure there has been a mismatch between the number of patients needing organs and the number of organs available (Gain et al. 2016).[1] This mismatch has persisted over time and is a feature of all organ transplant systems irrespective of their consent model opt-in, opt-out or mandatory choice (see chapter 2 in this book) – and irrespective of whether the system allows monetary compensation to organ donors or the families of dead donors. The mismatch is likely to increase as the indications for organ transplants continue to widen and bridging technologies become available which enable very ill patients to be stabilized and maintained while they wait for a transplant. This means that organs are a scarce, non-fungible resource and that allocation decisions have to be made concerning which of the many patients who need an organ should have priority when an organ becomes available. For life-saving organs, allocation decisions will inevitably mean that some patients receive organs and have their life extended, whereas others never receive an organ and die as a result of organ failure.

The difficulty determining an ethically justifiable way of allocating organs has generated a huge literature, and I don't pretend to present any new and truly original arguments in this chapter or to reference every important source on the topic. Every conceivable argument will already have been suggested, discussed and criticized somewhere in the literature (for an overview of the various arguments in the literature, see articles by Childress (1987, 1989, 2001) and Gutmann and Land (1997)). Nevertheless, there is value in providing a systematic account of the arguments and their ethical and pragmatic strengths and weaknesses.[2] While this may not allow us to design the

---

1 Bone marrow transplantation is also a form of organ donation, but issues about the allocation of bone marrow transplants fall outside the scope of this chapter because 1) bone marrow donation is almost always live donation, 2) bone marrow is a renewable resource, and 3) the scarcity in bone marrow availability is primarily due to problems in identifying a suitable donor and not due to the in principle unavailability of a donor.

2 A 'systematic account' here means an account based on a reasonably comprehensive review of the literature on the allocation of organs for transplant leading to a list of proposed, discussed and/or

perfect system of organ allocation, it will allow us to reject some suggested allocation criteria as unsustainable, identify the limitations of other criteria, and therefore narrow the area in which to search for a justifiable and defensible set of allocation criteria. As Calabresi and Bobbitt wrote more than 40 years ago in *Tragic Choices*, their seminal book on kidney dialysis and transplants, this chapter does not seek "to resolve tragic choices by means of discoveries of new methods, but to make it possible for us to get a clearer view of the state of affairs that troubles us" (1978: 195). Similarly, Childress writes:

> There is, I believe, a wide range of ethically acceptable policies, at least in principle; which policies should have priority will depend on considerations of ethical preferability and political feasibility. Excluding policies that would seriously violate fundamental ethical principles, society still has to choose policies that best express the whole constellation of ethical principles, including ideals, and that can actually be implemented. (1987: 86)

It is also important to note that the design and implementation of an organ allocation scheme in a particular country or region will inevitably be influenced by the basic structure of the health care system, and by the more general approach taken to allocation of health care resources and social resources in general in that system. When people decide to become organ donors in a well-governed health care system they decide to interact with an organ donation and transplant system, except in the relatively rare cases of directed living donation. Organ donation takes place in a complex network involving the potential donor, the recipient, the system, and the health care professionals in the system (Jonsen 2012). This means that the decisions people make to become donors, or to allow organ retrieval from their dead relatives, at least partly rely on their perception of the system and not only on their desire to help other people. A person who perceives the system as unjust or corrupt is probably less likely to become or remain a donor. This link between trust in the system and willingness to donate is also evidenced in a recent meta-synthesis of the qualitative literature on this topic (Shaw et al. 2013; Schwettman 2015). The system may also be seen as an embodiment of solidarity and notions of reciprocity, where people are willing to donate because they or their loved ones may at some point need an organ. If that is part of the motivation, discovering that the system is deliberately subverted and exploited by some actors may also undermine willingness to donate (Boulware 2007). Thus, as a precondition for maximizing donations, it is vital not only that the allocation system and its processes are fair, but also that they are seen to be fair by the population of potential donors. Perceptions of fairness may differ between different countries and health care systems. In some circumstances establishing robust, un-corruptible allocation processes may be more important than getting the allocation criteria absolutely right. The establishment of officially mandated and supported donation and transplant systems also means that transplantable organs become a social good. The system organizes and governs the transactions between donors, health care institutions and recipients on

---

actually used allocation considerations and criteria that can be ordered under and encompassed by a reasonably small number of headings, i.e. the list of allocative criteria presented in the section on 'allocative criteria'.

behalf of the community, and not as a set of commercial exchanges (Task Force on Organ Transplantation 1986). This entails that the generally accepted principles for the allocation of social goods apply prima facie to the allocation of organs, unless there are specific reasons to deviate from them.

2.   Allocative Criteria

Allocation of organs is in practice achieved through waiting list systems, where potential recipients for an organ are ranked according to a set of criteria. Some of the criteria are specific to the particular organ to be transplanted – e.g. size matters for paediatric transplantation of some organs, and immunological match matters for many – and some criteria are not specific to the organ but to the patient / recipient, such as time on the waiting list, or the urgency of the transplant need. Several criteria may be combined into one overall score to determine priority on the waiting list. For instance, the Lung Allocation Score (LAS), developed by the US Organ Procurement and Transplantation Network, is used both in the US and by Eurotransplant in Europe[3] to allocate lung transplants (OPTN 2020, Eurotransplant 2020). The LAS calculation looks simple:

10.1.F The LAS Calculation
The LAS calculation uses all of the following measures:
Waiting List Urgency Measure, which is the expected number of days a candidate will live without a transplant during an additional year on the waiting list.
Post-transplant Survival Measure, which is the expected number of days a candidate will live during the first year post-transplant.
Transplant Benefit Measure, which is the difference between the Post-transplant Survival Measure and the Waiting List Urgency Measure.
Raw Allocation Score, which is the difference between Transplant Benefit Measure and Waiting List Urgency Measure.
To determine a candidate's LAS, the Raw Allocation Score is normalized to a continuous scale of zero to 100.
The equation for the LAS calculation is:
$$LAS = 100*(PTAUC - 2*WTAUC + 730) / 1095 \text{ (OPTN 2020: 220)}$$

However, this apparent simplicity is deceptive. The above LAS formula is followed by 30 pages of instructions on how to calculate the PTAUC and the WTAUC based on a long list of clinical information including: Date of birth, Lung diagnosis, Height and Weight, Diabetes, Supplemental oxygen requirement, Six minute walk distance (6MWT), Pulmonary artery systolic pressure, Pulmonary artery mean pressure, Forced vital capacity, Serum creatinine, Mean pulmonary capillary wedge pressure, Functional status, Need for assisted ventilation, Current lowest and highest PCO_2, Bilirubin, Duration of ventilation, Coagulopathy, Extracorporeal support, and 6MWT*end-saturation (cp. Eurotransplant 2020).

---

3 Covering Austria, Belgium, Croatia, Germany, Hungary, Luxembourg, Slovenia, and The Netherlands.

A number of what we may call recipient-related allocative criteria have been discussed in the literature, although not all of these have ever been implemented in any officially adopted allocation system. The criteria can be broadly categorized as:

1	Medically related Criteria
a)	Medical Need
b)	Likelihood of Match
c)	Magnitude of Likely Medical Benefit
d)	Responsibility for Health State
2	Social Criteria
a)	Social Need
b)	Desert / Social Merit
c)	Future Social Contribution
d)	Time on Waiting List
e)	Wider Social Justice Issues
f)	Local or National Preference

Table 1: Recipient-related allocative criteria in organ donation

Many of the social criteria, apart from 'time on waiting list' and 'national preference,' were proposed and discussed early in the history of organ transplantation but have since fallen out of favour (Annas 1985). In the following, we will analyse the arguments for and against each of these criteria, and the problems in operationalizing them when moving from direct comparisons between a small number of potential recipients to a system that may have to allocate one organ within a pool of thousands of possible recipients.

2.1   Medical Criteria

The perhaps most intuitively appealing criterion is medical need. It seems prima facie obvious that we should allocate an available organ to the patient who has the greatest medical need, or at the very least that need should play a major role in our allocation decisions. Need is, however, not a simple concept, even if we restrict it to 'medical need'. The size of the medical need for an organ has at least two separable elements: 1) the severity of the current health state, and 2) the urgency of the transplant. That these may diverge can be seen if we consider a situation in which one patient is in a very bad, but stable, health state, while another patient is in a less serious health state now, but has the prognosis of an imminent deterioration leading to death. The first patient has a large need and therefore a strong claim to an organ even if that health state is currently stable, but so does the second patient, who needs the transplant urgently. The grounding of their need is just different. If we prioritize urgency too much, then stable but very ill patients will have difficulty getting transplants, and if we do not prioritize urgency enough, more people will die while on the waiting list.

Prioritization of urgency is illustrated in the rules for allocation of livers of Scandiatransplant, the transplant allocation organization for the Nordic countries and Estonia. These rules identify a class of 'High urgent calls' and specify that any available, suitable liver must be allocated to those patients: High urgent call (HU)

- An acute liver failure patient who is at a risk to die within few days (no prior liver disease)
- Need for re-transplantation within 2 weeks after transplantation (includes primary nonfunctioning graft)
- If several HU calls exist at the same time, the first one has priority over later HU call. This is also true if the second centre has a local donor
- Within 72 hours after HU call, every centre has an obligation to offer available livers for the recipient centre
- The first available donor liver with compatible AB0 blood group must be offered to recipients on HU call. (Scandiatransplant 2017a: 225)

A third, partly separable component of need is the availability of alternatives. In some circumstances an organ transplant it the best option for a patient, i.e. a kidney transplant is the best treatment option for many patients currently on dialysis, but there is at least one alternative, i.e. in this example staying on dialysis. Given the scarcity of organs we could argue that alternatives should always be pursued first, and that only patients for whom there are (no longer) any alternatives should be allocated an organ. But, such a policy is potentially counterproductive, because those patients who have run out of other options, e.g. dialysis or left ventricular assist devices, are likely to be much more ill than those who are stable on an alternative treatment, and therefore less likely to benefit from a transplant. There is also a considerable overlap between not having any other options and urgency. The likelihood of finding a matching organ for a particular recipient depends not only on the characteristics of the donor pool, but also on the degree to which a potential recipient has been immunologically sensitized to other tissue types than his or her own. Such sensitization can come about if the patient has had prior blood transfusions, previous transplants, or in some cases as a result of pregnancy and childbirth. The more tissue types a patient is sensitized to, the fewer organs will be a possible match for that patient. Highly sensitized patients may thus be 'stuck on the waiting list' indefinitely unless they get priority whenever an organ that matches their sensitization pattern becomes available. The magnitude of the likely medical benefit has traditionally been very important in the allocation of organs because long-term organ survival can only be achieved if the organ is not immunologically rejected by the recipient's body. Immunosuppression was not very advanced in the early days of organ transplantation, meaning that the tissue-type match between the donor organ and recipient was a very important factor in predicting organ survival and thus medical benefit. As immunosuppression methods have improved, the tissue-type match has become less important, and this has meant that other factors that may influence the medical benefit have become more prominent in discussions about allocative criteria, e.g. age, co-morbidity, ability to adhere to future treatment etc. Some of these other factors are potentially controversial because they may be seen to involve some form of problematic discrimination. For example, using age as a criterion for priority may be seen as ageist (on the general issue of using age as a resource allocation criterion, see Daniels 1988; Harris 1994; Callahan 1995; Williams 1997; Holm 2013; and chapter 12 in this book). Ability to adhere to future treatment is also a potentially problematic criterion: partly because it is not obvious how to assess this objectively; partly because some factors that might influence this ability, such as having cognitive deficits or being homeless, do not seem like the kind of conditions that should affect a person's claim to treatment for an important health need. One version of the ability-to-adhere argument focuses on persons whose behaviour have contributed to their current health state, and where the likelihood of long-term transplant success will be affected if they continue to behave in the same way. It is argued that such patients should be given lower priority, or not put on the waiting list at all, unless they cease their problematic behavior and there is some evidence that they won't start again. This argument is forward-looking: it does not justify lower priority because previous behaviour led to the transplant need, but because future similar behaviour would affect the likelihood of long-term medical benefit. This was for instance discussed in relation to the famous Manchester United and Northern Ireland footballer George Best, who received a liver transplant following liver failure caused by alcoholic liver cirrhosis. He was only put on the waiting list for a transplant after he became abstinent, but the media queried whether he would (or could) remain abstinent after the transplant (Murnane 2015). A possible consistency problem affects this kind of reasoning, because we do not seem to apply it across the board in health care (Douglas 2017). Playing many kinds of sports at elite level is a strong risk factor for ligament damage in the knee, and continuing to play at elite level after ligament surgery is an even stronger risk factor for a recurrence. However, we do not normally make it a condition of access to surgery that elite athletes give up their sport. It is important to distinguish this argument from the notion that a potential recipient's personal responsibility for being in a health state that requires an organ transplant reduces the strength of their claim to an organ. According to the latter argument, for instance, patients with alcoholic liver cirrhosis should have a lower priority on the waiting list for liver transplants, or should perhaps not be put on the waiting list at all. The patient who is deemed to carry some personal responsibility is often compared unfavourably to the 'innocent victim of disease'. In its pure form the personal responsibility argument is exclusively backward-looking, in contrast to the forward-looking ability-to-adhere argument. The argument has some intuitive appeal, but on closer inspection it is highly problematic. There are three main problems. The first two are deeply philosophical: we must first decide which kind of responsibility is relevant – causal responsibility, moral responsibility, or blameworthiness (see Holm 2008); then, we must decide how to apportion the relevant degree of responsibility or blame across a diverse range of actions, habits and lifestyles that have led to the need for a transplant. Where some are single, clearly autonomous acts, some may involve addiction or weakness of will (Douglas 2017), and some are lifestyles or habits formed either early in life and/or are common in the environment the person lives in.

Neither of these are trivial problems, since the causal networks leading to the final health state are often highly complex. The third problem is most often raised as a charge of arbitrariness: Why single out behaviour X as a case of personal responsibility leading to lower priority, when behaviours Y, Z etc. also generate bad health states and need for treatment? This charge can be general, or specific to organ transplants, and it is often supported by the observation that the behaviours that are singled out, such as alcohol abuse, smoking, or a sedentary lifestyle, are all to some degree already socially stigmatized.

2.2   Social Criteria

Social need, desert, merit and future social contribution have all been proposed as allocative criteria. Here, the idea is that we should, for instance, give (some) priority to patients who have many dependants, who have made a significant social contribution for which they deserve credit, or who are likely to make major contributions in the future. These proposals are problematic, partly because we usually do not apply them in other areas of health care, and partly because it is nearly impossible to define fair and non-arbitrary criteria for which social contributions should count as meritorious in this context. While we might be able to identify slackers who have contributed very little to anything, there is no simple metric by which we can compare entrepreneurial, sporting, political, homemaking and other prima facie valuable social contributions and decide who is most deserving overall. A particular type of the desert/merit/contribution argument focuses narrowly on contributions to the organ donation and transplant system itself. One version focuses on actual contribution and argues that persons who have been living donors should have priority on the waiting list if they ever need an organ. This seems straightforward: living donors have contributed significantly and have a legitimate expectation that society reciprocates in some way. But there are still issues that need to be resolved, especially in relation to whether having been a donor of one organ or part of an organ should give priority on all transplant lists, or just the list for the organ in question. I.e. should a live liver-lobe donor only have priority in relations to livers, or also in relation to kidneys, hearts etc.? Restricting priority to only the organ in question may seem natural, but it does require justification. One possible argument is that, by becoming a donor, the person has given up a good organ which could have saved them from needing the organ later, but this argument only works for paired organs and not if the condition leading to the need for a transplant would have affected both paired organs, as many conditions leading to kidney failure do. Thus, in many cases the donor who is now a potential recipient would still need a transplant even if they had not donated. Therefore, basing priority on the willingness to make a significant sacrifice for others would seem like a more solid argument, and that points towards priority on all waiting lists. Another version argues that persons who are merely willing to donate should get priority over persons who are not willing to donate. In practical terms this might mean that being on the donor register gives a person priority. This can be justified from considerations of reciprocity or solidarity, or as a way to deter 'free-riders' who are happy to accept the benefits of the social practice of donation and transplantation but not willing to contribute. Israel has implemented such a system, which gives priority not only to the willing donor but also to their family members (Quigley et al. 2012; Lavee/Brock 2012). Clearly, being willing to contribute as a donor at least potentially contributes to maintaining an effective donation and transplant system, so it is not directly affected by the relevance and arbitrariness concerns that undermine general merit and social contribution proposals. It is, however, affected by what is in some way the reverse problem: why single out this contribution among the many relevant contributions to the system. Signing up to the organ donor registry is not particularly onerous, and donating after death does not affect the donor's welfare, so the 'cost' to the donor is low, although the benefit to the recipient is large.[4] What is relevant to the donor's claim to priority is what they are willing to, or actually do, give up, and that is not much. Blood donors, tax payers, donors to relevant health charities, volunteers in the hospital and many others also contribute directly, and not as employees, to the possibility of having a donation and transplantation system, physically or financially or both; and some of these contributions are more burdensome than being on the donor register. So, why should they not count towards priority in organ allocation? The policy of also giving priority to family members of potential donors raises issues of justice. Why should those who do not have family members have their priority reduced? Giving priority to family members of potential donors also encourages strategic behaviour by those who have family members who can be predicted to potentially need an organ transplant in the future (Quigley et al. 2012; Lavee/Brock 2012).Time on the waiting list could be conceptualized as a medical criterion by making it a component of medical need. Just as your need increases if it is urgent, it increases if you have had to wait a long time and suffer the consequences of that wait. It is, however, perhaps more straightforward to see time on the waiting list as a social criterion, reflecting the view that society ought to (be able to) treat people at the point where their health needs occur. If society cannot provide treatment when a patient needs it and the patient has to go on a waiting list the strength of the claim to be provided treatment increases vis a vis society as time goes by and treatment is still not provided, and the comparative strength of the claim vis a vis other patients with a need for a transplant increases in the same way. This is supported by the intuitive appeal of the idea that if we have two identical patients on the waiting list and one has waited much longer than the other we should give an available organ to the patient who has waited the longest. If we accept this argument and give extra priority according to time on the waiting list, we need to be aware that there is some evidence that the decision concerning when to put a particular patient on the waiting list for a transplant may be potentially biased. It has, for instance been shown that white patients in dialysis are put on the waiting list earlier and more frequently than black patients in the USA. This has led the US Organ Procurement and Transplantation Network to move from time on waiting list to time in dialysis as the relevant criterion for priority for a kidney transplant (Zhang et al. 2018). Wider social justice issues are also potentially important when deciding on allocative criteria. If we find that a particular set of criteria lead to an unequal distribution of organs between age groups (where age does not affect outcome), ethnic groups, socioeconomic groups, or geographically defined groups etc. it raises the question whether these inequalities also constitute an injustice that should be rectified, and if so how rectification should be achieved. Organs for transplant are a social good distributed by official societal agents (see above); and if we have good reasons to think that equality in distribution is in general important between a specific set of groups, then those reasons transfer to distribution and allocation of organs. Some unequal distributions are at least partially explainable by differences in organ donation. In many countries there are, for instance differences in donation rates between different ethnic groups. Because tissue types are distributed differently in different ethnic groups, this may lead to a difficulty in

---

4 There may be costs to the family in that the hospital processes around the death of a known organ donor differs from the processes where organ donation is not taking place, but a lot can and should be done to minimize these differences.

finding well matched organs for potential recipients in those groups. But it is important to see that such group differences in donation rates cannot in themselves justify
group differences in transplantation rates. Being a member of a group with a low
donation rate does not affect the claim to equal treatment a patient would have as a
citizen and eligible beneficiary of a health care system. Even if the low donation rate in
the group is due to wilful refusal to donate and therefore ethically problematic, an
individual member of the group would not be responsible for how other group members acted. This does not mean that we should not target group differences in donation
rates and try to raise donation rates.[5] If group inequalities do exist, it may be necessary
in some cases to change the weighting of the allocation criteria that gives rise to the
differences. There is also strong evidence from the USA that the differences in transplantation rates between ethnic groups have many other and more problematic causes.
This evidence is summarized by Zhang et al. in relation to kidney transplants:

> [...] there are racial and ethnic disparities at each step of the kidney transplant process.
> Black patients are less likely to be referred for transplant, complete the evaluation
> process if referred, be placed on the waiting list, and receive a transplant compared to
> white patients. In addition, Hispanics have historically had lower transplant rates after
> waitlisting. Disparities are the result of many potential factors, such as poverty, geogra-
> phy, limited education about transplant, physician bias, and other system-level factors,
> such as federal policies that guide US organ allocation. (2018: 1937, references in original
> removed)

Similar problems can be found in many other countries and localities, including the
UK (Davies 2006). Donation and transplant systems are almost always geographically
bounded, and most often the boundaries follow existing internal or international
boundaries. This raises the question of the eligibility for organ allocation of recipients
who do not reside within the boundaries of the system. If the system retrieves organs
exclusively[6] from those who are resident, should it also allocate them exclusively to residents? If organs are unsuitable for anyone on the 'residents' waiting list', they should
clearly not be wasted but offered to neighbouring systems or to non-residents – but
that is the easy case where nothing is sacrificed by allocating the organ to a non-resident. The difficult questions are: 1) whether non-residents should be allowed on the
waiting list for organs; and if so, 2) whether they should receive the same priority as
residents? The organ allocation system in the USA originally implemented a rule that
only five per cent of available organs from dead donors could be used for transplantation of non-residents, but this hard limit has since been replaced by the publication
of an annual report on residence and citizenship status of recipients. In the first 19
months of operation of the new policy, less than one per cent of organs from dead
donors were transplanted into non-resident recipients (Glazier et al. 2014).

From a cosmopolitan point of view, residence should not matter, and we should
probably in principle introduce a global donation and transplant system. But this
is unlikely to happen any time soon, so we will have to answer the question for the

---

5 In all groups, as long as we have a scarcity of organs.

6 The rare organ may be retrieved from a tourist riding a motorcycle without a helmet, but for all practical purposes the donor pool comprises those who are ordinarily resident.

present context with multiple geographically bounded systems. The limited time an explanted organ can be kept viable for transplant will set practical limits on the possible geographical extension of organ sharing schemes, but these geographical time, and by implication distance, limits will not be co-extensive with national or regional borders. The question of the ethical relevance of national or regional borders therefore remains. On the one hand, this is a question of political philosophy; on the other hand, a matter of pragmatism.

Let us take the pragmatic argument first: if a large proportion of donated organs are allocated to non-residents this may undermine the willingness to donate, especially if these non-residents pay large amounts of money for the transplants and thereby enrich health care institutions and famous surgeons. If there is evidence that this is, or is likely to become, the case, there is an argument for controlling the access of non-residents to organ transplants. The argument in political philosophy concerns which of the many social goods a society/state distributes that can be legitimately restricted to the residents of that society (Cohen 2014). This question is still unresolved and subject to fundamental disagreements.In international transplant organizations, issues of justice may also arise if some member countries become net exporters of organs, and others net importers. This may undermine the support for the scheme over time, and some schemes have implemented 'payback' rules to mitigate these issues. An example is the payback scheme for livers in Scandiatransplant. Here, the center retrieving the organ must allocate it to patients elsewhere if they meet certain criteria, but it is guaranteed later payback in the form of an organ of a similar, specified quality. If the criteria for required export are fulfilled and the organ is exported, the following rule applies: "The organ is accepted and exported. Payback with first available ABO identical liver, quality according to written rules." (Scandiatransplant 2017b)

2.3   Are all Justifiable Allocation Criteria Compossible?

If more than one criterion is justifiably relevant to allocative decisions, the question arises whether the multiple criteria are compossible. Can we design a decision-making system which ensures that they are all fully satisfied at the same time, or will there necessarily be trade-offs between the criteria, so that not all are fully met? This has been discussed in relation to the criteria of medical need, likely medical benefit, time on waiting list, and wider social justice. Focusing only on the maximization of likely medical benefit as the basis for allocation will provide the biggest 'bang for the buck,' but it seems unfair in several respects (for other problems in pursuing this goal see Birch/Gafni 2006). Transplanting patients with urgent need, or larger needs because of co-morbidity, will often mean trading off some likely benefit because the success of the transplant is more uncertain. But these patients seem to have as strong a prima facie claim to an organ as any other patients, and potentially a stronger claim if they are unlikely to survive long enough to receive an organ in the future. Similarly, as already discussed above, focusing exclusively on likely medical benefit will often mean that patients belonging to ethnic minorities will be much less likely to receive a transplant than patients belonging to the majority population. This again seems deeply unjust; the prima facie claim of an ethnic minority patient is as good as the claim of any other patient. Other examples can be given where different fairness-related criteria may come into conflict. This indicates that unless we design an allocation system that only has one criterion, or one with a hierarchical set of criteria whereby lower criteria only come into play when the higher criteria have been fully (or in a sufficientarian system, sufficiently) met, then there will have to be trade-offs between criteria.

Because the criteria are based on very different ethical considerations, there is unlikely to be any 'in principle' solution to how such trade-offs should be evaluated. Let us for instance imagine that we have an additive point system in which priority is decided by adding the points achieved in four distinct criteria. We can model the effects of such a system with different point weights for each criterion and screen out those weightings that are dominated in the sense that one or more criteria will be less well met without the other criteria being more well met.[7] But we will still be left with a large set of weightings leading to widely differing allocation priorities, forcing us to make difficult decisions. What we really need is a convincing argument that, in this particular context, meeting Criterion X is twice as important as meeting Criterion Y, but it is difficult to see what such an argument could be.

Let us for instance look at the 2013 point system for allocating kidneys in the USA, where points are used to allocate priorities within four groups of waitlisted candidates.

Factor	Points Awarded
For qualified time spent waiting	1 per year (as 1/365 per day)
Degree of sensitization (CPRA)	0–202
Prior living organ donor	4
Pediatric candidate if donor Kidney Donor Profile Index (KDPI)*[8] <0.35	1
Pediatric candidate (age 0–10 yr at time of match) when offered a zero antigen mismatch	4
Pediatric candidate (age 11–17 yr at time of match) when offered a zero antigen mismatch	3
Share a single HLA-DR mismatch with donor	1
Share a zero HLA-DR mismatch with donor	2

Table 2: Priority point system for new kidney allocation (modified from Israni et al. 2014)

In this system some of the factors giving priority are related to medical need, some to likelihood of benefit, and one to prior contribution, but the number of points they each confer seem to be largely arbitrary. Why give one point per year on the waiting list

---

7 This could be put more formally as the point that any weighting of criteria that is not an actual Pareto optimal change from a 'no weighting' position is automatically ruled out as ethically unacceptable because such a weighting implies that someone will be harmed, without any additional benefit being gained by anyone else. Many weightings will lead to changes from the 'no weighting' position that are potentially Pareto optimal, e.g. some will be harmed and others benefited, but those who are benefited can fully compensate those who are harmed. Such weightings are not dominated by the no weighting position and can therefore not be a priori ruled out as ethically unacceptable.

8 KDPI predicts post-transplant survival of the organ. The KDPI ranges from 0.0–1.0 and a lower KDPI is better.

and not two? Why does having been a living donor only count for four points? And why does degree of sensitization dominate all other considerations? There are undoubtedly answers to these questions, but the important thing to note is that all of these answers are contestable.The observation above that we will always have to make difficult judgments, even if we can model the effects of a particular (change in an) organ allocation system, is evidenced by the change to the kidney allocation system (KAS) in the USA that produced the priority point system outlined above. The changes were made in order to reduce disparities between ethnic groups and to increase the chance of highly sensitized patients receiving an organ (Health Resources and Services Administration 2014). Modelling of the effects show that these objectives were very likely achieved to some degree, but that ethnic disparities remain. The modelling does, however, also indicate that the change led to fewer transplants in patients older than 50 years of age (Israni et al. 2014). Deciding whether the benefits of less ethnic disparity are worth the costs to older potential recipients is quite difficult to judge and may depend on the specific context in the USA.

One way of avoiding having to solve these issues is to argue that we should give up trying to achieve a complete ranking because 1) there are fundamental theoretical disagreements about what is just and fair, and 2) all weightings are to some degree arbitrary. Instead, we should decide what it is a reasonable benefit to gain from an organ transplant, either in terms of pure life-extension or some composite of life-extension and quality of life/welfare, and give everyone who passes the threshold of reasonable benefit in relation to a specific organ an equal chance to get that organ, for instance through a lottery (Savulescu 2002). (On the general use of lotteries as allocation mechanisms of social goods see Duxbury 2002). It is however not clear that this would solve the problem: while the proposal makes a compromise between allocation according to need and allocation according to likely benefit, it in no way encompasses other considerations that are at least potentially justifiable, such as length on waiting list or urgency. Another approach is to rely on the public's view of how these trade-offs should be made. This approach is problematic, however, even if we accept the premise that these matters should be decided by public or citizen opinion. The main problem is that there is good evidence that the public does not have one, univocal view on these matters, that the variation in views is at least partly correlated with respondent characteristics such as gender, race and age, and that the public endorses some allocation criteria that are ethically problematic, such as the 'worthiness' of recipients (Stahl et al. 2008; Tong et al. 2010; Umgelter et al. 2015; Oedingen et al. 2019).

3.   Organ Allocation Systems and the Incentive to Retrieve Organs

Promoting organ transplantation, having conversations with patients and families about donation, and retrieving organs from donors require financial and staff resources. Ethically speaking, institutions ought to see organ retrieval as an important activity simply because transplantation saves lives and relieves suffering, but this ethical incentive may not be enough to sustain institutional commitment. The transplant system therefore needs to create a systemic institutional incentive structure that makes organ retrieval an attractive activity. One way this has been implemented is by giving some priority to patients registered on the waiting list in the retrieving institution, or in the case of kidney donation, allowing the institution to retain one of the kidneys for transplant into the highest-ranked patient on the local waiting list. Other systems have operated 'payback' schemes, where the institution that provides an organ to the pool is guaranteed to receive a similar organ within a certain timeframe. Thus, the institution participates both in the costly and non-prestigious retrieval as well as in the lucrative and prestigious transplantation. Providing such local incentives for organ retrieval is distinct from the justice- and/or ownership-based considerations concerning local or national priority discussed above. Whether to implement such incentives in organ allocation systems depends primarily on the evidence for their effectiveness. If it can be shown that local incentives increase organ retrieval, we have an argument for introducing them. If it can be shown that they increase organ retrieval so much that everyone who would have got an organ without the local incentives in the system still gets an organ, we have a very strong argument, since no one has been made worse off and some have benefited from the introduction of the incentives (i.e. they lead to an actual Pareto-optimal change). Furthermore, since all of those who benefit from organ transplants are likely to belong to the Rawlsian group of 'the worst off' (Rawls 1971), any inequalities introduced by the incentives are unlikely to constitute a social injustice.

4.   Organ Allocation in the Future

In the future, we may reach a situation where it becomes possible to increase the number of available organs to a level that converts the organ allocation problem from one of material scarcity (i.e. lack of organs) to the much more common health care problem of financial scarcity. This might come about if we have an effective market in organs, through xenotransplantation (see chapter 16 in this book), or through the growing of organs from human stem cells in animals or completely ex vivo (see chapter 17 in this book). It is, however, unlikely to come about through an optimization of current practices of organ donation and retrieval. This means that although organs will be, or can be made available for transplant, they are likely to be priced according to the current pharmaceutical industry model of value-based pricing, and that they are therefore going to be (very) expensive. How should we think about organ allocation in this situation? The first thing to note is that our elaborate systems for organ allocation and sharing within countries and across borders will become redundant. But the allocative perspective will also change: The main difference is that in the current situation there will always be another potential recipient who can be helped and 'produce' medical benefit by getting the organ, and who has an almost as strong claim according to the criteria of the system. Because organs are non-fungible, giving an organ to one person therefore always involves not giving it to someone else and depriving that person of potentially life-saving benefits. Using money for a transplant does not in the same way directly deprive someone else of the benefits of a transplant: the alternative use of the resource might have been another organ transplant, but it might just as well have been hundreds of visits to a dental hygienist. If organs become easily available, we should therefore think of their allocation as a normal case of priority setting for expensive, potentially life-saving treatments. The patient needing an organ will be in the same position as the patient needing an expensive, potentially curative cancer treatment. The approach to this kind of priority setting varies between countries and health care systems, but a main difference to the current way of conceptualizing organ allocation is that the focus will move from thinking about how to rank individual patients in order of priority to thinking of delineating criteria that define the group of patients who will get access to a particular kind of transplant. In the UK, devising such criteria may be very dependent on incremental cost-effectiveness ratios and Quality Adjusted Life Years (QALY) calculations because this is the preferred method used by *The National Institute for Health and Care Excellence* (NICE). Whereas in Germany, pure effectiveness considerations will play a much more decisive role along the lines of the preferred method of the *Institut für Qualität und Wirtschaftlichkeit im Gesundheitswesen* (IQWiG). Despite these differences in approach, the changes in allocation approach are likely to have major clinical effects in all countries where organ transplant is financially possible within the overall financial envelope of the health care system. This will affect patients in different ways. Those patients who fall within the pre-defined groups of eligibility will have a much better experience. They will have a direct claim to be provided a transplant, and they will not experience the long and anxious wait on a waiting list but will instead be booked in for a planned, elective transplant. For those patients who fall outside the group of eligible patients as defined by the health care system, their situation will be more ambiguous. If they can afford it, they will be able to buy a transplant at a private hospital; but if they cannot, they may effectively be denied any chance of a transplant.

5.   Conclusion

The allocation of organs for transplant will continue to be an area of contention as long as there is a material scarcity of transplantable organs. This contention is intensified because allocation decisions are sometimes tragic choices that determine who gets a chance to live, and who must die. It is therefore fully understandable that there is a continuous push in the public debate and in academic work, including work in philosophy and ethics, for a principled solution that will once and for all provide a fair system of organ allocation. However, the analysis in this chapter shows that it is unlikely that a fair solution based only on principled considerations will ever be achieved. Although many suggested criteria for priority to receive an organ can be shown to be unjustifiable, especially some of the proposed social criteria, we are still left with a number of criteria that all have plausible ethical justifications – but justifications that do not flow from one, underlying master ethical principle. Furthermore, these justifiable criteria are not compossible because, when the criteria are applied to a large pool of potential transplant recipients, better fulfilling one criterion always means that another criterion is less fully met. A choice will therefore always have to be made about how to weigh different criteria, or to put it slightly differently, how to balance different criteria against each other. And such weighing and balancing will always be inherently contestable.

References

Annas, George J. (1985): "The Prostitute, the Playboy, and the Poet: Rationing Schemes for Organ Transplantation." In: American Journal of Public Health 75/2, pp. 187–189.

Birch, Stephen/Gafni, Amiram (2006): "The Biggest Bang for the Buck or Bigger Bucks for the Bang: the Fallacy of the Cost-Effectiveness Threshold." In: Journal of Health Services Research & Policy 11/1, pp. 46–51.

Boulware, L. Ebony/Troll, M. U./Wang, N-Y./Powe, N.R. (2007): "Perceived Transparency and Fairness of the Organ Allocation System and Willingness to Donate Organs: a National Study." In: American Journal of Transplantation 7/7, pp. 1778–1787.

Calabresi, Guido/Bobbitt, Philip (1978). Tragic Choices, New York: WW Norton.

Callahan, Daniel (1995): Setting Limits: Medical Goals in an Aging Society with 'a Response to My Critics'. Washington: Georgetown University Press.

Childress, James F. (1987): "Some Moral Connections Between Organ Procurement and Organ Distribution." In: Journal of Contemporary Health Law and Policy 3, pp. 85–110.

Childress, James F. (1989): "Ethical Criteria for Procuring and Distributing Organs for Transplantation." Journal of Health Politics, Policy and Law 14/1, pp. 87–113.

Childress, James F. (2001): "Putting Patients First in Organ Allocation: an Ethical Analysis of the US debate." Cambridge Quarterly of Healthcare Ethics 10/4, pp. 365–376.

Cohen, I. Glenn (2014): "Organs without Borders: Allocating Transplant Organs, Foreigners, and the Importance of the Nation-State." In: Law & Contemporary Problems 77/3, pp. 175–215.

Daniels, Norman (1988): Am I my Parents' Keeper?: An Essay on Justice Between the Young and the Old. New York: Oxford University Press.

Davies, Gail (2006): "Patterning the Geographies of Organ Transplantation: Corporeality, Generosity and Justice." In: Transactions of the Institute of British Geographers 31/3, pp. 257–271.

Douglas, Charles (2017): "Addiction Medicine Ethics: Relapse, No Lapse and the Struggle to Treat Addicts Like Everyone Else." In: Internal Medicine Journal 47/10, pp. 1121–1123

Duxbury, Neil (2002): Random Justice: On Lotteries and Legal Decision-Making, Oxford: Oxford University Press.

Eurotranplant (2020): "LAS: Information for Professionals." Available at: http://www.eurotransplant.org/wp-content/uploads/2020/01/LAS_professionals.pdf (accessed June 28, 2020)

Gain, Philippe/Jullienne, Rémy/He, Zhiguo/Aldossary, Mansour/Acquart, Sophie/Cognasse, Fabrice/ Thuret, Gilles (2016): "Global Survey of Corneal Transplantation and Eye Banking." In: JAMA Ophthalmology 134/2, pp. 167–173.

Glazier, A. K./Danovitch, G. M./Delmonico, F. L. (2014): "Organ Transplantation for Nonresidents of the United States: a Policy for Transparency." In: American Journal of Transplantation 14/8, pp. 1740–1743.

Gutmann, Thomas/Land, Walter (1997): "The Ethics of Organ Allocation: the State of Debate." In: Transplantation Reviews 11/4, pp. 191–207.

Harris, John (1994): "Does Justice Require that We Be Ageist?" In: Bioethics 8/1, pp. 74–83.

Health Resources and Services Administration (2014): "The New Kidney Allocation System (KAS) Frequently Asked Questions." Available at: https://optn.transplant.hrsa.gov/media/1235/kas_faqs.pdf (accessed June 28, 2020)

Holm, Søren (2008): "Parental Responsibility and Obesity in Children." In: Public Health Ethics 1/1, pp. 21–29.

Holm, Søren (2013): "The Implicit Anthropology of Bioethics and the Problem of the Aging Person." In: I. Martje Schermer/Wim Pinxten (eds), Ethics, Health Policy and (Anti-)Aging: Mixed Blessings, Dordrecht: Springer, pp. 59–71.

Israni, Ajay K./Salkowski, Nicholas/Gustafson, Sally/Snyder, Jon J./Friedewald, John J./Formica, Richard N./Wang, Xinyue/Shteyn E./Cherikh, W./Stewart D./Samana, C. J./ Chung, A./Hart, A./Kasiske, B. L. (2014): "New National Allocation Policy for Deceased Donor Kidneys in the United States and Possible Effect on Patient Outcomes." In: Journal of the American Society of Nephrology 25/8, pp. 1842–1848.

Jonsen, Albert R. (2012): "The Ethics of Organ Transplantation: A Brief History." In: AMA Journal of Ethics 14/3, pp. 264–268.

Lavee, Jacob/Brock, Dan W. (2012): "Prioritizing Registered Donors in Organ Allocation: an Ethical Appraisal of the Israeli Organ Transplant Law." In: Current Opinion in Critical Care 18/6, pp. 707–711.

Murnane, Barry (2015): "George Best's Dead Livers: Transplanting the Gothic into Biotechnology and Medicine." In: Justin D. Edwards (ed.), Technologies of the Gothic in Literature and Culture, London: Routledge, pp. 123–136.

Newton, Joshua D. (2011): "How Does the General Public View Posthumous Organ Donation? A Meta-Synthesis of the Qualitative Literature." In: BMC Public Health 11, pp. 791. DOI: 10.1186/1471-2458-11-791

Oedingen, Carina/Bartling, Tim/Mühlbacher, Axel C./Schrem, Harald/Krauth, Christian (2019): "Systematic Review of Public Preferences for the Allocation of Donor Organs for Transplantation: Principles of Distributive Justice." In: The Patient – Patient-Centered Outcomes Research 12/5, pp. 475–489.

OPTN – Organ Procurement and Transplantation Network (2020): "OPTN Policies Effectives as of April 3 2020." Available at: https://optn.transplant.hrsa.gov/media/1200/optn_policies.pdf (accessed June 28, 2020)

Quigley, Muireann/Wright, Linda/Ravitsky, Vardit (2012): "Organ Donation and Priority Points in Israel: an Ethical Analysis." In: Transplantation 93/10, pp. 970–973.

Rawls, John (1971): A Theory of Justice, Cambridge, MA: Harvard University Press.

Savulescu, Julian (2002): "How Do We Choose Which Life to Save? Equality of Access or a Fair Go?" In: Current Paediatrics 12/6, pp. 487–492.

Scandiatransplant (2017a): "Liver Exchange and Pay Back Rules – revised Oct. 04, 2017." Available at: http://www.scandiatransplant.org/organ-allocation/NLTG_Exchange_payback_rules_Dec_2017.pdf (accessed June 28, 2020)

Scandiatransplant (2017b): "Liver Exchange and Pay Back Rules – revised Dec. 1, 2017." Available at: http://www.scandiatransplant.org/organ-allocation/Flow_NLTG_Exchange_payback_rules_oct_2017.pdf (accessed June 28, 2020)

Schwettmann, Lars (2015): "Decision Solution, Data Manipulation and Trust: The (Un-)Willingness to Donate Organs in Germany in Critical Times." In: Health Policy 119/7, pp. 980–989.

Shaw, David/Neuberger, James/Murphy, Paul (2013): "Lessons from the German Organ Donation Scandal." In: Journal of the Intensive Care Society 14/3, pp. 200–201.

Stahl, James E./Tramontano, A. C./Swan, J. S./Cohen, B. J. (2008): "Balancing Urgency, Age and Quality of Life in Organ Allocation Decisions – What Would you do? A Survey." In: Journal of Medical Ethics 34/2, pp. 109–115.

Task Force on Organ Transplantation (1986): Organ transplantation: Issues and Recommendations, Washington.

Tong, Allison/Howard, Kirsten/Jan, Stephen/Cass, Alan/Rose, John/Chadban, Steven/ Allen, Richard D./Craig, Jonathan C. (2010): "Community Preferences for the Allocation of Solid Organs for Transplantation: a Systematic Review." In: Transplantation 89/7, pp. 796–805.

Umgelter, Katrin S./Tobiasch, Moritz/Anetsberger, Aida/Blobner, Manfred/Thorban, Stefan/ Umgelter, Andreas (2015): "Donor Organ Distribution According to Urgency of Need or Outcome Maximization in Liver Transplantation. A Questionnaire Survey Among Patients and Medical Staff." In: Transplant International 28/4, pp. 448–454.

Williams, Alan. (1997): "Intergenerational Equity: an Exploration of the 'Fair Innings' Argument." In: Health Economics 6/2; pp. 117–132.

Zhang, Xingyu/Melanson, Taylor A./Plantinga, Laura C./Basu, Mohua/Pastan, Stephen O./ Mohan, Sumit/Howard, David H./Hockenberry, Jason M./Garber, Michael D./Patzer, Rachel E. (2018): "Racial/Ethnic Disparities in Waitlisting for Deceased Donor Kidney Transplantation 1 Year After Implementation of the New National Kidney Allocation System." In: American Journal of Transplantation 18/8, pp. 1936–1946.

10. Allocating Organs
Altruism and Reciprocity

Peter Sykora

1.   Introduction

Would you give one of your kidneys to a stranger? This is a title of the online version of the article published in the *New Scientist* on June 21, 2017.[1] The article describes the new trend of increasing numbers of living donors who are giving their spare kidney to save the life of someone they have never met. There are more such donors than one would have expected, but they are still far from enough. It was initially expected that organs from deceased donors (cadaveric donors) would be able to satisfy the demand for transplant organs. However, because the gap between demand and supply of transplant organs did not close, it soon became clear that organ donation would also have to be extended to living donors (Munson 2007). Thanks to advances in the development of effective immunosuppressive drugs and tissue cross matching tests, transplant organ donation from genetically unrelated donors became medically feasible. In directed donation an organ is donated to a specific individual – a family member or friend, in contrast to non-directed donation that anonymous stranger is a donor of organ to any person who needs it (cf. Veach and Ross 2015; and chapter 8 in this book). Such directed living organ donations have been extended from biologically related family members (parent, sibling, offspring, grandparent, grandchild, aunt, uncle, niece, nephew) to emotionally related persons (e.g. spouse, in-laws, adopted parent or child, friend) (see chapter 7 in this book).

While donating a kidney to a family member or a loved one is understandable, giving it to a completely unrelated stranger might seem suspicious. Until recently, physicians, ethicists and policy makers were reluctant to support unrelated living organ donations. As Gohh et al. note, such donors were considered to be "an impenetrable taboo" (2001: 619); but this attitude is slowly changing. Some countries have relaxed their organ procurement policies to also allow non-directed organ donations, but such transplantations from living donors still represent only a marginal number of living donations (see chapter 8 in this book).

---

1 https://www.newscientist.com/article/mg23431310-900-would-you-give-one-of-your-kidneys-to-a-stranger/#ixzz6IdddqBLN. (accessed March 31, 2020).

In last two decades living donors have become an important source of transplant organs. The average worldwide proportion of live kidney donors to all kidney donors (live and deceased) is about 42 per cent (for comparison, in the USA it is 28 per cent, in the European Union 20 per cent) (Domínguez-Gil/Matesanz 2018: 18, 31, 46). In countries with a low cadaveric organ procurement rate, and which have difficulties raising it (for example, due to unwillingness to change from an opt-in to an opt-out procurement policy), the increase in living donations is crucial. In countries like Israel, the Netherlands, the UK and the USA, living kidney donations have become the most important alternative to deceased kidney donations.

People who risk their own life to save the life of another are generally considered to be heroes. Accordingly, awareness-raising campaigns often use heroic images and narratives when appealing to ordinary people to become live organ donors. As Hansen et al. have pointed out in their analysis of posters used in such campaigns, the moral appeal of heroic donors is that they are "elevated to the level of a superhero in every-day life" (2018: 6). Images used in such campaigns usually directly refer to the comic hero Superman. The superhero image and narrative have also been recently used in the Europe-wide awareness-raising campaign organized by the European Union during the 2018 "European Day for Organ Donation and Transplantation". The leading slogan of the campaign was "Be ready to save lives, become a superhero!" and it referred to popular superheroes.[2]

Since the gap between demand and supply of transplant organs is permanently high, it is reasonable to ask whether appealing to heroic organ donors is enough to solve the shortage of transplant organs. While one might argue that all is needed is to improve the efficacy of campaigns to increase donor numbers, some commentators are proposing more radical changes to the whole philosophy of organ donation. After six decades of experience with the current organ procurement system, a growing number of voices argue that the policy of altruistic donations has reached its limits; it is too idealistic and needs to be replaced with a more realistic model. According to these proponents, most of whom are economists, the organ market should sooner or later reach an equilibrium between the demand and supply of transplant organs, just like any other commodity (Nelson 1991; Thorne 2006; Beard et al. 2013).

However, since the early days of transplantation practice, the world-wide attitude have been almost universally against the commercialization of transplant organs. This attitude does not seem likely to change in foreseeable future.[3] Indeed, in recent years the stance against the commodification of human organs has been strengthened in the form of measures against organ trafficking at the national as well as international level, while arguments that a legal organ market would eliminate the black market in human organs have not been widely accepted (see chapter 11 in this book).

The debate about the finding new ways to solve the inefficiency of the altruistic model is often framed as a dichotomy or moral dilemma, in which there is a choice between a moral but ineffective altruistic model on the one hand, and a morally con-

---

2 https://www.edqm.eu/en/news/be-ready-save-lives-become-superhero-say-yes-organ-tissue-and-cell-donation;   https://video.repubblica.it/dossier/lucca-comics-2019/lucca-comics-chiese-a-11-anni-di-essere-assunto-da-magic-oggi-e-il-designer-delle-carte-da-gioco/347231/347814?ref=vd-auto&cnt=1. (accessed January 16, 2020).

3 The only exception is Iran, where financial incentives for kidney donation are officially permitted.

tested but (presumably) effective commodification model on the other. In the words of Gillespie: "A vocal alternative to the status quo policy of altruism is a market-based approach: pay people for their organs." (2019: 101)

In my view, it is misleading to frame the debate on organ shortage as a simple dichotomy between altruistic and non-altruistic alternatives, where the non-altruistic alternative usually means accepting some form of payment for transplant organs, including an organ market.

In the following, I explore the possibility of organ donation based on indirect reciprocity, which might overcome the conceptual deadlock between altruism and commodification. My main goal is to ethically justify an organ donation policy in which donations are indirectly reciprocated. I focus on kidney exchange transplantations, whereby, to overcome biological obstacles, donor/recipient pairs exchange kidneys. Kidney exchange is considered to be the most important innovation in living organ donations in recent years. In general, kidney exchanges are presumed to be fully compatible with the altruistic model: all donors involved in kidney exchanges seem to be altruistically motivated. In contrast, I argue here that kidney exchange is not compatible with the altruistic model, since the motivations of donors cannot be considered to be (purely) altruistic, and in fact indirect reciprocal relations are set up between donors and recipients. I further argue that kidney exchange might nevertheless be ethically justified if indirect reciprocity is morally accepted.

In the following, I begin by describing the background to the organ shortage crisis and the importance of living organ donations, in particular kidney exchange programs. This is followed by a brief overview of kidney exchange schemes. Next, I revisit and analyze the ambiguities of altruism, reciprocity, exchange, and market as these concepts are used in organ donation discourse. Such analysis will prepare the ground for further analysis of kidney exchange as an example of indirect reciprocity. Finally, I present my argument that kidney exchange can be ethically justified on the condition that indirect reciprocity is accepted as an additional moral principle alongside altruism.

2.   Transplant Organ Shortage and Kidney Exchange Innovation

2.1   Chronic Shortage of Transplant Organs

Over the past fifty years, the transplantation of human organs has become a global practice. From a medical point of view, it is a great success story; the only limiting factor is the number of available transplant organs. Unfortunately, the disproportion between organ supply and demand, especially for kidney transplantations, continues to widen. Even though the number of transplantations has increased in recent years, the number of transplant candidates has increased even faster. For example, in the US between 1991 and 2017, the number of transplants has increased by 121 per cent and organ donors by 137 per cent. However, over the same period the number of people on the waiting list has increased by 396 per cent. As of January 2019, there were 113.000 people on the waiting list, with 20 people each day waiting for a transplant.[4] The situa-

---

4   https://www.organdonor.gov/statistics-stories/statistics.html (accessed June 29, 2020)

tion is similar in Europe: in 2016 over 142.000 patients in the Council of Europe member states were registered on a waiting list (an increase of about ten per cent compared to 2013); every day, 19 patients die in Europe waiting for a transplant.[5]

In order to increase the number of available organs, health care professionals have become more open to accepting living donors, although they were initially reluctant to follow this path because of the specific ethical difficulties related to living donors. Living donors can donate a kidney, a liver lobe, a pancreas segment, and recently a lung lobe. The highest demand is for kidneys, which together with liver represent about 88.2 per cent of all solid organ transplantations (kidney 64.9 per cent and liver 23.3 per cent). Since 2000, the global number of living kidney donations increased rapidly from 7.676 to 32.085.[6]

It is broadly accepted that the shortage of available organs for transplantation is chronic. However, not everyone agrees that the current altruistic model has reached its limits and must be replaced. Defenders of the current system of organ procurement argue that full potential of the altruistic model has not been reached, and that there is a lot of scope to improve its efficiency. For example, Jawoniyi et al. (2018), based on their systematic review of literature on the organ donation/procurement from deceased donors published between 2005–2015, concluded that if the web of factors responsible for limiting the procurement of transplant organs was adequately addressed, there would be enough organs to meet all transplantation needs. Of the various factors they identified in their meta-analysis, the most important were health care professionals' attitudes toward, and experience of, the organ donation and transplantation process. However, Spain, which for years has had the highest rate of organ procurement and is referred as a model for other countries to follow (the so called Spanish model), is far from being self-sufficient in organ supply. This probably illustrates the limits of altruistic model for the cadaveric donation scheme (Matesanz et al. 2017).

2.2   Kidney Exchange Schemes

Kidney paired donations, also known as kidney paired exchange or just kidney exchange (KE), are probably the most important recent innovation in the policy of organ procurement, and they have already significantly increased living kidney donations over the last two decades (Veale et al. 2009). In principle, KE is ingeniously simple: put together emotionally connected pairs of potential donors and recipients, who are deeply motivated but unfortunately immunologically incompatible, and arrange them in such a way that a donor from one donor/recipient pair donates a kidney to an unrelated but immunologically compatible recipient from another such donor/recipient pair. The idea of KE was already discussed as early as the 1970s. In 1997, Ross with collaborators proposed a pilot study of the clinical and ethical aspects of paired kidney exchanges, which stimulated discussion and later implementation of KE in transplantation practices (Ross et al. 1997).

---

5   https://www.edqm.eu/en/news/european-day-organ-donation-and-transplantation-eodd-2018-aware ness-campaign-starts. (accessed March 3, 2020)

6   http://www.transplant-observatory.org/download/2017-activity-data-report/ (accessed March 3, 2020.

The simplest form of KE is a kidney swapping between two donor/recipient pairs (so called two-way exchange): a donor from each pair provides a kidney to an immunologically compatible recipient the other pair. However, kidney exchange can also be arranged between more than two pairs, for example between three and four pairs (three- or four-way exchange). These are examples of closed KE schemes because they involve a closed circle of kidney exchanges – the donor from the last donor/recipient pair donates kidney to the recipient from the first pair. In practice, the number of donor/recipient pairs that can be arranged in this way is quite limited.

The first kidney exchange in the world was performed in South Korea in 1991, and three- and four-way exchanges began there in 1995. In 1999, the first kidney exchange was performed in Europe (Switzerland), and in 2000 in the USA. In 2002, the Paired Donation Consortium was set up in the USA, and it started to organize kidney exchanges on a bigger scale between transplant programs across the country (Wallis et al. 2011).

An important step towards a more efficient form of kidney paired exchange was developed by Montgomery et al. under the title "domino paired kidney donation" (2006: 419) or kidney exchange chain (KE chain), which was later implemented with a great success in the USA. According to this scheme, a non-directed stranger donor is matched with pools of incompatible donor/recipient pairs which otherwise would not be able to exchange kidneys among themselves. The unpaired stranger donor (also called altruistic donor) gives a kidney to a recipient in the first incompatible donor/recipient pair; the donor from that pair then donates a kidney to a recipient in the next incompatible donor/recipient pair, thus initiating a chain of matches between incompatible donor/recipient pairs. The domino effect multiplies the number of transplants. The donor from the last matching donor/recipient pair in this domino sequence could donate to the first eligible recipient from the waiting list, which would close this matching sequence (closed KE chain). Alternatively, the altruistic stranger donor could become a bridge donor who later initiates a new KE chain.

Bridge donors agree in advance to donate his/her kidney, not when his/her loved one in the incompatible pair receives a kidney transplant, but later to a recipient in another incompatible donor/recipient pair: this is the first pair in the new chain KE. The bridge donors 'bridge' or 'link' two distinct KE chains, merging them into a larger chain. This innovative variation, called 'NEAD' (never ending altruistic donor) chain, was first proposed in 2007 (Rees et al. 2009). Bridge donors could also be altruistic stranger donors (unrelated non-directed living donors)[7] who instead of donating a kidney to a waiting list may link two domino chains, or they may link unexpected breaks in a chain, as when a matching donor from incompatible donor/recipient pair decides to withdraw (see also chapter 8 in this book). The utilization of bridge donors has dramatically multiplied the number of transplants performed. Using bridge donors, donation chains can theoretically be unlimited ('never ending'); in practice, the longest transplantation chain to date has surpassed 100 kidney donations (Cook 2018).

---

7 According to a new classification proposed by ELPAT (Ethical, Legal, and Psychosocial Aspects of Transplantation, a section of the European Society for Organ Transplantation), such donations are better referred to as unspecified donations (Dor et al. 2011).

KE chains have attracted widespread media coverage, including a front-page story in the New York Times[8] and nation-wide prime-time broadcasting on TV promoting the idea of KE to general public. According to Healy and Krawiec, kidney exchange, and in particular NEAD chains, "in some ways [NEAD chain] resembles a form of *generalized exchange* (italics in original) an ancient and widespread instance of the norm of reciprocity [...] as the obligation to 'pay it forward' rather than the obligation to reciprocate directly with the giver." (2012: 103) However, they argue it differs in some important details from generalized exchange: (for example, a NEAD chain is open, it does not cycle back, it occurs between pairs rather than individuals, and it is carefully organized instead of spontaneously emerging). Importantly, in their analysis of NEAD, Healy and Krawiec do not treat kidney exchange as a market exchange but rather as a social exchange phenomenon, and they point out that "imaginary of solidarity and collective commitment generated through a chain of gifts has been important to the success of NEAD chains" (ibid: 104). If two persons are involved in reciprocal interactions, we talk about dyadic reciprocity. But if interactions involve a third party, either a number of people in a complicated network of reciprocal interactions, or an institution (e.g. a health insurance company), we talk about indirect reciprocity in organ donation (for indirect reciprocity mechanisms, see Ferguson 2015: 214–215).

The latest innovation in kidney exchange is the global kidney exchange (GKE) program (Rees et al. 2017), which extends the pool of incompatible donor/recipient pairs to the developing world. In general, GKE's philosophy is designed to overcome both immunological and poverty barriers in transplantation. There are many end-stage renal diseases in developing countries where no funds for KE programs are available to patients even though there are potential donor/recipient pairs. Two possible GKE schemes have been suggested. First is a simple two-way kidney exchange between two incompatible donor/recipient pairs: a donor from a developing-world pair donates a kidney to a recipient in a pair from developed world and vice versa. Up to that point, this would be an international kidney exchange. However, in addition, transplant and long-term care for the kidney recipient in the developing-world pair is paid for by funds from developed country. This produces an apparent win-win situation: in the developed country, the health care insurance system saves money because transplantation is cheaper than long-term dialysis; in the developing country, the recipient would not have been able to receive a transplant kidney even if they had an immunologically compatible donors, because without extra funding the local health care insurance does not cover transplantation and post-transplantation health care costs. The second mechanism of GKE schemes is when a donor from a pair in the developing world initiates a KE chain by donating a kidney to a recipient in a pair in developed world (Rees et al. 2017). Thereby, the health insurance funds of all involved recipients can be combined to finance the transplantation costs for the recipient in the pair from the developing world. However, GKE is highly controversial because it involves a transfer of finances from incompatible donor/recipient pairs in developed countries to donor/recipient pairs in developing countries.

---

8 https://www.nytimes.com/2012/02/19/health/lives-forever-linked-through-kidney-transplant-chain-124.html?_r=0 (accessed June 29, 2020)

3.   Altruism and Reciprocity: Theoretical Foundations

3.1   Prolegomena to All Models of Organ Donation Based on Reciprocity

The altruistic model of organ donation is often said to be chronically ineffective and therefore should be replaced by some model of organ selling. This implies there are only two options: either the organ donor acts purely altruistically, or they receive money to donate. I consider such a dichotomy to be misleading and harmful to efforts to increase donor numbers.

Instead, I suggest a third alternative regarding how to deal with the organ shortage – one based on indirect reciprocity. Such a model would not be altruistic (although it would incorporate altruistic organ donation), but neither would it be based on commercialization of organ procurement. The idea of using reciprocity to motivate organ donation and thus dramatically increase donor numbers is not new. It is based on a model of human behavior, which assumes that organ donations will significantly increase if the organ procurement policy is set up in such a way that it is in a person's self-interest to commit to organ donation.

For example, Nadel and Nadel (2005) proposed that the US system of organ procurement be changed so that those who committed to donating an organ after death (the USA has an opt-in system) would receive priority on a waiting list, or live kidney donors would also receive priority if they later needed a transplant organ. The major complaint about a reciprocity policy was already formulated for a similar reciprocity proposal a decade earlier by the US federal organ procurement authority (UNOS): it inherently compromised the altruism of the existing organ procurement policy. Nadel and Nadel counter that "priority policy would actually represent a form of 'reciprocal altruism'" (ibid: 320), a concept used in both evolutionary biology and experimental economics. However, their proposal has never been accepted.

Several similar policies based on reciprocity have been suggested. For example, Kolber (2003) has suggested a model of priority incentives for opt-in system of deceased organ donation. According to this proposal, registered adult organ donors are given some priority should they need an organ themselves. Such a system has been implemented in Israel (Lavee et al. 2010; Zaltzman 2018). A more radical version of this model has been suggested by Tabarrok (2002: 107), who has dubbed it "no-give, no-take". According to this model, signing the organ donor card would be a necessary condition for entry into the pool of potential organ recipients. Critics have argued that such a system is in fact equivalent to buying organ transplantation insurance.

The vast majority of proposals that involve some reciprocity for organ donations have not been implemented (Israel's abovementioned priority system is one of few exceptions). The main reason is that they challenge principles and values of organ donation at a much deeper level than their proponents may realize. At first glance, it may seem that such policy proposals are just pragmatic compromises between the two extremes of altruism and commercialization; it should therefore be enough to defend them on the grounds that they will save more lives. Why then have proposed reciprocity policies not been welcomed even though they promised higher rates of organ donation without the introduction of an organ market? Answering this question requires re-examination of a founding principle of the altruistic model and carefully analysis of the relationship between altruism, reciprocity, and commercialization. I believe that many proposed reciprocity policies have failed because they have not included such analysis, and furthermore they use terms such as altruism, reciprocal altruism, reciprocity, exchange, and market ideologically and imprecisely. In what follows, I analyze kidney exchange from the indirect reciprocity and altruism perspectives. This will prepare the ground for my argument that KE cannot be ethically justified within the framework of altruistic model.

3.2   Genuine Altruism, Quasi Altruism, and Reciprocity

Let us begin by examining the relationship between altruism and reciprocity. What is obvious from the start is that the boundaries between altruism and reciprocity are blurred, as are the boundaries between reciprocity and commerce, as we will later see. The understanding of altruism in organ donation has been confusing from the very beginning. In his seminal book *The Gift Relationship*, Titmuss (1970) refers to blood donation as a form of altruistic gift-giving: a selfless behavior without any expectation of repayment, in contrast to the blood procurement policy in the USA, which was partially based on blood purchasing. Since that time, the gift metaphor, as a synonym for non-commercial altruistic giving, has dominated narratives on blood, and later organ procurement policies (Childress 1986). Unfortunately, Titmuss conflates two different meanings of the gift term (Sykora 2009): the gift as a voluntary act of pure generosity (as in a charity donation or the giving of alms), and the gift as a tool of negotiating social relations. For Titmuss, who was inspired by Mauss's concept of gift (Mauss 1954), the act of giving blood is voluntary, altruistic, and unilateral, without any obligation to reciprocate. This is how most lay people and health care professionals continue to understand the term 'gift' in relationship to organ donation (Sharp/Randhawa 2014). However, the Maussian gift is nothing like this. Rather, it involves the triple obligations: to give, to accept, and to reciprocate. Despite his misunderstanding of the Maussian gift, Titmuss argues that altruistic blood donation transcends the given material thing itself, becoming what Mauss has called a 'total social fact' (*fait social total*) – an activity with symbolic, economic, axiological, political, legal and religious implications, when subjective as well as objective aspects of a thing are interwoven together. Titmuss uses his understanding of Maussian gift relations as a paradigm for the creation of non-commercial "islands" (for health care systems and education) inside the modern free-market economy society. I believe that Mauss would be excited by kidney exchange policies, which would be exactly what he had in mind when he was referring to the total social act. But as we saw, Maussian gift relations are based on reciprocity and obligations. Jurgen de Wispelaere calls them "quasi-altruistic social transfers", which are very valuable in society, but they "do not fit the analytical category of an altruistic act precisely because their motivation is not a fundamental concern for the other but rather a Humean enlightened self-interest" (2004: 11–12).[9] And de Wispelaere immediately adds that "[o]nce we accept the distinction between altruism and quasi-altruism, many apparent cases of altruistic behaviour turn out not to properly fit the definition" (ibid: 12). That is, to be 'pure,' 'genuine,' 'strong' altruism, in con-

---

9 According to Hume, enlightened self-interest is when someone serves their own interests by considering and serving the interests of others. Thus, motivated by self-interest, we keep our promises to others in order to ensure that others also keep their promises to us in the future (cf. Cohon 2018).

trast to quasi-altruism, an act must be motivated only by a desire to benefit someone other than oneself (Kraut 2018).

For moral philosophers who treat altruism as a moral principle, altruistic acts should be impartial.[10] Thus, transplant organs should be given to anybody who needs one, as is the case in unrelated, non-directed organ donations (donors as altruistic strangers). Giving a transplant organ to a loved one is not impartial. But helping emotionally related people is very natural human behavior; it can hardly be classified as immoral, although it is not altruistic according to the impartialistic definition. Crouch and Elliott blame the notion that the human agent is independent, disengaged from others, for producing "an inadequate picture of the human agent *within the family*" (italics in original), because "being devoted to the family and its members is a source of deep meaning and value in our lives and the lives of those around us" (1999: 283). As they conclude, the interests of a family member are bound with the interests of the family and its members. But Ross et al. argue that intrafamilial donations, although they are still worthy of moral praise, are not altruistic, because "they serve the interests of recipient as well as the interests of the family" (2002: 419). By contrast, Daar (2002) replies that intrafamiliar organ donations are altruistic because altruism does not negate every element of self-interest. He believes that Ross et al. do not take into consideration that even altruistic strangers, "the purest of altruist", may "have their own equally binding sense of intimacy, obligation, and duty" (2002: 425) to unrelated recipients.

The debate between Ross et al. and Daar started with the aim of determining whether unrelated and related living donor should be on the same ethical level, but it soon became an inquiry into the nature of altruistic organ donation itself. It is a good illustration of how difficult it is to differentiate between 'pure' and 'not-so-pure' altruistic behavior.

3.3   The Paradox of the Altruistic Donation Model

It is generally agreed within the transplantation community that the current organ procurement policy, which has operated for more than a half a century, was "founded on the pillars of altruism" (Dalal 2015: 45), whereby organ donations from both deceased and living donors must be purely altruistic.

Unrelated non-directed living donors who donate organs (mostly kidney) anonymously to a stranger on the waiting list are consistent with such a definition of altruism, and this is the reason why they are often called 'Good Samaritan donors', 'altruistic strangers', or 'altruistic donors'. As Daar (2002) points out, if altruism is the most acceptable basis for organ donation, then altruistic strangers should be the most acceptable donors. But they are not. In fact, for a long time they were not accepted as donors at all, and this attitude has only recently changed, and only in some countries. Are they saints (biblical 'Good Samaritans'), or are they crazy? Conversely, does it mean that so-called related and directed living donors – donors who are emotionally related to the recipient – are not altruistic, or not altruistic enough? A careful reading of the

---

10 "It is characteristic of modern moral thought to see impartiality as a requirement of, if not a fundamental component of, morality." (Jollimore 2020)

following text from *The Transplantation Ethics* reveals difficulties with basing various forms of organ donation on altruism:

Finally, some transplant programs *even* began to consider *purely altruistic* live donors of kidneys to strangers when donors had no expectation of *any reward beyond the satisfaction* of helping another human being in need. Because we do not want to imply that those who donate to family members and friends are not also *in some sense 'altruistic'* [...]" (Veach/Ross 2015: 187–188, my italics).

The word 'even' here refers to the beginning of the practice of accepting altruistic strangers, who had previously not been allowed to donate organs. Without a doubt, donors to strangers may be classified as "purely altruistic"; there is no even theoretical possibility that they, anonymous donors, not knowing recipients of their kidney, could be rewarded by them. However, although there is no reward from recipients, donors may receive a psychological reward in form of "satisfaction" – simply feeling good for saving somebody else life, or a boost to his/her own self-esteem. Finally, saying that the donation of a kidney to a loved one is also "in some sense 'altruistic'" indicates that there is a perception of different levels of altruism, that the giving kidney to a stranger is more altruistic than giving it to an intimate.

But isn't it a paradox that theoretically ideal altruistic organ donation has been seen for a long time as pathological behavior, and altruistic strangers have been refused by the medical practitioners because their mental health was questioned (today, even though altruistic donors are accepted in principle, a part of their selection involves psychosocial tests). Some critics of the stranger donors refer to "the dark side of altruism" (Flescher/Worthen 2007: 31). For example, the famous case of Zell Krawinsky, a millionaire who against the wishes of his wife donated a kidney to a stranger, has been much discussed in a literature (ibid: 31–42).

Munson (2007) offers an interesting interpretation of this discussion, arguing that the debate between Ross et al. 2002 and Daar rests on a misunderstanding of the role of altruism in organ donation. According to Munson, altruism "is not a moral basis for allowing living donors"; it is "a value, but it is neither a duty nor an ethical principle, and it is a mistake to look to it to justify donation policies" (ibid: 224). Altruism may serve as an explanation of donor's motives, but it is not the moral norm for allowing donation because "a misanthrope who wants to become a donor is as acceptable as a philanthropic superstar" (ibid: 224). It is important to note that there are several ethical principles and societal values on which organ donation is based: not only altruism, but also respect for the human dignity, autonomy, equity, and justice (see also chapter 11 in this book). It is the special status that the human body holds which has, historically and today, informed many of the general public's moral intuitions against commodification of human organs.

Munson thus supports the distinction between altruism defined by motivations and altruism defined by outcome – what I have called, respectively, the narrow concept of altruism, used by ethicists and philosophers, and the broad definition, used by behavioral scientists and biologists (Sykora 2009). Others simply differentiate between motivational altruism and action/practice altruism (Moorlock et al. 2014: 134).

The crucial problem with motivational altruism is epistemological: we are not able to see the true motivations behind a particular, apparently altruistic, behavior. We can only infer indirectly from the outcome of the behavior and its context whether there is even a small theoretical possibility that that behavior could somehow be reciprocated.

Therefore, anonymous unrelated non-directed donors are called altruistic because it is impossible to imagine how this could be reciprocated or what benefit donors could have. By contrast, there are many ways in which an emotionally related donor would benefit from donating a kidney to a loved one (for example, not suffering the loss of the loved one, or being able to share a full partnership life, which is not possible when one partner is undergoing hemodialysis). Moorlock et al. (2014) criticize using motivational altruism as a criterion of altruistic donation precisely because of these epistemic difficulties (among other things); it is nearly impossible for transplantation staff to establish true altruistic motivations of donors.

3.4   The Janus-Face like Character of Altruistic Motivation: Internal/Psychological Reciprocity

In their book *The Altruistic Species*, Flescher and Worthen (2007) relate a story to illustrate the essence of psychological egoism, the enlightened self-interest philosophical theory in ethics.

The story goes like this: Abraham Lincoln, yes, that Abraham Lincoln, once argued with a fellow passenger on his way in coach across the country that all men were prompted by selfishness to do good. His fellow passenger strongly disagreed with him. By chance, they passed over a small bridge that spanned a slough. As they crossed, they heard a terrible noise made by an old sow because her piglets had got into the slough and were in danger of drowning. Lincoln immediately called out to the driver to stop for a moment. He jumped out, rescued the piglets from the mud, and placed them on the bank. When he returned, his fellow passenger said: "What have you done is absolutely against what you have just said. How did your selfishness prompt your behaviour to save these little pigs?" Lincoln's answer was that what he has done was the very essence of selfishness: "I should have had no peace of mind all day had I gone on and left that suffering old sow worrying over those pigs. I did it to get peace of mind." (ibid.: 87–88).

It has long been known that the motivations of blood, tissue, and organ donors are mixed and complex. For example, several distinct types of motives were identified among unrelated bone marrow donors, among them empathy-related motives, positive feeling (improving self-esteem), idealized helping, social obligation, and the most common (45 per cent) were exchange-related motives (donor's hope that they or their family were in a similar situation as recipients, others would do the same for them) (Switzer et al. 1997).

Based on previous works which revealed that both intended and actual blood donations increase positive mood in donors, Ferguson et al. (2008) tested the hypothesis that blood donation is more an act of benevolence than altruism. Three studies, carried out on about 1.500 subjects in total, supported their hypothesis. According to the benevolence hypothesis, both donors and recipients gain: the donor receives a personal reward (feeling good about themselves), and recipients receive a donation (ibid.: 328).

There is some experimental evidence that altruistic acts such as charitable donations involve some kind of reciprocity in form of a psychological, emotional reward. For example, in one study 19 participants could choose to either endorse or oppose societal causes by anonymously deciding to donate or refrain from donating to real charitable organizations. As they chose, their brain activity was measured by functional magnetic resonance imaging (fMRI). The authors of this study found that "the mesolimbic reward system is engaged by donations in the same way as when monetary rewards are obtained" (Moll 2006: 15623). But maybe the difference between rare unrelated non-directed donors representing genuine altruistic donors (heroic donors) and more common "less altruistic" donors to love ones is a consequence of another psycho-sociological parameter: the individual perception of social distance. Psychological experiments with altruistic kidney donors classified as extreme altruists revealed that they do not perceive social distance between self and others (Vekaria et al. 2017). In other words, they perceive others as themselves ('Love thy stranger as thyself'). If this is true, then "such blurred self-other distinctions would require a conceptual revisiting of altruism, because an overlap of one's self- and other-concepts would leave no space for other-regarding preferences" (Kalenscher 2017: 2).

It could be that such hyper altruism is one extreme of the normal distribution of humans' proclivity to cooperate, with extreme egoism, misanthropism, at the other extreme. The vast majority would be represented by area around the average corresponding to 'cooperator' or 'reciprocator'.

In another study, Marsh et al. (2014) used structural and magnetic resonance imaging (fMRI) in conjunction with behavioral tasks to explore 19 extraordinary altruists who had volunteered to donate a kidney to a stranger. They found that extraordinary altruists have larger right amygdala as well as enhanced responsiveness to fearful facial expressions. It is known that reduced amygdala and reduced responsiveness to fearful facial expressions have been observed in psychopathic individuals. They concluded that such variation in neural anatomy and functioning can be seen as a continuum, with extraordinary altruists at the one extreme and unusually callous egoists, antisocial psychopaths, at the other. The authors speculate that "[e]xtraordinary altruism in humans may be associated with variations in established neuro-cognitive phenomena that support social responsiveness and caring for others' welfare" (Marsh et al. 2014: 15039). Commenting on these findings, Greene stresses that "the observed differences between altruists and controls are matters of degree and not stark categorical differences (Greene 2014: 14967).

Such a hypothesis on altruism would perfectly accord with the model of reciprocity, which I suggested for cell, tissue, and organ donations (Sykora 2009, 2011). Here, the simple categorical dualism between altruism and market exchange based on self-interests is replaced by a continuum.

There is no doubt that cultural, ethical, and social norms stimulate cooperative human behavior. However, evolutionary psychologists and experimental economists have suggested that there are also inner biological propensities for reciprocal behavior which are responsible for our species-specific ability to be involved in very complex acts of cooperation, including indirect reciprocal interactions (Nowak/Sigmund 2005; Bowles/Gintis 2011). If there are such propensities for reciprocal behavior, as empirical research (see for example Farrel 2015) might suggest, then a nudging approach could be used to exploit these propensities in the design of more effective organ procurement policies. It is surprising that until recently almost no attention has been paid to reciprocity in public policy designing (Oliver 2017, 2019). Although, the fathers of the nudge theory, Thaler and Sunstein (2008), have already speculated about encouraging higher rate of cadaveric organ donation by changing opt-in policy to mandated choice based on our cognitive biases. However, they ignore the bioethical complexity of the issue (see chapter 3 in this book). It is yet to be empirically verified whether nudging in organ donation could use human propensities for reciprocal behavior. A much stronger criticism of the use of neurobiological proclivities to reciprocal behavior to design more efficient organ donation policies is that they are reductionist and deterministic (Campbell 2009: 21–23). But this is a strawman argument since human proclivities towards a particular behavior can hardly be equated with biological determinism.

A review of 23 studies on public attitudes to various organ procurement policies (Hoeyer at al. 2013) has found that there is broad public support for some kind of reciprocity to be a part of organ donation policies, but not so much for financial incentives or payments for organ donation. The metastudy revealed that there is a general preference for new non-financial reciprocity policies, such as removing disincentives, over policies based on financial incentives such as cash payments. Interestingly, an important factor was whether remuneration was perceived as expression of fairness (thus a form of reciprocity) or as an incentive.

3.5 Reciprocity, Exchange, and Market

The common understanding of reciprocity (reciprocate, reciprocal) implies "a relation (as in each other)", "a mutual or equivalent exchange or a paying back of what one has received ('reciprocated their hospitality by inviting them for a visit')", "mutual, joint, shared" (Concise Oxford Dictionary 1999: 1002).[11] The language, semantics, is of a great importance here, because it frames the discourse in a particular way. For example, there is a big difference between referring to kidney swapping between pairs as 'kidney exchange' (typical in the USA) or 'kidney sharing' (in Europe).

Although an organ market is generally considered to be immoral, several authors argue that a system which would provide financial rewards to donors is morally justified, especially in case of living donors, who put themselves at a non-trivial health risk (e.g. Radcliffe-Richards et al. 1998; Dijk/Hilhorst 2007). Many authors propose a softer alternative of a regulated market. In the so-called ethically regulated organ market, organs would be bought from donors for a fair price by a non-profit organization; however, the organs would not be sold to recipients but instead allocated according to medical criteria. Money for buying organs would come from health insurance companies and charities (Erin/Harris 2002).

But the principal objection to any kind of market, regulated or unregulated, is that it transforms human organs into commodities – and it is not acceptable to commodify the human body because of its inherent dignity (see also chapter 11 in this book).

One of the biggest problems with the use of reciprocity as a basis for organ donation policy is that it is usually equated with exchange, in particular market exchange. And if market exchange is not allowed for organ procurement, then organ procurement based on reciprocity should not be allowed. But this argument is not valid because reciprocity should not be equated with market exchange. For sociologists and anthropologists, exchange, along with reciprocity, have much broader meanings. Indeed, they are considered to be the basis on which the entire social and ethical life of civilization rests. Social exchange theory describes human social behavior from the perspective

---

11 Cp. https://www.merriam-webster.com/dictionary/reciprocate (accessed June 29, 2020).

of social exchange and reciprocity; the exchange of goods at the market is just a very small part of it (Cook/Rice 2006).

Indirect reciprocity plays a crucial role in human societal solidarity, and it is behind many modern welfare state policies, such as the tax, pension, and health care systems. Komter has explored the relationship between the gift giving and solidarity, asking whether they are any similarities "[B]etween donating blood and being a union member?" (2006: 203). In her study she noticed that when respondents expressed motives for gift giving that they believed were purely altruistic – friendship, love, gratitude, respect, loyalty, or solidarity – they may have had a strategic aim. According to Komter's analysis, reciprocity is a key and most effective factor in "creating the cement of society" because reciprocity is "the elegant combination of self-interested concerns with the requirements of social life" (ibid).

And finally, modern economists also see reciprocity in a much wider context than just a synonym for the exchange of goods. For example, according to renowned economist Serge-Christophe Kolm (2006), it has become common after WWII to distinguish three types of economic systems: exchange (referring to market exchange), redistribution, and reciprocity. In his comprehensive study on reciprocity from the economic point of view, he refers to reciprocity as "one of the main basic social relations that constitute societies" (ibid.: 375). Thus reciprocity "consists of being favorable to others because others are favorable to you" (ibid.).

4.   Altruism, Kidney Exchange, and Reciprocity in Transplantation Medicine

4.1   Is Kidney Exchange Morally Wrong because it is not Altruistic?

Having shown how confusing the use of concept of altruism in transplantation ethics could be, I now turn to the analysis of the kidney exchange concept from the perspective of altruism. Altruism is by definition an ethical barrier to commodification of human organs; altruistic organ donation is usually understood as the antithesis to buying and selling human organs. Obviously, commercial relations between seller and buyer are not based on altruism but on self-interest. Critics of KE argue that this system is not based on altruism: although kidneys are not exchanged for money, they are still exchanged, in what amounts to a form of kidney barter. This is a form of non-monetary market, and therefore KE is a commodification of kidneys.

In the USA, the question of whether KE procedures can be introduced at transplantation centers is not just ethical, it is also legal. Would KE be compatible with the federal organ donation legislation (The National Organ Transplant Act, NOTA), which bans organ markets? Therefore, opponents of the KE scheme, such as Menikoff, see it as "a quasi-contractual arrangement", and although "no money changes hands," it is "a step toward for-profit transactions, and it threatens to undermine the organ donor system" (1999: 28), which is based on altruistic donation. However, after several years of debate, legislators finally declared that KE procedures were compatible with the NOTA (an amendment to the NOTA declaring it was fully compatible with KE had to be added). With this change, proponents of organ markets now argue that because kidney exchange procedures are legal, kidney markets should be too. Such an argument, of course, is also used by critics of KE, who argue that the system's market-like character means that it should *not* be legalized.

The word exchange in the term "kidney paired exchange" is the main reason that KE could be so easily classified as barter. Because economists classify barter as a form of trade, critics of KE argue that although it involves no selling and buying, it is in fact a form of kidney market: "From an economic point of view, a kidney exchange is one of the purest forms of trade." (Sönmez/Ünver 2017: 681).

Even if we do not agree that kidney barter is a form of trade, we still encounter an ethical problem because of the reciprocal relations underpinning KE. For defenders of genuine altruism in organ donation, KE represents the gradual slide down the slippery slope towards an organ market and the commodification of the human body. In their view, the pragmatic and utilitarian justifications cannot counterbalance the abandoning of the ethical principle of altruism.

4.2   Towards Indirect Reciprocity Model

Minerva et al. (2019) argue against the accusation that the GKE program is unethical because it is a form of organ trafficking and involves exploitation of the poor, coercion, and the commodification of transplant organs. They defend GKE as non-commercial, arguing that any money involved is used solely to cover the cost of the transplantation, not to buy organs. They also refer to the altruistic motivation of all donors participating in GKE to help a loved one; *a fortiori* GKE cannot be considered to be a form of organ sale: "[T]he motivation of all donors involved in the GKE, whether in high income or low income countries, is not financial gain, but altruistic: to help a loved one to survive kidney failure." (ibid.: 1776).

In kidney exchange, a donor does not directly donate to a loved one but to an unrelated recipient in another donor/recipient pair. However, because they donate on the condition that their loved one receive a kidney in return, their primary motivation is not to help an unrelated person but rather their loved one. In KE the formula could be: 'You give your kidney to my loved one and I'll give my kidney to your loved one', a variation of "You scratch my back and I'll scratch yours" – a classic expression of reciprocal altruism.

There is empirical support for the claim that reciprocity, not altruistic giving, is fundamental to KE programs. According surveys, most KE donors would not be likely to donate to their respective recipients without a kidney being designated to their partners. As Toews et al. point out: "Donation through kidney paired donors is done in exchange for – and with expectation of – a reciprocal kidney donation and transplantation." (2017: 1996) In fact, one of the reasons why two- or three-way KE are performed simultaneously is so that donors do not have the chance to withdraw after their loved one receives their transplant.

The Nuffield Report on the Human Body (2011), prepared by the highly respected the UK Nuffield Council on Bioethics, is clear about the reciprocal character of KE: kidney exchange is underpinned by the "value of reciprocity", the donor/recipient pairs enter "a reciprocal arrangement" (ibid: 121). The Report documents a significant shift in organ and tissue donation discourse from pure altruism to the acceptance of some forms of reciprocity – since there is a close connection between reciprocity and solidarity, and solidarity and altruism are seen as overlapping concepts.

5.   Conclusion

The current system of organ procurement based on altruistic organ donation is considered by many to be "a qualified failure" (Satel et al. 2014: 217), and the most common suggested solution is to replace it with some form of organ market scheme. I have argued that we need to stop thinking in this dichotomy, and I have proposed a new approach to the organ shortage problem based on indirect reciprocity. Such a model would not be altruistic (although it would incorporate altruistic organ donation), but neither would it be based on commercialization of organ procurement.

I argue here that the fundamental human propensities for reciprocal behavior (explored by experimental economists and behavioral psychologists) could become an important part of the complex motivations behind organ donation, and could dramatically increase the number of donors. If the organ procurement policy is set up so that it would be in a person's self-interest to commit to organ donation, this should translate into higher organ procurement and therefore more transplantations. The blurred line between reciprocity and market exchange is probably the main reason why various new policy proposals to stimulate motivation through some kind of reciprocity are viewed with great distrust and fear of organ commercialization.

The borderline between altruism and reciprocity is also blurred. I have explored here the ambiguity of altruistic motivations, and the relationship between altruism and reciprocity in both unrelated non-directed living donors (heroic altruistic donors) as well as emotionally related directed living donors. Complex motivations of emotionally related directed donors, who are willing to give organs to a loved one but not to a stranger, involve an important aspect of reciprocity, in which genuine concern for the well-being of the loved person merges with self-interest.

Next, I analyzed indirect reciprocal relations between donors and recipients from immunologically incompatible donor/recipient pairs participating in KE transplantation programs. KE is a very successful innovation in living organ donation with great potential to increase the organ procurement rate. In my interpretation, the very essence of kidney exchange policy is indirect reciprocal relations between donors and recipients (with important exception of bridge donors).

The concept of altruism has been used recently to defend GKE programs from the accusation that they are a kind of organ market, organ trafficking (Minerva et al. 2019). The authors argue that GKE cannot be organ trafficking because all donors involved in GKE have altruistic motivations (to help a loved one). I agree that GKE is not an organ market, but not because kidney donation in KE is altruistic; rather, there is no organ selling and buying in GKE or other forms of KE. I argued KE programs are an example of a reciprocal donation model, not an altruistic one. This raises a question: Can KE be ethically justified if it is not based on altruistic organ donation? I argued that it can, but indirect reciprocity has to be at first accepted as a moral practice.

Because the concept of altruism is often used vaguely, and ideologically, I started by revisiting and rethinking the roots of the concept's ambiguities. I call this exploration a prolegomena for any future proposals of organ procurement policies based on reciprocity.

After some preliminary clarification of the relationship between altruism, reciprocity, and exchange, I focused on kidney exchange. I had two reasons: First, kidney exchange transplantations are the most important recent innovation in the policy of organ procurement and have great potential. Second, the moral status of kidney exchange is controversial. Although they have been accepted in some countries, after several years of discussion, as being compatible with the altruistic model of organ donation, their critics argue that they are a form of organ barter; and since economists consider barter to be a form of non-monetary market, kidney exchanges are not compatible with altruistic model and should not be allowed.

By contrast, I argued that organ donation based on indirect reciprocity can be ethically justified, outlining the kind of analysis that is required for such a justification. I have focused on living organ donations, but I believe that philosophy of organ donation based on indirect reciprocity is also applicable to deceased organ donations. Once indirect reciprocity is accepted to be as moral as altruism, then various new organ procurement policies based on indirect reciprocity, both from living or deceased donors, will be accepted and implemented.

Acknowledgments

I would like to thank both anonymous reviewers for their insightful comments on the paper, which have helped me improve the work.

This work was supported by VEGA No. 1/0563/18 grant from the Ministry of Education, Slovak Republic.

References

Beard, T. Randolph/Kaserman, David/Osterkamp, Rigmar (2013): The Global Organ Shortage: Economic Causes, Human Consenquences, Policy Responses, California: Stanford University Press.

Bowles, Samuel/Gintis, Herbert (2011): A Cooperative Species: Human Reciprocity and Its Evolution, Oxford: Oxford University Press.

Campbell, Alastair V. (2009): The Body in Bioethics. New York: Routledge-Cavendish.

Childress, James F. (1986): "The Gift of Life. Ethical problems and Policies in Obtaining and Distributing Organs for Transplantation." In: Critical Care Clinics 2/1, pp. 133–148.

Cohon, Rachel (2018): "Hume's Moral Philosophy." In: Edward N. Zalta (ed.), The Stanford Encyclopedia of Philosophy. Available at: https://plato.stanford.edu/archives/fall2018/entries/hume-moral/ (accessed June 29, 2020)

The Concise Oxford Dictionary (1999), Oxford: Clarendon Press.

Cook, Karen/Rice, Eric (2006): "Social Exchange Theory." In: John DeLamater (ed.), Handbook of Social Psychology, Dordrecht: Springer, pp. 53–76.

Cook, Harrison (2018): "Nation's Longest Kidney Transplant Chain Surpasses 100 donations." In: Becker' Clinical Leadership and Infection Control. Available at: https://www.beckershospitalreview.com/quality/nation-s-longest-kidney-transplant-chain-surpasses-100-donations.html. (accessed March 31, 2020)

Crouch, Robert A./Elliott, Carl (1999): "Moral Agency and the Family: the Case of Living Related Organ Transplantation." In: Cambridge Quarterly of Health Care Ethics 8, pp. 275–287.

Daar, Abdallah S. (2002): "Strangers, Intimates, and Altruism in Organ Donation." In: Transplantation 74/3, pp. 424-426.

Dalal, Aparna R. (2015): "Philosophy of Organ Donation: Review of Ethical Facets." In: World Journal of Transplant 5/2, pp. 44–51.

De Wispelaere, Jurgen (2004): "Altruism, Impartiality and Moral Demands." In: Jonathan Seglow (ed.), The Ethics of Altruism, London: Frank Cass, pp. 11–12.

Dijk, van Gert/Hilhorst, Medard T. (2007): "Financial Incentives for Organ Donation. An Investigation of the Ethical Issues." In: Centre for Ethics and Health (ed.), Ethics and Health Monitoring Report, The Hague.

Domínguez-Gil, Beatriz/Matesanz, Rafael (eds.) (2018): "Newsletter Transplant: International Figures on Donation and Transplantation 2017." In: European Directorate for the Quality of Medicine and Health Care 23, pp. 1–86. Available at: http://www.ont.es/publicaciones/Documents/NewsleTTER%202018%20final%20CE.pdf. (accessed March 31, 2020)

Dor, Frank J./Massey, Emma K./Frunza, Mihaela/Johnson, Rachel/Lennerling, Annette/Lovén, Charlotte/Mamode, Nizam/Pascalev, Assya/Sterckx, Sigrid/Van Assche, Kristof/Zuidema, Wilij C./Weimar, Willem (2011): "New Classification of ELPAT for Living Organ Donation." In: Transplantation 91/9, pp. 935–938.

Erin, Charles A./Harris, John (2003): "An Ethical Market in Human Organs." In: Journal of Medical Ethics 29, pp. 137–138.

Farell, Anne-Maree (2015): "Addressing Organ Shortage: are Nudges the Way Forward?" In: Law, Innovation and Technology 7/2, pp. 253–282.

Ferguson, Eamonn/Farrell, Kelly/Lawrence, Claire (2008): "Blood Donation is an Act of Benevolence Rather Than Altruism." In: Health Psychology 27/3, pp. 327–336.

Ferguson, Eamonn (2015): "Mechanism of Altruism Approach to Blood Donor Recruitment and Retention: a Review and Future Directions." In: Transfusion Medicine 25/4, pp. 211–226.

Flescher, Andrew M./Worthen, Daniel L. (2007): The Altruistic Species. Scientific, Philosophical, and Religious Perspectives of Human Benevolence, Philadelphia/London: Templeton Foundation Press.

Gillespie, Ryan (2019): "What Money Cannot Buy and what Money Ought not Buy: Dignity, Motives, and Markets in Human Organ Procurement Debates." In: The Journal of Medical Humanities 40, pp. 101–116.

Gohh, Reginald Y./Morrissey, Paul E./Madras, Peter N./Monaco, Anthony P. (2001): "Controversies in Organ Donation: the Altruistic Living Donor." In: Nephrology Dialysis Transplantation 16, pp. 619–621.

Greene, Joshua (2014): "From Fear Recognition to Kidney Donation." In: Proceedings of the National Academy of Sciences of the United States of America 111/42, pp. 14966–14967.

Hansen, Solveig L./Eisner, Marthe I./Pfaller, Larissa/Schicktanz, Silke (2018): "Are You In or Are You Out?! Moral Appeals to the Public in Organ Donation Poster Campaigns: A Multimodal and Ethical Analysis." In: Health Communication 23/8, pp. 1020–1034.

Healy, Kieran/Krawiec, Kimberly D. (2012): "Custom, Contract, and Kidney Exchange." In: Duke Law Journal 62/3, pp. 102-126.

Hoeyer, Klaus/Schicktanz, Silke/Deleuran, Ida (2013): "Public Attitudes to Financial Incentive Models for Organs: a Literature Review Suggests that it is Time to Shift the Focus from 'Financial Incentives' to 'Reciprocity'." In: Transplant International 26/4, pp. 350–357.

Jawoniyi, Oluwafunmilayo/Gormley, Kevin/McGleenan, Emma/Noble, Helen Rose (2018): "Organ Donation and Transplantation: Awareness and Roles of Healthcare Professionals – A Systematic Literature Review." In: Journal of Clinical Nursing 27, pp. e726–e738.

Jollimore, Troy (2020): "Impartiality." In: Edward N. Zalta (ed.), The Stanford Encyclopedia of Philosophy. Available at: https://plato.stanford.edu/archives/sum2020/entries/impartiality/ (accessed June 29, 2020)

Kalenscher, Tobias (2017): "Love Thy Stranger as Thyself." In: Nature Human Behaviour 1/0108. DOI: 10.1038/s41562-017-0108.

Kolber, Adam Jason (2003): "A Matter of Priority: Transplanting Organs Preferentially to Registered Donors." In: Rutgers Law Review 55, pp. 671–739.

Kolm, Serge-Christophe (2006): "Introduction to the Economics of Giving, Altruism and Reciprocity." In: Serge-Christophe Kolm/Jean Mercier Ythier (eds.), Handbook of the Economics of Giving, Altruism and Reciprocity, Volume 1, North Holland: Elsevier, pp. 1–122.

Komter, Aafke E. (2006): Social Solidarity and the Gift, Cambridge: Cambridge University Press.

Kraut, Richard (2018): "Altruism." In: Edward N. Zalta (ed.), The Stanford Encyclopedia of Philosophy. Available at: https://plato.stanford.edu/archives/spr2018/entries/altruism/ (accessed June 29, 2020)

Lavee, Jacob/Ashkenazi, Tamar/Gurman, Gabriel/Steinberg, David (2010): "A New Law for Allocation of Donor Organs in Israel." In: The Lancet 375, pp. 1131–1133.

Marsh, Abigail A./Stoycos, Sarah A./Brethel-Haurwitz, Kristin M./Robinson, Paul/VanMeter, John W./Cardinale, Elise M. (2014): "Neural and Cognitive Characteristics of Extraordinary Altruists." In: Proceedings of the National Academy of Sciences of the United States of America 111/42, pp. 15036–15041.

Matesanz, Rafael/Domínguez-Gil, Beatriz/Coll, Elisabeth/Mahíllo, Beatriz/Marazuela, Rosario (2017): "How Spain Reached 40 Deceased Organ Donors per Million Population." In: American Journal of Transplantation 17, pp. 1447–1454.

Mauss, Marcel (1954): The Gift, London: Routledge.

Menikoff, Jerry (1999): "Organ Swapping." In: The Hastings Center Report 29, pp. 28–33.

Minerva, Francesca/Savulescu, Julian/Singer, Peter (2019): "The Ethics of the Global Kidney Exchange Programme." In: The Lancet 394/10210, pp. 1775–1778.

Moll, Jorge/Krueger, Frank/Zahn, Roland/Pardini, Matteo/De Oliviera-Souza, Ricardo/Grafman, Jordan (2006): "Human Fronto-mesolimbic Networks Guide Decisions about Charitable Donations." In: Proceedings of the National Academy of Sciences of the United States of America 103, pp. 15623–15628.

Montgomery, Robert A/Gentry, Sommer E/Marks, William H/Warren, Daniel S/Hiller, Janet/Houp, Julie/Zachary, Andrea A/Melancon, J Keith/Maley, Warren R/Rabb, Hamid /Simpkins, Christopher/Segev, Dorry L (2006). "Domino paired kidney donation: a strategy to make best use of live non-directed donation." Lancet 368, pp. 419-21.

Moorlock, Greg/Ives, Jonathan/Draper, Heather (2014): "Altruism in Organ Donation: an Unnecessary Requirement?" In: Journal of Medical Ethics 40, pp. 134–138.

Munson, Ronald (2007): "Organ Transplantation." In: Bonnie Steinbock (ed.), The Oxford Handbook of Bioethics, Oxford: Oxford University Press, pp. 211–239.

Nadel, Mark S./Nadel, Carolina A. (2005): "Using Reciprocity To Motivate Organ Donations." In: Yale Journal of Health Policy, Law, and Ethics 5/1, pp. 293–325.

Nuffield Council on Bioethics (2011): Human Bodies: Donation for Medicine and Research, London.

Nelson, Mark T. (1991): "The Morality of Free Market for Transplant Organs." In: Public Affairs Quarterly 5, pp. 63–79.

Nowak, Martin A./Sigmund, Karl (2005): "Evolution of Indirect Reciprocity." In: Nature 437, pp. 1291–1298.

Oliver, Adam (2017): "Do Unto Others: On the Importance of Reciprocity in Public Administration." In: The American Review of Public Administration 48, pp. 279–290.

Oliver, Adam (2019): Reciprocity and the Art of Behavioural Public Policy, Cambridge: Cambridge University Press.

Radcliffe-Richards, Janet/Daar, Abdallah S./Guttmann, Ronald D./Hoffenberg, Raymond/Kennedy, Ian/Lock, Martin/Sells, Robert A./Tilney, Nicholas (1998): "The Case for Allowing Kidney Sales. International Forum for Transplant Ethics." In: Lancet 351/9120, pp. 1950–1952.

Rees, Michael A./Kopke, Jonathan E./Pelletier, Ronald P. et al. (2009): "A Nonsimultaneous, Extended, Altruisic-Donor Chain." In: New England Journal of Medicine 360, pp. 1096–1101.

Rees, Michael A./Dunn, Ty B./Kuhr, Christian S./Marsh, Christopher L./Rogers, Jeffrey/Rees, Susan E./Cicero, Arrigo/Reece, Laurie J./Roth, Alvin E./Ekwenna, Obi/Fumo, David E./Krawiec, Kimberly D./Kopke, Jonathan E./Jain, Samay/Tan, Miquel/Paloyo, Siegfredo R. (2017): "Kidney Exchange to Overcome Financial Barries to Kidney Transplantation." In: American Journal of Transplantation 17, pp. 782–790.

Ross, Lainie F./Rubin, David T./Siegler, Mark/Josephson, Michelle. A./Thistlethwaite, Richard/Woodle, E. Steve (1997): "Ethics of a Paired-Kidney-Exchange Program." In: The New England Journal of Medicine 336, pp. 1752–1755.

Ross, Lainie F./Glannon, Walter/Josephson, Michelle A./Thistlethwaite, J. Richard Jr. (2002): "Should all Living Donors be Treated Equally?" In: Transplantation 74/3, pp. 418–421.

Satel, Sally/Morrison, Joshua C./Jones, Rick K. (2014): "State Organ-Donation Incentives under the National Organ Transplant Act." In: Law & Contemporary Problemss 77, pp. 217–252.

Sharp, Chloe/Randhawa, Gurch (2014): "Altruism, Gift Giving and Reciprocity in Organ Donation: A Review of Cultural Perspectives and Challenges of the Concepts." In: Transplantation Reviews 28, pp. 163–168.

Siegal, Gill/Bonnie, Richard J. (2006): "Closing the Organ Gap: A Reciprocity-Based Social Contract Approach." In: Journal of Law, Medicine and Ethics 34, pp. 415–423.

Sönmez, Tayfun/Ünver, Utku M. (2017): "Market Design for Living-Donor Organ Exchanges: an Economic Policy Perspective." In: Oxford Review of Economic Policy 33, pp. 676–704.

Sýkora, Peter (2009): "Altruism in Medical Donations Reconsidered: the Reciprocity Approach." In: Michael Steinmann/Peter Sýkora/Urban Wiesing (eds.), Altruism

Reconsidered: Exploring New Approaches to Property in Human Tissue, Aldershot: Ashgate, pp. 13–50.

Sýkora, Peter (2011): "Altruism: Reciprocity/Solidarity Approach." In: Willem Weimar/ Michael A. Bos/Jan J. Van Busschbach (eds.), Organ Transplantation: Ethical, Legal and Psychosocial Aspect. Expanding the European Platform, Lengerich/Berlin: Pabst, pp. 365–369.

Switzer, Galen E./Dew, Mary A./Butterworth, Victoria A./Simmons, Roberta G./ Schimmel, Mindy (1997): "Understanding Donor's Motivations: A Study of Unrelated Bone Marrow Donors." Social Science & Medicine 45/1, pp. 137–147.

Tabarrok, Alexander (2002): "The Organ Shortage: A Tragedy of the Commons." In: Alexander Tabarrok (ed.), Entrepreneurial Economics: Bright Ideas from the Dismal Science, Oxford: Oxford University Press, pp. 107–113.

Thaler, Richard H./Sunstein, Cass R. (2008): Nudge: Improving Decisions about Health, Wealth, and Happiness, New Haven: Yale University Press.

Thorne, Emanuel D. (2006): "The Ecomonics of Organ Transplantation." In: Serge-Christophe Kolm/Jean Mercier Ythier (eds.), Handbook of the Economics of Giving, Altruism and Reciprocity 2, Amsterdam: Elsevier, pp. 1335–1370.

Titmuss, Richard M. (1970): The Gift Relationship: From Human Blood to Social Policy, London: Allen and Unwin.

Toews, Maeghan/Giancaspro, Mark/Richards, Bernadette/Ferrari, Paolo (2017): "Kidney Paired Donation and the Valuable Consideration Problem." In: Transplantation 101, pp. 1996–2002.

Veach, Robert M./Ross, Lainie F. (2015): Transplantation Ethics, 2nd edition, Washington: Georgetown University Press.

Veale, Jeffrey L./Capron, Alexander/Nassiri, Nima/Danovitch, Gabriel/Gritsch, H. Albin/Waterman, Amy/Del Pizzo, Joseph/Hu, Jim C./Pycia, Marek/McGuire, Suzanne/Charlton, Marian/Kapur, Sandip (2009): "Vouchers for Future Kidney Transplants to Overcome 'Chronological Incompatibility' Between Living Donors and Recipients." In: Transplantation 101, pp. 2115–2119.

Vekaria, Kruti M./Brethel-Haurwitz, Kristin M./Cardinale, Elise M./Stoycos, Sarah A./ Marsh, Abigail A. (2017): "Social Discounting and Distance Perceptions in Costly Altruism." In: Nature Human Behaviour 1/0100, https://doi.org/10.1038/s41562-017-0100.

Wallis, C. Bradley/Samy, Kannan P./Roth, Alvin E./Rees, Michael A. (2011): "Kidney Paired Donation." In: Nephrology Dialysis Transplantation 26, pp. 2091–2099.

Zaltzman, Jeffrey (2018): "Ten Years of Israel's Organ Transplant Law: is it on the Right Track?" In: Israel Journal of Health Policy Research 7/1, pp. 1–3.

11. Selling Organs
Dignity as a Further Concern

Zümrüt Alpınar-Şencan

1. Introduction: Occurrence of the Problem

Over the past few decades, transplantation has become a unique cure and successful treatment for people suffering from an end-stage organ failure. The demand for organs for transplantation is increasing daily, with ever-growing waiting lists of patients in need of an organ to regain their health.[1]

The shortage of organs is a major global health problem. Apart from systems of postmortem organ donation aiming to increase the number of organs donated after death, living donation is an alternative for people who are waiting for a suitable organ to be transplanted. Although it is a promoted social practice, living donation does not solve the problem brought about by the shortage of organs. Many factors influence both living and deceased donation rates, such as the religious stance and cultural reasons as well as a mistrust in the health care system, ignorance about the organ donation system (Irving et al. 2012) and a lack of awareness regarding the importance of donating organs. Due to the insufficient number of donated organs and the high demand for new organs to be transplanted, new solutions to get over this scarcity come to the fore. To increase the number of organs donated, financial incentives are used, such as tax reductions, payments covering funeral expenses made to the donor's family as well as nonfinancial incentives, such as giving priority to patients on waiting lists who have signed a donor card, as is the case in Israel (Statz 2006; Levy 2018). Because of the shortage, people suffering from end-stage organ failure started to look for organs abroad, which led to an international trade in organs involving commercial transactions (Shimazono 2007). The concern over the purchase of organs is expressed by World Health Assembly's 2004 and 2010 resolutions (WHA 57.18 and WHA 63.22). In May 2010, the sixty-third World Health Assembly endorsed the World Health Organizations (WHO)'s Guiding Principles on Human Cell, Tissue and Organ Transplantation that forbade organ selling and urged its member states to take measures to prevent commercial organ transactions. Maximization of postmortem organ donation is

---

1 Based on OPTN (The Organ Procurement and Transplantation Network) data of April 15, 2019. In the United States of America, for example, as of January 2019, there are more than 113.000 people on the waiting list. In 2018, 36.528 transplants were performed, based on OPTN data as of January 16, 2019.

also promoted as an ethically acceptable alternative for addressing the organ shortage. Many countries banned commercial transactions of organs, however, because of the demand, the illegal trafficking and trade in organs is pushed further underground.

2.   Organ Trade is a Fact

The scarcity of organs and the growing ease of Internet communication led to transplant tourism[2] and organ trafficking[3]. Even though comprehensive, precise data about organ trafficking is not available, according to a WHO report, it is estimated that nearly around 10.000 illegal kidney transplantations take place every year (Campbell/ Davison 2012). The fact of organ trade has been reported from various countries and regions in the last decades: in Indonesia, for instance, people waiting for a kidney transplant refer to online social media (i.e. Facebook) to look for 'donors' with a price range from 9270US$ to 32.430US$ (Shelton et al. 2018). In a paper by Yosuke Shimazono (2007), it is reported that some websites offer "transplant packages" for people waiting for an organ, which include kidneys, lungs, livers, pancreases or hearts with a range from 70.000US$ to 160.000US$. Such websites are used to attract foreign recipients (i.e. patients) to have their transplantations in China, Pakistan and the Philippines (ibid). These transactions cannot be said to be profitable for the *donors*. For instance, whereas the patients travelling to China, Pakistan or to India pay up to 200.000US$ to purchase a kidney, the *donor* is paid around 5000US$ or even less (Campbell/Davison 2012). It has been reported that the recipients from Australia, Europe, the Middle East and the United States pay up to 40.000US$ to obtain a kidney from a Pakistani, who is paid about 1000US$ to 2000US$ (Garwood 2007: 6). Due to the civil war in Syria, it was reported that refugees, who fled to Lebanon, sold their kidneys to brokers for 7000US$ in order to survive, which were purchased by the customer for 15.000US$ (Putz 2013). Recently, Egypt is a growing center for organ trafficking, in which African refugees are the victims of illegal organ harvesting (Baraaz 2018; Columb 2019).

It is not only the recipients that move globally, but also the live *donors*. For instance, in the mid-1990s, some Israeli patients travelled to Turkey to have their operations when they were matched with *donors* from Moldova, Romania and Russia (Scheper-Hughes 2003; Rohter 2004). In 2014, police broke an organ trafficking ring, in which Vietnamese were brought to China to sell their kidneys (Tram/Tung 2014).

---

2   "Travel for transplantation [which 'is the movement of persons across jurisdictional borders for transplantation purposes'] becomes transplant tourism, and thus unethical, if it involves trafficking in persons for the purpose of organ removal or trafficking in human organs, or if the resources (organs, professionals and transplant centers) devoted to providing transplants to non-resident patients undermine the country's ability to provide transplant services for its own population." (The Transplantation Society and International Society of Nephrology 2018: 2–3)

3   "Trafficking in persons for the purpose of organ removal is the recruitment, transportation, transfer, harboring, or receipt of persons, by means of the threat or use force or other forms of coercion, of abduction, of fraud, of deception, of the abuse power or of a position of vulnerability, or of the giving or receiving of payments or benefits to achieve the consent of a person having control over another person, for the purpose of the removal of organs." (The Transplantation Society and International Society of Nephrology 2018: 2)

In the media, it is reported that black market transactions are taking place in some private hospitals, performed by professional surgeons to this day. In a *Guardian* article, David Smith (2010) reports that a South African hospital, Netcare, which is the largest private hospital network in South Africa and the United Kingdom, "took part in an international scam that allegedly saw poor Brazilians and Romanians paid 6000US$ (3840£) for their kidneys to be transplanted to wealthy Israelis". In 2003, it emerged that this hospital network was taking part in organ trafficking:

> Investigators said Brazilians who passed a medical checkup were flown to South Africa, where their kidneys were extracted for transplants into Israeli patients. [...] It is believed more than 100 illegal kidney transplants were performed at Netcare's St. Augustine Hospital in the eastern coastal city of Durban in 2001 and 2002. (Bryson 2010)

In a more recent article, it is reported that by bribing doctors and government officials, a broker flew the British patients to India and Nepal to have their illegal kidney transplants in private hospitals (Kelly 2019).

Journalist Haroon Siddique (2011) reported that a Turkish doctor was arrested on suspicion of illegally procuring kidneys and transplanting them to patients in exchange for high financial gains. The EU prosecutor Jonathan Ratel stated that "poor people were lured to Pristina 'with false promise of payments' for their kidneys and patients from Canada, Germany, Poland and Israel paid up to 90.000€ (76.400£) for the black-market kidneys" (ibid).

All these cases show the cruel and devastating phenomena of organ trafficking and transplant tourism, the desperation of both patients and vendors, and demonstrate how black markets work globally. In order to avoid such black markets and the undesirable harm and exploitation that results from illegal organ markets, some have proposed to establish legally regulated organ markets. It is stated that having legal markets is a way to avoid the scarcity of the transplantable organs and to protect the vendors.

3.   An Overview of the Moral Arguments in the Debate

As Budiani-Saberi and Delmonico point out, "the commercial transaction is a central aspect of organ trafficking; the organ becomes a commodity and financial considerations become the priority for the involved parties instead of the health and well-being of the donors and recipients" (2008: 926). Buying and selling human organs raises ethically challenging questions and moral concerns. As Alpinar-Sencan et al. (2017) point out, the arguments in the debate offered by the opponents are mostly founded on contingent factors, such as the possible undesirable outcomes, the motives or reasons for participating and the conditions under which the practice takes place. The generally adopted principles of biomedical ethics, namely autonomy, beneficence, non-maleficence, justice, and plausible moral concerns, such as the protection of the vulnerable, mostly guide such claims (Radcliffe-Richards 2013; Biller-Andorno/Alpinar 2014). More specifically, the objections to organ markets address harm, exploitation, coercion and its plausible effects on social values, whereas the proponents argue that none of the objections would necessarily apply in a fairly regulated market.

In this section, an overview of the moral arguments in the debate will be presented by explaining the moral concerns raised by a regulated organ market.

3.1   Harm and Benefit

The harm argument is one of the strongest objections levelled against organ selling. The main concern is that the vendors will be exposed to harm by being subjected to unnecessary risk and pain in exchange for money. How the money would influence the quality of the transplantation is one of the main concerns. Many quantitative and qualitative studies reveal the undesirable consequences of transplant tourism and black markets for the organ vendor, which will be briefly referred to below.

Organ vendors would be likely to suffer from ill health as a result of having an organ (generally a kidney) harvested. It is stated by Scheper-Hughes (2003) that studies considering vendors in India, Iran, the Philippines and Moldova showed that vendors of kidneys suffer from chronic pain and ill health (see also, Naqvi et al. 2007; Zargooshi 2001a; Goyal et al. 2002; Budiani-Saberi/Delmonico 2008; Padilla 2009). Those who were interviewed in Brazil, Turkey, Moldova and Manila stated that they had not seen a doctor or been treated after the operation's first year, even at the hospitals where the operations took place. Some of them were ashamed to appear in public clinics while others feared receiving bad news, since they might not be able to afford the required medication and treatments (Scheper-Hughes 2003).

Here, one can raise a question whether the medical outcomes of commercial transaction would be worse for the 'donor' compared to non-commercial practice. Although the practice, that is, the extraction of an organ, is the same, it is the conditions under which the operation takes place and the quality of the follow-up care that make the difference, leading the commercial donors to suffer from a worse condition after operation compared to noncommercial donors. It should be noted that living (non-commercial) donation is not risk-free either: the quality of the life of the donor could be decreased and the donor might suffer from function losses. According to some studies, this is not necessarily the case (Beavers et al. 2001; Reese et al. 2015). However, some studies showed that among some diverse subpopulations (i.e. underrepresented minority groups) donor groups showed more likelihood of post-donation complexities, such as hypertension and kidney failure (Lentine/Patel 2012; Lentine/Segev 2013). Receiving full medical reimbursement and life-long follow-up care provision is crucial (Morgan and Ibrahim 2011), which also points to the influence of the socio-economic condition of the donor.

Although most concerns are raised about the outcomes of this practice regarding the vendors, some of these studies' focus is on the graft survival rates and patients' (i.e. receivers') health conditions after having their transplantations abroad. Most of these studies show that the outcomes of overseas (commercial) transplants are lower than expected by showing that those patients had a more complex post-transplantation course with higher incidence of acute rejection and infectious complications (Cohen 2009; Alghamdi et al. 2010; Rizvi et al. 2009a; Rizvi et al. 2009b). This outcome is likely because the quality of the organ obtained from the poor vendor is likely to suffer in a market setting. Some others argued that it is not necessarily hazardous for the patient to have a kidney transplant abroad (either commercial or not) *only if* the patients come back with some information about the operation they had and have an early postoperative period, which is an important factor in influencing the graft-survival rates (Geddes et al. 2008).

In addition to the outcomes showing how the vendors' and recipients' health conditions are influenced, the possible undesirable outcomes related to the vendors' socio-economic conditions should also be considered.

In addition to harm based on health conditions, it is also highly doubtful whether the vendors would benefit financially from the transaction, as proponents of market schemes argue. Studies show that there is a decrease or no improvement in the vendors' economic conditions. For instance, according to a study by Naqvi et al. (2007), despite being one of the largest centers of commerce centers for kidney transplantation, kidney vendors in Pakistan had no economic improvement in their lives, contrary to their expectations (see also, Zargooshi 2001a; Goyal et al. 2002; Scheper-Hughes 2003; Budiani-Saberi/Delmonico 2008; Padilla 2009; Cohen 2009; Rizvi et al. 2009b). Furthermore, since the vendors do not get sufficient postoperative care, they could not work effectively and hence suffered from unemployment (Zargooshi 2001a; Scheper-Hughes 2003). This promotes or even strengthens the cycle of debt and poverty the vendors are in and which they want to break through by participating in such transactions in the first place.

The vendors faced psychological problems, such as serious depression, a loss of self-respect, a sense of worthlessness and social isolation (Zargooshi, 2001a; Scheper-Hughes 2003; Budiani-Saberi/Delmonico 2008). Additionally, some of them regretted having been a vendor (Zargooshi 2001a; Zargooshi 2001b; Budiani-Saberi/Delmonico 2008; Padilla 2009). Thus, the harm produced is not limited to vendors' deteriorated health and financial status, but also includes psychological and social harm. "Although many individuals have benefited from the ability to purchase the organs they need, the social harm produced to the donors, their families, and their communities gives sufficient reason for pause." (Scheper-Hughes 2003: 1647)

Contrary to these facts reported, both by the quantitative and qualitative studies, on a theoretical level, some claim that harmful outcomes could only be avoided by a legal, regulated market system (Kishore 2005; Daar 2006; Khamash/Gaston 2008), which means that the sales are performed under good, regulated conditions (Wilkinson 2003: 107–108; Radcliffe-Richards 2013: 48–58). In addition, it is claimed that compared to donation, sale is not more dangerous or risky and the mere fact of payment does not add any danger (Wilkinson 2003: 108). It is also argued that giving permission for organ markets would increase the range of options for financial gain open to oneself, which would be seen as an opportunity for those people to widen their limited options (Radcliffe-Richards et al. 2006).

Another hypothesis that might be considered is that regulation of the market would increase the number of organs available. This assumption might be true regardless of the quality of the organ obtained in an unregulated global market considering many desperate people's willingness to sell one of their kidneys to get out of their situation (Biller-Andorno/Alpinar 2014). However, it is doubtful whether people in a developed country with a good social security system would participate in such transactions if there were a regulated market, as a study held in Switzerland shows (Rid et al. 2009).

Very generally, opponents of organ selling claim that the ban on this practice should be kept in place due to the harmful outcomes for both vendors and recipients involved in the practice of organ selling. However, proponents generally argue that if the conditions are bettered and the practice is performed under good, regulated conditions, the harm could be avoided and the risk kept to a minimum.

3.2   Exploitation and Justice

Another concern is the danger of exploiting poor and vulnerable people, who are more likely to participate in such transactions as a last resort, to end their desperation. Some claim that having a market for human organs would lead to the exploitation of vulnerable and socio-economically disadvantaged people (Budiani-Saberi/Delmonico 2008; Tsai 2010). It should be noted that in this context and in biomedical context in general, vulnerable people stands for being "exposed to potentially harmful circumstances [...] and socioeconomically impoverished. Those who are easily susceptible to intimidation, manipulation, coercion, or exploitation are commonly classified among the vulnerable" (Beauchamp/Childress 2009: 89). Exploitation, very generally, means taking unfair advantage of others to benefit from their resources, labor and efforts.

The purchase of human organs is considered exploitative because financial considerations come to the fore in such transactions and it is very likely that mostly poor people would offer their organs for sale.[4] That is why, in the first place, the fifty-seventh World Health Assembly (WHA) in May 2004 urged its member states to "take measures to protect the poorest and vulnerable groups from 'transplant tourism' and the sale of tissues and organs" (WHA 57.18: 50). Some empirical studies also show this is the case: typically, the vendors had either decided to sell their kidneys to pay their debts, to get some money immediately (Goyal et al. 2002; Phadke/Anandh 2002; cf. Naqvi et al. 2007; Cohen 2009; Rizvi et al. 2009b) or to get out of their desperate situation (Zargooshi 2001b; Scheper-Hughes 2003; Budiani-Saberi/Delmonico 2008). In response, some argue that only with unregulated markets would exploitation continue to occur, in which only the poor sell and the rich afford the organ (Daar 2006). This states that organ selling cannot be argued to be inherently exploitative, but can be claimed to be so under certain conditions and this is not necessarily the case when it is performed under good, regulated conditions (Radcliffe-Richards 2013: 70–74; Brennan/Jaworski 2016: 20, 148). However, the practice might be argued to be "intrinsically exploitative", since it takes advantage of the desperate situation of potential victims to get their organs in exchange for money, and therefore treat body parts as if they were "sealable objects" (Andorno 2017: 123).

While it is argued that organ trade causes inequality and injustice by targeting the vulnerable and impoverished (Phadke/Anandh 2002; Delmonico 2009; Rizvi et al. 2009b), it is claimed that with a regulated market exploitation would be avoided (Cherry 2005). Erin and Harris (2003) argue that it is possible to have an ethical market if there is one national, governmental purchaser and where organs are distributed according to medical priority only. However, such assumptions should be examined closely by review of empirical data. Iran, for instance, adopted a legal, regulated model in 1988 and it seems to have eliminated the waiting lists (Ghods/Savaj 2006; Rizvi et al. 2009b). Although studies show that even those from lower socio-economic class can be recipients (Ghods/Savaj 2006), the system might leave out very poor patients suffering

---

4   This issue can be regarded as a modern capitalist route for organ flow "from South to North, from Third to First World, from poor to rich" (Scheper-Hughes 2000: 193).

from the final stage of kidney failure, who have to wait for deceased donors (Rizvi et al. 2009b). However, Kishore (2005) rightly points out that the problem is scarcity and that if the demand for organs could be satisfied by offering them for sale but still no action is being taken to legalize it, then inequity may occur. This will lead to unfairness between people and the risk of exploitation of the vulnerable will still be there. Considering it is not likely that a materially well off person will offer his kidney for sale (Rid et al. 2009), the poor will generally take part in such transactions. This will lead to exploitation of economically vulnerable people. Hence, whether it is regulated or not, it might be argued that organ sales could benefit the rich only and exploit the poor.

3.3 Autonomy and Coercion

Whether the option to sell an organ enhances one's autonomy or constrains it is an ongoing debate. Autonomy used here in the personal sense, meaning, very basically, being "free from both controlling interference by others and from certain limitations such as an inadequate understanding that prevents meaningful choice" (Beauchamp/Childress 2009: 99). To give an organ freely, as in donation, requires "genuine and well-informed choice [...] and excludes vulnerable persons who are incapable of fulfilling the requirements for voluntary and knowledgeable consent" (WHO 2010: Commentary on Guiding Principle 3: 4). This emphasizes the importance of autonomous choice in participating in the practice. However, when money is involved, concerns are raised regarding the voluntariness of participation. To summarize, opponents generally argue that organ selling is coercive because economically vulnerable people are *forced to sell* their organs to get out of their desperate situations or are *more likely* to participate in such transactions, which they would otherwise prefer not to make (Zargooshi 2001b; Scheper-Hughes 2003; Budiani-Saberi/Delmonico 2008). Hence, since selling is based on coercion (Phadke/Anandh 2002, Budiani-Saberi/Delmonico 2008; Rizvi et al. 2009b), the consent for such a transaction is claimed to be involuntary and problematic (Phadke/Anandh 2002; Scheper-Hughes 2003; Tsai 2010).

On the contrary, proponents of a legal organ market emphasize that people are autonomous and rational subjects; therefore, they are responsible for their choices and actions, and should be respected by others in light of their choices (Cherry 2005). Even in a desperate economic situation, it is argued that kidney vendors deliberately choose to act in a certain way; hence they act autonomously (Gill/Sade 2002; Taylor 2005). Some claim that it is wrong to say that some people cannot decide for themselves (Savulescu 2003; Kishore 2005). If there were legal organ markets, Taylor (2005) claims, a typical vendor would not suffer from impaired autonomy.

Although it is not considered to be wrong to claim that financial pressure has an erosive effect on one's consent, it is also argued that forbidding the person to sell one of her kidneys could be more harmful than allowing her to sell it, since that would undermine the person's autonomous consent (Wilkinson/Garrard 1996). However, the ban on organs' sale does not diminish the person's autonomy considering the decision to sell is unlikely to be made autonomously or willingly and freely (Biller-Andorno/Alpinar 2014).

3.4   Social Values

Concerns are also raised about the possible erosive effects of human organ markets on social values. Such values are the ones that all citizens agree upon rationally and reasonably to live in a society together and should be respected and protected by the government (Cohen 2002: 59–60). The worry regarding the selling of organs is about how the practice of donation would be affected by involving money and how it would affect the parties involved in such transactions (WHO 2010: Commentary on Guiding Principle 5: 5). The most common argument given against selling, and promoting live donation is founded on promotion of the socially desirable values. This requires a moral distinction between donating and selling.

At first sight, the difference between the two practices is the payment involved in the case of the latter. How money could change the value of the practice is mostly related to the purity of the motivation. The motivation of the donor is altruism in the first case, whereas in the latter the motivation might not be *pure*[5]. Therefore, some opponents argue that allowing sales would violate socially desirable values such as altruism, interconnectedness and solidarity, which are required to keep society together (Cohen 2002: 61–62). Some other opponents stated that it would lead to a decrease in altruistic acts (Phadke/Anandh 2002; Danovitch/Leichtman 2006; Rothman/Rothman 2006), which would jeopardize the sense of being a community (Titmuss 1997 [1970]), and would have an erosive effect on the norm of giving (Sandel 2012: 123–124). Proponents, on the other hand, argue that allowing sales would not necessarily lead to such a decrease, since it would not exclude the possibility of free donation (Wilkinson 2003: 113) and none of these necessarily occurs (Wilkinson/Garrard 1996; Radcliffe-Richards 2013). However, the possibility of obtaining an organ, such as a kidney, from a stranger in exchange for money is more tempting than burdening a relative instead (Scheper-Hughes 2009: 11).

3.5   Is There a Further Concern?

Although the arguments in favor of and against organ selling are thoughtful and sophisticated, it could be claimed that they are either (a) derived from generally accepted principles or plausible moral concerns, such as autonomy, exploitation or the need to protect the vulnerable, etc. without further inquiry or (b) *in some way* dependent upon the contingent factors. With regard to (a), all the arguments that are presented against the allowance of organ selling are to support an uncomfortable, strong moral feeling or a general opposition against the practice without any good justifications and moral reasoning (Radcliffe-Richards 2013). With regard to (b), it might be argued that *if* these contingent factors were adjusted appropriately, then all these arguments against organ selling *could be* defeated or reformulated (Wilkinson 2003; Cherry 2005). However, it seems plausible to claim that even if the circumstances

---

5 It should be noted here that any act of donation or giving away an organ might not be argued to be purely altruistic, which is stated by Kishore (2005: 363) as well. There might be some other strong motivations to donate an organ to a relative, such as pursuing "happiness (to avoid loneliness and the thought of living without the dearest one), possible benefits (i.e. socio-psychological benefits) and outcomes (i.e. saving the life of the receiver)" (Alpinar-Sencan 2016: 26 [footnote]).

under which the practice takes place are bettered, still an intuitive notion regarding the wrongness of offering human organs for sale for transplantation purposes is raised. Thus, independently of the contingent factors, some philosophical questions come to the fore requiring qualified moral reasoning: What is wrong with the practice itself? How can we evaluate the moral permissibility of organ selling independently of contingent factors that are adjustable? The arguments, which try to find an answer to these questions, refer to dignity.

4.   What's at Stake? Dignity as a Promising Approach

> We do not find an explicit definition of the expression 'dignity of the human person' in international instruments or (as far as I know) in national law…. When it has been invoked in concrete situations, it has been generally assumed that a violation of human dignity can be recognized even if the abstract term cannot be defined. 'I know it when I see it even if I cannot tell you what it is.' (Schachter 1983: 849)

As the quotation above clearly puts it, the term (human) dignity appears quite frequently in European and international legal documents (United Nations 1948; Council of Europe/United Nations 2009) as well as in national laws and constitutions. We also come across this term in academic discussions quite frequently and in popular culture. Although references to (human) dignity are quite frequent, it is not clear what is meant by dignity. The meaning and the content of the term is vague, thus consensus cannot be achieved easily. However, its violations are quite recognizable. Generally, it appears to be an inviolable and inalienable value to be protected, which guarantees the proper respect for the bearers of it.

Such vagueness in the meaning of the term raises suspicions with regard to its content. In the contemporary philosophical literature, there is an ongoing debate to determine whether dignity has any specific content, which would show either that the concept of dignity is valid *or* that it is just rhetoric. In legal documents and laws, as mentioned above, and sometimes even to justify a particular point of view in debates, dignity is referred to as a valuable concept, but it is not clearly defined.

Contradictory viewpoints appear concerning the term's specific content. Very generally, on the one hand, it is argued that dignity can be used interchangeably with the principles of 'respect for autonomy' (Macklin 2003) and 'respect for the person' (Pinker 2008) without any loss in the content. On the other hand, dignity is acknowledged as an absolute, intrinsic, metaphysical property possessed by all human beings regardless of any contingent properties (Nordenfelt 2004; Sulmasy 2009). Such an idea of dignity is systematically developed in the philosophical writings of Immanuel Kant in *The Metaphysics of Morals* (MM) and in his *Groundwork for the Metaphysics of Morals* (G), in which he argued that persons have dignity just by virtue of being human, since they have faculty of reason (MM 6: 434–6: 435; G 4: 434–4: 436). This forms the basis of human rights (Schachter 1983; Gewirth 1992) and morality (Kass 2002). Some authors describe different ideas of dignity in addition to intrinsic dignity, which are not absolute but can be lost and gained. These are, generally speaking, dependent on the results of the subjects' deeds, on the virtues, skills and talents that the persons have, on acting in accordance with the society's expectations or on the persons' positions or social ranks (Nordenfelt 2004; Schroder 2008; Sulmasy 2009).

These discussions often stay at a very general and theoretical level. The violations of dignity are quite recognizable even though a consensus could not be easily achieved on a unique definition of dignity, as stated in the quotation at the beginning of this subsection. A satisfactory notion of dignity would be able to reveal violations of it concerning certain practices and acts, and thus should be associated with occurrences in social life (Kaufmann et al. 2011: 1–2). Thus, we have to look for instances of its violation (Stoecker 2011: 11). In that sense, the practice of organ selling provides us with an important context for exploring the meaning and plausible function of dignity. This would be helpful to find a more general intuitive idea of dignity and to explore its plausible role in the debate.

Beyleveld and Brownsword (2004, 1998) classified the dignity-based arguments as dignity as empowerment and dignity as a constraint, which emphasizes the link between dignity and autonomy. The first view emphasizes dignity's function as reinforcing the claims of self-determination. This approach supports the argument that dignity is a redundant concept in the debate, since respect for autonomy would be sufficient to authorize organ selling. This states that dignity is a 'useless concept', as argued by Macklin (2003) and Pinker (2008). However, this approach falls short of explaining the concern raised above (Alpinar-Sencan et al. 2017). The latter view, on the other hand, functions as a constraint on one's autonomous choices. This approach supports the idea that there could be limits to one's autonomy regarding certain practices. A promising approach in the debate draws upon a *social* notion of dignity, which offers the most plausible understanding of dignity in the debate by explaining why organ selling is considered to involve violations of dignity (Alpinar-Sencan 2014; Alpinar-Sencan et al. 2017).

There are differing dignity-based arguments in the organ selling debate in particular and to make such a claim requires a systematic discussion (Alpinar-Sencan et al. 2017). After having critically evaluated both the negative and positive features of each approach, a successful understanding of dignity was developed; that is, a social account of dignity (ibid). In the following, very briefly, I will refer to the mentioned account. It should be noted that this account is inspired by Samuel J. Kerstein's (2009) approach, but it differs from it by emphasizing that a stringent and coherent account of dignity should not be limited to perceiving certain classes of people as lacking value whenever they perform an unfavorable act.

Some practices are (intuitively) thought to be or, as Sandel in his 2012 book points out, carry an inherent property of being degrading or humiliating, independent of whether the subject chooses to act autonomously and regardless of the external conditions. Thus, some acts are necessarily degrading and condemned even when practiced under fair, regulated conditions (e.g. as in a legal market). The violation of dignity occurs when people are symbolically perceived and treated in certain ways that are incompatible with their worth, that is their dignity. The allowance of practice of organ selling is argued to pose threats to human dignity by symbolizing the view that some lack worth, which is believed to be possessed by human beings equally from birth. By 'symbolizing', it is meant that the affected persons do not have less worth than others do by participating in such transactions, but they might be perceived to be so. Having an organ market, even though regulated, presents such a case in which a degrading view of the persons is promoted. It should be noted that we could not measure how strong a tendency or an idea about seeing people in a specific way was induced. However, there are empirical, qualitative studies that seem to indicate there is such a tendency to see others as lacking dignity (i.e. as if they were worthless and inferior to others) whenever they perform unfavorable acts (Zargooshi 2001a).

The main concern regarding organ selling is that the practice "inherently runs the risk of promoting the idea that some persons have less worth than others, or even that their worth is comparable to a price" (Alpinar-Sencan et al. 2017: 190). This also explicates the concern raised by WHO Guiding Principles (2010) regarding payment for cells, tissues and organs. "Such payment conveys the idea that some persons lack dignity, that they are mere objects to be used by others." (Commentary in Guiding Principle 5: 5) Such an approach to dignity significantly explains what is wrong with regard to such practices and raises an awareness of the need for global prohibitions of such practices.

It might be argued that this is a semiotic objection towards markets considered noxious or immoral in general. For instance, some argue that it is necessary to revise the meaning assigned to such markets and pay attention to the benefits and usefulness (i.e. outcomes) of markets wherever a clash occurs between outcomes and such objections (Brennan/Jaworski 2015, 2016). However, if it is considered that organ selling is wrong independently of contingent factors, then it is also wrong in a regulated market. Indeed, it is dignity's constraining function, supporting the widely held belief that the practice is wrong independently of any contingent factors and the probable consequences of a fair, regulated market.

Before concluding, a final question might be raised: do we need to refer to dignity to support the prohibition of organ markets? This hints at a potential redundancy concerning the concept. It might be stated that referring to real life situations as well as arguments concerning exploitation,[6] vulnerability and fairness would provide enough evidence to prohibit the practice or even to raise global awareness. However, they fall short of demonstrating the significance of the 'seeing people as if they had a price' thesis. The scope of the referred approach is broader; that is, it is unlikely to be limited to those who are economically vulnerable. Hence, it presents us different and better reasons to support global prohibition demonstrating the distinct function of dignity.

---

6 Exploitation argument might be connected to dignity debate; since it can be argued that the concept of dignity is linked to non-instrumentalization of people, as exploitation can be argued to instrumentalize people by reducing their body parts to marketable objects (Andorno 2017). Such an argument is mounted on Kantian grounds. There are many Kant-inspired arguments in this specific debate. As I argued elsewhere, by referring to Kant's distinction between price and dignity (G 4: 434–4: 436) and by adopting Nicole Gerrand's (1999) paper, in which she offers the most plausible reading of Kant's arguments, in a Kantian framework, no compelling argument can be given against organ selling (Alpinar-Sencan 2016). Besides, instrumentalization can also be referred to on the other side of the debate: One might argue that paying for organs avoids instrumentalization of the vendor, since the transaction offers him a fair deal instead. As mentioned earlier, organ transactions can be exploitative, however as the term implies, the exploitative feature of the practice can be limited to those economically vulnerable and this cannot be simply avoided.

5.   Conclusion

This chapter presents a brief sketch of the moral arguments in the contemporary debate on organ selling. After briefly explaining the occurrence of the problem and presenting global trafficking of organs under the real-world conditions, basic lines of the moral arguments, which are founded on concerns regarding harm and benefit, exploitation and justice, autonomy and coercion as well as social values are given. Then a further concern regarding the practice is introduced, which presents a dignity-based objection to organ selling. Due to the qualitative and quantitative studies conducted and the consensus on organ selling being exploitative and coercive, some might argue that a reference to dignity is not needed to arrive a policy prohibiting organ selling, but actually dignity has a very functional role in the debate. It presents even better reasons to prohibit the practice and supports the intuitive notion that the practice is believed to be wrong independently of any contingent factors.

Acknowledgments

I would like to thank Roberto Andorno and Juha Räikkä, who have seen an earlier version, for their valuable comments and suggestions.

References

Alghamdi, Saad A./Nabi, Zahid G./Alkhafaji, Dania M./Askandrani, Sumaya A./Abdelsalam, Mohamed S./Shukri, Mohamed M./Eldali, Abdelmoneim M./Adra, Chaker N./Alkurbi, Lutfi A./Albaqumi, Mamdouh N. (2010): "Transplant Tourism Outcome: A Single Center Experience." In: Transplantation Journal 90/2, pp. 184–188.

Alpinar-Sencan, Zümrüt (2014): "A Social Understanding of Dignity: A Promising Approach in the Organ Selling Debate." In: Bioethica Forum 7/4, pp. 148–154.

Alpinar-Sencan, Zümrüt (2016): "Reconsidering Kantian Arguments against Organ Selling." In: Medicine, Health Care and Philosophy 19, pp. 21–31.

Alpinar-Sencan, Zümrüt/Baumann, Holger/Biller-Androno, Nikola (2017): "Does Organ Selling Violate Human Dignity?" In: Monash Bioethics Review 34, pp. 189–205.

Andorno, Roberto (2017): "Buying and Selling Organs: Issues of Commodification, Exploitation and Human Dignity." In: Journal of Trafficking and Human Exploitation 2, pp. 119–127.

Baraaz, Tamara (2018): "Illegal Organ Harvesting is Rampant in Egypt, and Refugees are the Main Target." In: Haaretz. Availabe at: https://www.haaretz.com/middle-east-news/egypt/.premium.MAGAZINE-illegal-organ-harvesting-is-rampant-in-egypt-and-refugees-are-the-main-target-1.6492013 (accessed June 29, 2020)

Beauchamp, Tom L./Childress, James F. (2009): Principles of Biomedical Ethics, 6th ed., New York: Oxford University Press.

Beavers, Kimberly L./Sandler, Robert S./Fair, Jeffrey H./Johnson, Mark W./Shrestha, Roshan (2001): "The Living Donor Experience: Donor Health Assessment and Outcomes after Living Donor Liver Transplantation." In: Liver Transplantation 7/11, pp. 943–947.

Beyleveld, Deryck/Brownsword, Roger (1998): "Human Dignity, Human Rights, and Human Genetics." In: The Modern Law Review 61/5, pp. 661–680.

Beyleveld, Deryck/Brownsword, Roger (2004): Human Dignity in Bioethics and Biolaw, 2nd ed., Oxford: Oxford University Press.

Biller-Andorno, Nikola/Alpinar, Zümrüt (2014): "Organ Trafficking and Transplant Tourism." In: Henk A M J ten Have/Bert Gordijn (eds.), Handbook of Global Bioethics, Dordrecht: Springer, pp. 771–783.

Brennan, Jason/Jaworski, Peter Martin (2015): "Markets without Symbolic Limits." In: Ethics 125, pp. 1053–1077.

Brennan, Jason/Jaworski, Peter Martin (2016): Markets without Limits: Moral Virtues and Commercial Interests, New York: Routledge.

Bryson, Donna (2010): "Netcare, South African Hospital, Charged in Organ Trafficking." In: Huffington Post. Available at: http://www.huffingtonpost.com/2010/09/16/netcare-south-african-hos_n_719128.html (accessed June 29, 2020)

Budiani-Saberi, Debra A./Delmonico, Francis L. (2008): "Organ Trafficking and Transplant Tourism: A Commentary on the Global Realities." In: American Journal of Transplantation 8/5, pp. 925–929.

Campbell, Denis/Davison, Nicola (2012): "Illegal Kidney Trade Booms as New Organ Is 'Sold Every Hour.'" In: The Guardian. Available at: http://www.theguardian.com/world/2012/may/27/kidney-trade-illegal-operations-who (accessed June 29, 2020)

Cherry, Mark J. (2005): Kidney for Sale by Owner: Human Organs, Transplantation, and the Market, Washington: Georgetown University Press.

Cohen, Cynthia B. (2002): "Public Policy and the Sale of Human Organs." In: Kennedy Institute of Ethics Journal 12/1, pp. 47–64.

Cohen, David J. (2009): "Transplant Tourism: A Growing Phenomenon." In: Nature Clinical Practice. Nephrology 5/3, pp. 128–129.

Columb, Seán (2019): "Organ Trafficking in Egypt: 'They Locked Me In and Took My Kidney'." In: The Guardian. Available at: https://www.theguardian.com/global-development/2019/feb/09/trafficking-people-smugglers-organs-egypt-mediterranean-refugees-migrants (accessed June 29, 2020).

Council of Europe/United Nations (2009): Trafficking in Organs, Tissues and Cells and Trafficking in Human Beings for the Purpose of the Removal of Organs. Strasbourg.

Daar, Abdallah S. (2006): "The Case for a Regulated System of Living Kidney Sales." In: Nature Clinical Practice Nephrology 2/11, pp. 600–601.

Danovitch, Gabriel M./Leichtman, Alan B. (2006): "Kidney Vending: The 'Trojan Horse' of Organ Transplantation." In: Clinical Journal of the American Society of Nephrology 1/6, pp. 1133–1135.

Delmonico, Francis L. (2009): "The Implications of Istanbul Declaration on Organ Trafficking and Transplant Tourism." In: Current Opinion in Organ Transplantation 14/2, pp. 116–119.

Erin, Charles A./Harris, John (2003): "An Ethical Market in Human Organs." In: Journal of Medical Ethics 29/3, pp. 137–138.

Garwood, Paul (2007): "Dilemma over Live-Donor Transplantation." In: Bulletin of the World Health Organization 85/1, pp. 5–6.

Geddes, Colin C./Henderson, Andrew/Mackenzie, Pamela/ Rodger, Stuart C. (2008): "Outcome of Patients from the West of Scotland Traveling to Pakistan for Living Donor Kidney Transplants." In: Transplantation 86/8, pp. 1143–1145.

Gerrand, Nicole (1999): "The Misuse of Kant in the Debate about a Market for Human Body Parts." In: Journal of Applied Philosophy 16/1, pp. 59–67.

Gewirth, Alan (1992): "Human Dignity as the Basis of Rights." In: Michael J. Meyer/ William A. Parent (eds.), The Constitution of Rights: Human Dignity and American Values, Ithaca: Cornell University Press, pp. 10–28.

Gill, Michael B./Sade, Robert M. (2002): "Paying for Kidneys: The Case against Prohibition." In: Kennedy Institute of Ethics Journal 12/1, pp. 17–45.

Ghods, Ahad J./Savaj, Shekoufeh (2006): "Iranian Model of Paid and Regulated Living-Unrelated Kidney Donation." In: Clinical Journal of American Society of Nephrology 1/6, pp. 1136–1145.

Goyal, Madhav/Mehta, Ravindra L./Schneiderman, Lawrence J./Sehgal, Ashwini R. (2002): "Economic and Health Consequences of Selling a Kidney in India." In: Journal of the American Medical Association 288/13, pp. 1589–1593.

Irving, Michelle J./Tong, Allison/Jan, Stephen/Cass, Alan/Rose, John/Chadban, Steven/Allen, Richard D./Craig, Jonathan C./Wong, Germaine/Howard, Kirsten (2012): "Factors that Influence the Decision to be an Organ Donor: A Systematic Review of the Qualitative Literature." In: Nephrology Dialysis Transplantation 27/6, pp. 2526–2533.

Kant, Immanuel (1996 [1797]: The Metaphysics of Morals, New York: Cambridge University Press.

Kant, Immanuel (2002 [1785]): Groundwork for the Metaphysics of Morals, New York: Oxford University Press.

Kass, Leon R. (2002): Life, Liberty and The Defense of Dignity: The Challenge for Bioethics, New York: Encounter Books.

Kaufmann, Paulus/Kuch, Hannes/Neuhäuser, Christian/Webster, Elaine (2011): "Human Dignity Violated: A Negative Approach – Introduction." In: Paulus Kaufmann/Hannes Kuch/Christian Neuhäuser/Elaine Webster (eds.), Humiliation, Degradation, Dehumanization: Human Dignity Violated, Dordrecht: Springer, pp. 1–5.

Kelly, Tom (2019): "Revealed: Hundreds of Britons who Buy Kidneys on the Black Market from Overseas Traffickers Charging £ 30.000 in a bid to Avoid NHS Waiting Lists are Coming Back with Deadly Diseases such as HIV and Hepatitis." In: Mail Online News January. Available at: https://www.dailymail.co.uk/news/article-6613407/Hundreds-Britons-buy-KIDNEYS-black-market-overseas-traffickers-charging-30-000.html (accessed June 29, 2020)

Kerstein, Samuel J. (2009): "Kantian Condemnation of Commerce in Organs." In: Kennedy Institute of Ethics Journal 19/2, pp. 147–169.

Khamash, Hasan A./Gaston, Robert S. (2008): "Transplant Tourism: A Modern Iteration of an Ancient Problem." In: Current Opinion in Organ Transplantation 13/4, pp. 395–399.

Kishore, R. R. (2005): "Human Organs, Scarcities, and Sale: Morality Revisited." In: Journal of Medical Ethics 31/6, pp. 362–365.

Lentine, Krista L./Patel, Anita (2012): "Risks and Outcomes of Living Donation." In: Advances in Chronic Kidney Disease 19/4, pp. 220–228.

Lentine, Krista L./Segev, Dorry L. (2013): "Health Outcomes Among Non-Caucasian Living Kidney Donors: Knowns and Unknowns." In: Transplant International 26/9, pp. 853–864.

Levy, Mélanie (2018): "State Incentives to Promote Organ Donation: Honoring the Principles of Reciprocity and Solidarity Inherent in the Gift Relationship." In: Journal of Law and the Biosciences 5/2, pp. 398–435.

Macklin, Ruth (2003): "Dignity Is a Useless Concept." In: British Medical Journal 327/7429, pp. 1419–1420.

Morgan, Benjamin R./Ibrahim, Hassan N. (2011): "Long-Term Outcomes of Kidney Donors." In: Arab Journal of Urology 9/2, pp. 79–84.

Naqvi, Syed Ali Anwar/Ali, Bux/Mazhar, Farida/Zafar, Mirza Naqi/ Rizvi, Syed Adibul Hasan (2007): "A Socioeconomic Survey of Kidney Vendors in Pakistan." In: Transplant International 20/11, pp. 934–939.

Nordenfelt, Lennart (2004): "The Varieties of Dignity." In: Health Care Analysis 12/2, pp. 69–81.

Organ Procurement and Transplantation Network (2020): "Organ Donor Statistics." Available at: https://www.organdonor.gov/statistics-stories/statistics.html (accessed June 29, 2020)

Padilla, Benita S. (2009): "Regulated Compensation for Kidney Donors in the Philippines." In: Current Opinion in Organ Transplantation 14/2, pp. 120–123.

Phadke, Kishore D./Anandh, Urmila (2002): "Ethics of Paid Organ Donation." In: Pediatric Nephrology 17/5, pp. 309–311.

Pinker, Steven (2008): "The Stupidity of Dignity: Conservative Bioethics' Latest, Most Dangerous Ploy." In: The New Republic 238, pp. 28–31.

Putz, Ulrike (2013): "Lebanese Black Market: Syrian Refugees Sell Organs to Survive." Spiegel Online. Available at: https://www.spiegel.de/international/world/organ-trade-thrives-among-desperate-syrian-refugees-in-lebanon-a-933228.html (accessed June 29, 2020)

Radcliffe-Richards, J./Daar, A. S./Guttmann, R. D./Hoffenberg, R./Kennedy, I./Lock, M./Sells R. A./Tilley, N./for the International Forum for Transplant Ethics (2006): "The Case for Allowing Kidney Sales." In: Helga Kuhse/Peter Singer (eds.), Bioethics: An Anthology, 2nd ed., Oxford: Blackwell, pp. 487–490.

Radcliffe-Richards, Janet (2013): The Ethics of Transplants: Why Careless Thought Costs Lives, 1st paperback ed., Oxford: Oxford University Press.

Reese, Peter P./Boudville, Neil/Garg, Amit X. (2015): "Living Kidney Donation: Outcomes, Ethics, and Uncertainty." In: The Lancet 385/9981, pp. 2003–2013.

Rid, Annette/Bachmann, L. M./ Wettstein, V./Biller-Andorno, Nikola (2009): "Would You Sell a Kidney in a Regulated Kidney Market? Results of an Exploratory Study." In: Journal of Medical Ethics 35/9, pp. 558–564.

Rizvi, Syed Adibul Hasan/Naqvi, Syed Ali Anwar/Zafar, Mirza Naqi/Mazhar, Farida/ Muzaffar, Rana/Naqvi, Rubina/Akhtar, Fazal/Ahmed, Ejaz (2009a): "Commercial Transplants in Local Pakistanis from Vended Kidneys: A Socio-Economic and Outcome Study." In: Transplant International: Official Journal of the European Society for Organ Transplantation 22/6, pp. 615–621.

Rizvi, Syed Adibul Hasan/Naqvi, Anwar Syed Ali Anwar/Zafar, Mirza Naqi/Ahmed, Ejaz (2009b): "Regulated Compensated Donation in Pakistan and Iran." In: Current Opinion in Organ Transplantation 14/2, pp. 124–128.

Rohter, Larry (2004): "The Organ Trade: A Global Black Market; Tracking the Sale of a Kidney On a Path of Poverty and Hope." In: The New York Times. Available at: http://www.nytimes.com/2004/05/23/world/organ-trade-global-black-market-tracking-sale-kidney- path-poverty-hope.html (accessed June 29, 2020)

Rothman, S. M./Rothman D. J. (2006): "The Hidden Cost of Organ Sale." In: American Journal of Transplantation 6/7, pp. 1524–1528.

Sandel, Michael J. (2012): What Money Can't Buy: The Moral Limits of Markets, New York: Farrar, Straus and Giroux.

Savulescu, Julian (2003): "Is the Sale of Body Parts Wrong?" In: Journal of Medical Ethics 29/3, pp. 138–139.

Schachter, Oscar (1983): "Human Dignity as a Normative Concept." In: The American Journal of International Law 77/4, pp. 848–854.

Scheper-Hughes, Nancy (2000): "The Global Traffic in Human Organs." In: Current Anthropology 41/2, pp. 191–224.

Scheper-Hughes, Nancy (2003): "Keeping an Eye on the Global Traffic in Human Organs." In: The Lancet 361/9369, pp. 1645–1648.

Scheper-Hughes, Nancy (2009): "The Tyranny and the Terror of the Gift: Sacrificial Violence and the Gift of Life." In: Economic Sociology_The European Electronic Newsletter 11/1, pp. 8–16.

Schroeder, Doris (2008): "Dignity: Two Riddles and Four Concepts." In: Cambridge Quarterly of Healthcare Ethics 17/2, pp. 230–238.

Shelton, Tracey/Arifah, Iffah Nur/Renaldi, Erwin (2018): "Kidneys for Sale: Cash-Strapped Indonesians turn to Facebook to Sell Organs." In: ABC News. Available at: https://www.abc.net.au/news/2018-10-12/kidneys-for-sale-cash-strappled-indonesians-turn-to-facebook/10364676 (accessed June 29, 2020)

Shimazono, Yosuke (2007): "The State of the International Organ Trade: A Provisional Picture Based on Integration of Available Information." In: Bulletin of the World Health Organization 85/12, pp. 955–962.

Siddique, Haroon (2011): "Turkish Doctor Arrested over Organ Traffic Allegations." In: The Guardian January 12. Available at: http://www.theguardian.com/world/2011/jan/12/turkish-doctor-organ-traffic (accessed June 29, 2020)

Smith, David (2010): "South African Hospital Firm Admits 'Cash for Kidney' Transplants." In: The Guardian November 10. Available at: http://www.theguardian.com/world/2010/nov/10/south-africa-hospital-organ-trafficking (accessed June 29, 2020)

Statz, Sarah E. (2006): "Finding The Winning Combination: How Blending Organ Procurement Systems Used Internationally Can Reduce The Organ Shortage." In: Vanderbilt Journal of Transnational Law 39/5, pp. 1677–1709.

Stoecker, Ralf (2011): "Three Crucial Turns on the Road to an Adequate Understanding of Human Dignity." In: Paulus Kaufmann/Hannes Kuch/Christian Neuhäuser/ Elaine Webster (eds.), Humiliation, Degradation, Dehumanization: Human Dignity Violated, Dordrecht: Springer, pp. 7–17.

Sulmasy, Daniel P. (2009): "Dignity and Bioethics: History, Theory, and Selected Applications." In: Edmund D. Pellegrino/Adam Schulman/Thomas W. Merrill (eds.), Human Dignity and Bioethics, Notre Dame: University of Notre Dame Press, pp. 469–501

Taylor, James Stacey (2005): Stakes and Kidneys: Why Markets in Human Body Parts Are Morally Imperative, Aldershot: Ashgate.

Titmuss, Richard M. (1997 [1970]): The Gift Relationship: From Human Blood to Social Policy, New York: The New Press.

The Transplantation Society and International Society of Nephrology (2018): "The Declaration of Istanbul on Organ Trafficking and Transplant Tourism (2018 Edition)." Available at: http://www.declarationofistanbul.org/ (accessed June 29, 2020)

Tram, Mai/Tung, Thanh (2014): "Vietnam Police Probe Paid Kidney 'Donors' for Hint of Trafficking." In: Thanh Nien News, April 29. Available at: http://www.thanhnien-news.com/society/vietnam-police-probe-paid-kidney-donors-for-hint-of-trafficking-25267.html (accesed June 29, 2020).

Tsai, Daniel Fu Chang (2010): "Transplant Tourism from Taiwan to China: Some Reflection on Professional Ethics and Regulation." In: The American Journal of Bioethics 10/2, pp. 22–24.

United Nations (1948): "The Universal Declaration of Human Rights." Available at: http://www.un.org/en/documents/udhr/ (accessed June 29, 2020)

Wilkinson, Stephen/Garrard, Eve (1996): "Bodily Integrity and the Sale of Human Organs." In: Journal of Medical Ethics 22/6, pp. 334–339.

Wilkinson, Stephen (2003): Bodies for Sale: Ethics and Exploitation in the Human Body Trade, London: Routledge.

World Health Organization (2004): Fifty-Seventh World Health Assembly: Resolutions and Decisions, Annexes. Geneva, 17–22 May, pp. 1–78. Available at: http://apps.who.int/gb/ebwha/pdf_files/WHA57/A57_REC1-en.pdf (accessed June 29, 2020)

World Health Organization (2010): Sixty-Third World Health Assembly: Resolutions and Decisions, Annexes. Geneva, 17–21 May, pp. 1–150. Available at: http://apps.who.int/gb/ebwha/pdf_files/wha63-rec1/wha63_rec1-en.pdf (accessed June 29, 2020)

World Health Organization (2010): "WHO Guiding Principles on Human Cell, Tissue and Organ Transplantation." In: Transplantation 90/3, pp. 229–233.

Zargooshi, Javaad (2001a): "Quality of Life of Iranian Kidney 'Donors.'" In: The Journal of Urology 166/5, pp. 1790–1799.

Zargooshi, Javaad (2001b): "Iranian Kidney Donors: Motivations and Relations with Recipients." In: The Journal of Urology 165/2, pp. 386–392.

12. Selecting Donors and Recipients
The Role of Old Age

Mark Schweda & Sabine Wöhlke

1. Introduction

When Carlton Blackburn, a retired teacher from Texas, died from a brain hemorrhage just nine days before his 93rd birthday, he became the oldest postmortal organ donor in the United States: his liver was successfully transplanted to a 69-year old woman with end stage liver disease (US Department of Health and Human Services 2012). A year later, an 83-year-old dialysis patient in the US received a living kidney donation from an 84-year-old friend. After three years, the donor as well as the recipient were healthy and leading active lives. The "world's oldest donor-recipient solid organ transplantation" (Mistry et al. 2010: 534) had been a success.

These examples appear to be symptomatic: as a consequence of historically unprecedented demographic aging in nearly all Western countries, questions of old age and intergenerational relations are receiving more and more attention in medicine and health care as well as in the relevant public, bioethical, and health policy debates. This trend also becomes manifest in the field of organ donation and transplantation medicine: as average life expectancies and population age increase, so does the age of organ donors and recipients. In 2018, one third of all organ donors and over 62 per cent of recipients in the US were over the age of 50. In the area covered by Eurotransplant, the largest European organization coordinating organ allocation in Austria, Belgium, Croatia, Germany, Hungary, Luxemburg, the Netherlands, and Slovenia, the median age of donors increased from 45 to 55 between 2000 and 2018 (Eurotransplant 2018: 18). In Germany alone, the average age of donors and recipients has risen from 33 and 42 years, respectively, to 52 and 51 years over the last 30 years.[1]

These developments also raise new questions in the ethical debate on organ donation. For example, the increasing life expectancy and population age lead to a growing demand for transplantable organs and thus intensify concerns about 'organ scarcity' and fuel controversies about the efficient use and just distribution of available donor organs between the generations (Cuende et al. 2007; Goldstein 2012). In this context, old age is discussed as a criterion for organ allocation in postmortal donation, fostering controversial proposals for age-based rationing of medical resources for the sake

---

1 Own statistical analysis of Eurotrasplant data (1988–2018).

of younger age groups (Reese et al. 2010). At the same time, older people are emerging as a largely untapped source of donor organs that could help to expand the donor pool. In addition, they also become incorporated into new systems of more efficient and fair utilization of the available donor organs. For example, older adults are targeted as a separate subgroup of donors and recipients in 'old for old'-schemes such as the Eurotransplant Senior Programme (ESP), or they are addressed as 'end-users' of organs with a limited lifetime in so-called domino donations (Montgomery et al. 2006).

Similar developments can also be observed in the context of living organ transplantation. Here, age and intergenerational relations within the family have traditionally played a prominent role in setting moral expectations and decisions regarding organ donation. In recent years, however, the moral significance and economy of age and intergenerational relations in the field of living donation appear to be changing. Earlier qualitative research suggested that traditional life plans and family roles made donations from parents, and especially mothers, to their minor children appear almost natural and self-evident (Zeiler et al. 2010). In the meantime, increasing life expectancies and new, more ambitious expectations and projects for the second half of life may challenge and transform the moral norms underlying traditional attitudes and decisions. Thus, recent qualitative studies indicate the growing frequency of living donations from middle-aged adults to their older relatives as a new paradigm of intra-familial care and solidarity (Kaufman/Fjord 2011; Kaufman et al. 2009).

Against this backdrop, our contribution explores the ways in which age matters in the context of organ donation. In order to illustrate the development and variety of procedural and institutional approaches, we first outline the history and organization of organ donation and transplantation with regard to aging and old age in different countries. In addition, we also provide a brief overview of the medical state of the art in transplantation medicine regarding the transfer of donor organs from or to older people. On this basis, we then describe the emerging ethical debate on the role of age in organ donation and attempt to systematize the relevant ethical aspects and arguments regarding postmortal and living donation. We conclude by highlighting the most important issues and questions and arguing for further empirical research as well as ethical deliberation on age and organ donation. Crucially, more information and critical reflection on traditional age stereotypes are needed. In a recent representative survey in Germany, almost half of the respondents wrongly assumed there were an upper age limit for organ donation (Caille-Brillet et al. 2019: 88). Indeed, many older Germans still do not even hold a donor card because they consider themselves too old and their organs unsuitable for transplantation (Caille-Brillet et al. 2015: 17, 60).

2.   History and Organization of Organ Donation and Transplantation from or to Older People

Allocation rules for the limited number of available donor organs have been developed since the mid-20th century. In this context, social factors such as age have been frequently proposed as rationing criteria. Historically, one of the starting points of the debate was the Admission and Policy Committee of the Seattle Artificial Kidney Center (Veatch/Ross 2015). In the 1960s, when the availability of dialysis machines was still low, this committee of doctors and citizens established rules for access to dialysis

(Alexander 1962). Besides medical factors, criteria included a sense of responsibility and emotional maturity, compliance, proximity of place of residence to the clinic, adequate financial resources, and a certain value for the community (Feuerstein 1995; following Attali 1981: 224–225). A further criterion was being between 17 and 50 years of age. Here, almost all types of non-medical criteria that were significant in later organ transplantation debates were already present.

In the US-American context, concerns about inefficiency and age-discrimination in the kidney allocation system go back to the 1990s (Veatch/Ross 2015). Indeed, between 1994 and 2000, only 0.3 per cent of the kidney recipients in the United States were older than 75 at the time of transplantation and 6.4 per cent were aged between 60 and 75 (Macrae et al. 2005). As a result of a reform of the system originally implemented by the United Network for Organ Sharing (UNOS) in 2002, the allocation method for kidneys now divides donors into two categories: standard criteria donors (SCDs) and expanded criteria donors (ECDs). ECD kidneys derive from donors older than 60 years and from donors 50 to 59 years with co-morbidities. Introduced in 2014, participation in this reformed allocation scheme is voluntary because one can choose whether to be listed for the ECD kidneys (opt in). The system is particularly advantageous for older people but less attractive for younger candidates, who often have other conditions that reduce waiting time in any case. Therefore, the vast majority of those on the ECD waiting list are older candidates. For older people, an advantage of this new system is that it uses an age-matching formula whereby recipients are entitled to kidneys from donors who are no more than 15 years younger or older (Veatch/Ross 2015, 340–341). Indeed, due to an aging population, the average age of postmortal kidney donors and recipients has risen in the US in recent years. Today, patients older than 65 make up 21.9 per cent of all kidney recipients.[2]

Within Europe, different regulations regarding age and organ donation exist. For example, Norway has a comparatively liberal policy, organized via the Scandinavian network Scandiatransplant. Patients for kidney transplantation are accepted following an individual medical evaluation without any formal upper age limit (Heldal et al. 2008). In other European countries, the indication for transplantation has been expanded for older people since the 1990s, and the age for both donors and recipients has been lifted. Under the purview of Eurotransplant, a special program for kidney transplantation from older donors to older recipients was established in 1999 – the Eurotransplant Senior Program (ESP). ESP was designed to reduce the waiting time of older patients and to achieve a higher efficiency in the use of kidneys from older donors (Smits et al. 1998). The program allocates organs between donors and recipients who are 65 years and older and does not permit these older candidates to receive younger kidneys (Frei et al. 2008; Boesmüller et al. 2011). For the first two years, participation of transplantation centers was voluntary. Since 2001, the ESP has become part of the Eurotransplant Kidney Allocation System (EKTAS) (Smits et al. 2002). Germany, the Netherlands and Belgium are the most important contributors (Doxiadis et al. 2004). Using regional allocation based on waiting time and blood group only, regardless of human leukocyte antigens (HLA) match, a short cold ischemic time (CIT) and thus a good primary organ function could be achieved (Bentas et al. 2008). The treating physicians in the transplantation centers have the responsibility to carry out the details of the program and to obtain informed

---

2 Source: OPTN data from 2019: https://optn.transplant.hrsa.gov/ (accessed March 18, 2021)

consent. ESP leads to significantly reduced waiting times and enhances the chance for older patients to receive a renal graft (Frei et al. 2008).

In Austria, Belgium, Luxembourg and Slovenia, kidneys from ESP donors are allocated to ESP recipients from the reporting centers' local waiting list. In the Netherlands and Croatia, kidneys from ESP donors are allocated to ESP recipients according to the national waiting list.[3] In Germany, kidneys from ESP donors are allocated to ESP recipients by the national organ procurement organization, the German Organ Transplantation Foundation (Deutsche Stiftung Organtransplantation (DSO)). Kidneys from ESP donors are first allocated to ESP recipients registered within the same country area as the donor and then to ESP recipients registered within other sub-regions.[4] Due to the current low donor rate in Germany, waiting times in the ESP program are significantly longer than when the program was first introduced, at present over 3.6 years on average (Heldal et al. 2008). Still, this is significantly shorter than in the standard allocation system, where patients on the waiting list may have to wait for over ten years. Older patients therefore benefit from ESP. However, recipients over the age of 65 must choose between ESP or standard allocation (EKTAS) without ESP; a simultaneous listing for both programs is not possible (Heemann/Renders 2018). Overall, the percentage of kidney recipients over the age of 65 rose from 3.6 per cent to 19.7 per cent between 1991 and 2007, and the proportion of kidney donors over 64 rose from 2.3 per cent to 18.1 per cent during the same period (de Fijter 2009). Since the beginning of the ESP, the average age of donors and recipients increased by two years in both groups (see Figure 1). In addition, the figures show that the drop in organ donation rates also affected the 'old-for-old' program. This decline was repeatedly attributed to public mistrust in the system, although this explanation is controversial (Schicktanz et al. 2017).

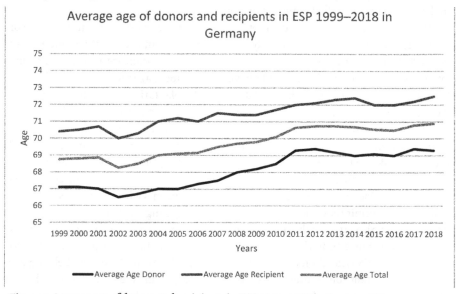

Figure 1: Average age of donors and recipients in ESP 1999–2018 in Germany (Source: Eurotransplant 2019)

---

3 https://www.eurotransplant.org/cms/index.php?page=esp (accessed March 18, 2021)

4 https://www.eurotransplant.org/cms/index.php?page=esp (accessed March 18, 2021)

Regarding living organ donation and transplantation, it is harder to determine both the role and relevance of age as well as changes in average donor and recipient age. Living donation is usually not organized within the framework of larger institutional structures but rather handled in local and regional contexts. In many countries such as Austria, Finland, France, Germany, or Hungary, living donation is restricted to family members and perhaps close friends and thus does not require any intermediate distributing organizations (Lopp 2013: 89). Legal regulations vary between different countries, but age does not seem to play a prominent role. In several countries – e.g., Austria, Germany, the Netherlands, Italy, and Spain – living donation is only allowed from the age of 18, but there are no upper age limits (ibid: 78). However, advanced age may become an issue in the context of specific living donation schemes, such as cross-over or chain donations, which imply some idea of equity or proportionality between donors and recipients. Due to the fragmented nature of living organ donation, there are often no central registries. As a consequence, large-scale and reliable sociodemographic figures on donor and recipient ages are frequently hard to obtain. Qualitative studies indicate that the practice of organ donation from adult children to their older parents or between older spouses may be becoming more relevant (Kaufman et al. 2009; Heldal et al. 2008). Statistics from the US show that living kidney donors have become older over recent decades (Hart et al. 2019). The annual number of living kidney recipients over 65 has almost tripled in the last 20 years, their proportion rising from 6.2 per cent in 2000 to 18.7 per cent in 2019 (November).[5]

3.   Medical Aspects of Organ Donation and Transplantation of Older People

Special transplantation programs for older people have been existing for more than 20 years. As a result, the age cutoff used to study outcomes in older patients varies between different studies. In general, patient and transplant survival are the essential parameters for success after transplantation. Most research on the ESP analyzes the initial function of the transplanted kidney in relation to the cold ischemia period, recipient age, and dialysis duration. Yet, the factors that predict clinical outcomes in older transplant patients have not yet been fully determined (Hebert et al. 2019).

Overall, older patients benefit from organ transplantation. In the US and Europe, a survival advantage for older people (>60 years) vis-a-vis patients on the waiting list who remain on dialysis could be observed (Heldal et al. 2008). Compared to dialysis, organ transplantation doubles the life expectancy of older people (Frei et al. 2008). Survival improves after the first year in patients between 60–74 years with a predicted increased life expectancy of five years and a 61 per cent reduction in long-term mortality risk (Oniscu et al. 2005; Rao et al. 2007). Even in ESP kidney transplantation, the quality of life and the survival rate are significantly better than in patients of the same age who are dialyzed (Fritsche et al. 2003).

Nevertheless, donor age obviously has a significant impact on the success of transplantation. Overall, patients who are transplanted within ESP still have the lowest five-year survival rate. EKTAS-patients who received older transplants have a similarly

---

5 Source: OPTN data from 2019: https://optn.transplant.hrsa.gov/ (accessed March 18, 2021)

poor transplant survival rate. The rate is more favorable when older patients receive younger organs (Schulte et al. 2018). Schamberger and colleagues (2018) also found a correlation between the smoking status of the donor and the survival of the transplant in ESP patients. Regarding living organ donation, several studies point out that carefully selected older kidney donors provide good organs and do not face a higher risk of death than younger donors (Reese et al. 2014; Wu et al. 2008).

From the very beginning of ESP, it became apparent that most recipients had a delayed graft function. A few had a spontaneous graft function, and some had no function admission (Schlieper et al. 2003). Despite 'immunosenescense', an age-associated deterioration of the immune system that is hoped to reduce pharmacological immunosuppression and improve allograft or even xenograft tolerance, the risk of acute rejection must be considered (Rickert/Markman 2018). Acute rejection in older patients is often associated with a worse graft survival and lower patient survival. Frei and colleagues (2008) show that most rejections among older patients occur during the first six months, with less than three per cent more than one year after transplantation. Increased kidney immunogenicity from older donors as well as the HLA mismatches and the poorer ability of older kidneys to recover from tissue damage are the main causes of a poorer graft survival of older patients (Schamberger et al. 2018).

As potential recipients, older patients clearly pose certain physiological challenges. McAdams-DeMarco and colleagues (2017) point out that transplantations in older patients often coincide with frailty, which is associated with delayed graft function, longer hospital stays, higher readmission rates, immunosuppressive intolerance, and mortality. Moreover, severe cognitive impairment could increase the risk of poor outcomes and require the provision of strong social support after transplantation (Hebert et al. 2019). A primary cause of mortality in older organ recipients is severe infections after transplantation. At the beginning of the ESP, 51 per cent of patients suffered from serious infections, and more than 50 per cent of all deaths could be attributed to infection events (Frei et al. 2008). Another problem arises from a high mortality rate due to the longer dialysis time before transplantation. Older patients with a shorter waiting time perform better in terms of survival and organ function than patients with long-term dialysis prior to kidney transplantation (Smits et al. 2002). Hence, careful preliminary examinations of older patients for comorbidities are deemed necessary to help minimize early morbidity and mortality after transplantation. Overall, however, age per se is not considered a limiting factor in organ transplantation anymore (Zhou et al. 2008; Heldal et al. 2008).

4.   Ethical Implications of Old Age in Organ Donations

The biomedical expert discourse on old age and organ donation mainly focuses on considerations of medical efficiency and success. However, as the overview on the historical development and current state of the art in transplantation medicine indicates, the relevant empirical assumptions need to be clarified, continuously critically examined, and updated in light of medical progress. Otherwise, outdated information and unfounded prejudices regarding the feasibility and success of transplantation from or to older people may bias medical decision-making processes and health policy regulations. In addition to these seemingly objective scientific aspects, an ethical perspective must also reflect the moral significance of the underlying conceptions and criteria of efficiency and success. In particular, their utilitarian underpinnings must be made explicit and weighed against other ethical principles such as individual autonomy and distributive justice (Ladin/Hanto 2011).

4.1   Postmortal Donation, Organ Allocation, and Distributive Justice

From the point of view of distributive justice, there has been comparatively little systematic ethical consideration and discussion of the moral significance of age in organ donation and allocation. As far as postmortem donation is concerned, general debates on old age as a criterion for resource allocation seem to play a role in this context, too. Some prominent ethical arguments in favor of age rationing – that is, the limitation of access to health care based on age – have also been applied in the field of organ allocation (Veatch 2002: 339–340)

Utilitarian arguments often refer to aspects of cost-efficiency (Meier-Kriesche et al. 2005). There has been a long discussion about the unfair implications of using cost-efficiency measures as criteria for the allocation of medical interventions. A prominent case is the concept of quality-adjusted life years (QALYs), which systematically disadvantages older people due to their limited average life expectancy (Tsuchiya 2000). Similar concerns about ageism have also been raised regarding proposals to use such assessment instruments in the context of organ transplantation. One example is the life years from transplant (LYFT) approach to allocate donor kidneys to those patients with the greatest potential survival benefit (for allocation principles, see also chapter 9 in this book). While LYFT would definitely extend the lives of kidney recipients, it would at the same time discriminate against older people by restricting their chances of obtaining a kidney transplant (Reese et al. 2010).

Another argument in favor of age rationing, the so-called 'natural lifespan' account, is based on communitarian considerations. It states that after a fulfilled life of about 80 years, extensive and expensive life sustaining interventions should be withheld in favor of good care and palliative treatment (Callahan 1987). This perspective is sometimes extended to the field of organ donation because transplantation medicine is widely seen as the epitome of advanced medical technologies (Callahan 1992). However, an application of the 'natural lifespan account' would require the definition of a sharp chronological cut-off age for organ transplantation that would be hard to justify and would ultimately appear arbitrary (Veatch 2002: 339). Indeed, at closer inspection, the natural lifespan account seems to presuppose a certain traditional notion of an adequate temporal extension and structure of human life without further explanation (Schweda 2017).

A prominent liberal-egalitarian argument is the 'prudential lifespan account.' It holds that if each person had to distribute a total amount of medical resources over their entire lifespan without knowing their actual age and state of health, it would be reasonable for everyone to allot the bulk to young and middle age instead of later life (Daniels 1988). Similar considerations have also been alluded to in the discussion of age in organ allocation (Kilner 1988). However, the 'prudential lifespan account' does not provide any concrete criteria to identify the specific claims different age groups may have for donor organs (Veatch 2002: 340). Moreover, against the backdrop of increasing average life expectancies, the prudence of the underlying rationale for apportioning limited health care resources such as donor organs may be called into question (Schweda 2017).

Finally, the so-called 'fair innings' argument appeals to the common intuition that it makes a moral difference whether someone still has their whole life in front of them or has already completed a full lifespan. The approach suggests that it can be fair to give priority to younger people when it comes to lifesaving medical care and limit access for those who have already arrived at old age (Harris 1985: 94). Analogous arguments have also been formulated regarding the just distribution of donor organs (Persad et al. 2009). Thus, it could be argued that the prioritization of younger people in the allocation of donor organs would help to ensure equal opportunities for everyone to complete a full life cycle (Veatch 2002: 341). However, in times of increasing life expectancies and more promising prospects and ambitious expectations for later life, it appears less than clear when a life can actually be regarded as completed (Schweda 2017).

These general lines of argument also play a role in the discussion of more concrete aspects of allocation policies and programs. Thus, Veatch and Ross (2015: 335) argue that serious moral problems can arise if the graft survival time of organs from older donors is shorter than the normal life expectancy of their recipients or, conversely, if older recipients have a lower life expectancy than the organs they receive from younger donors. Against this backdrop, they consider a certain age matching between donors and recipients ethically justified. At the same time, however, Veatch and Ross (2015) point out that insufficiently reflected age-based algorithms can have adverse effects. Thus, if age became a criterion for prioritization, older patients might end up having a higher chance of receiving a donor organ than younger patients: they would not only receive the organs that are regularly assigned to them but also those that have previously been rejected by younger potential recipients. In order to avoid such inadvertent detrimental effects, Veatch and Ross argue for organ allocation based on age difference between donor and recipient rather than a categorical cutoff for older persons. Evaluating recent formulas for taking age into account in organ donation, they argue that need over a lifetime should have priority over present need (Veatch/Ross 2015: 351). With regard to the ESP in particular, they criticize that the old-for-old practice restricts patient autonomy and does not promote principles of utility and justice that could justify such a restriction (ibid: 341; also see Süsal et al. 2020).

4.2   Living Donation, Familial Responsibilities, and Autonomous Decision Making

When it comes to the topic of living organ donation, the moral significance of age appears even more complex and less discussed. In contrast to the focus on distributive justice in postmortal donation, the ethical debate on living donation concentrates on questions of donors' voluntariness and self-determination. Especially in the family context, these questions are frequently intertwined with matters of age, parental and filial claims and responsibilities, and intergenerational relations between organ donors and recipients (Schweda/Wöhlke 2013; Lock/Crowley-Makota 2008).

Several socio-empirical studies have highlighted how traditional, often gendered family roles and relationships play into decision-making processes for living organ donation, posing challenges to the implementation of individualistic conceptions of personal autonomy and informed consent. This not only holds true for cultures with a traditionally strong inclination towards family decision making and moral duties based on kinship (Lee 2015), but also for late-modern Western societies (Wöhlke 2015; Crombie/Franklin 2007; Crouch/Elliot 1999). In particular, the responsibility of parents – especially mothers – to donate to their children often seems to be considered almost natural and self-evident, all the more so when minor children are concerned (Schweda/Wöhlke 2016; Zeiler et al. 2010).

However, recent ethnographic research conducted in the United States also indicates the increasing relevance and changing moral implications of age and generational roles and relations in this context. Due to advancing medical possibilities, increasing life expectancies and changing expectations regarding later life and intrafamilial care relationships, there appears to be a trend toward living organ donation from young or middle-aged persons to their older relatives. Adult children in their thirties, forties, and fifties feel inclined to donate an organ to their parents in their sixties and seventies in order to keep them alive, to express their gratitude, or to 'give something back' (Kaufman et al. 2009). In turn, the respective members of this older generation often seem to feel obliged to accept the offered organ donation in order to comply with what has become routine medical practice and to be around some time longer for the sake of their descendants (ibid.). The consequence seems to be a shift in the 'moral economy' of living organ donation between the generations of a family: what once may have appeared morally inappropriate or even 'unnatural' seems to be becoming more and more common, commendable, or even appropriate (ibid.).

From an ethical point of view, the question of the voluntariness and appropriateness of these decisions deserves closer inspection and clarification. Thus, according to Kaufman et al. (2009), the decisions of patients and health care professionals about life-extending medical interventions such as organ transplantation are usually influenced by the routine pathways of treatment, the pressures of the technological imperative, and the growing normalization, ease, and safety of treating ever older patients. The respective studies indicate that "the standard use of medical procedures at ever older ages trumps patient-initiated decision making" (ibid.: 175). This could be ethically problematic as it may undermine well-informed, deliberate and autonomous choice regarding living organ transplantation. In addition, the chances and risks for the organ recipient must also be continually evaluated and reconsidered in light of the risks for the living organ donor. The provision of adequate information about risks as well as graft and patient survival is crucial for well-informed and autonomous decisions on both sides (Cooper et al. 2011). Finally, the question of living organ donation between members of different generations within the family also touches upon the intensifying ethical debate on family obligations and especially mutual intergenerational (parental and filial) claims and responsibilities (Crouch/Elliot 1999; Lindemann Nelson/Lindemann Nelson 1995).

4.3 The Moral Relevance of Concepts of Age and Aging

In the debate on both postmortal and living transplantation, positions and arguments regarding organ donation are apparently intertwined with morally loaded ideas of aging, the individual life course, and intergenerational roles and relations. They rely on certain images of old age, age norms, and social obligations, and they touch upon more general controversies about care responsibilities, transfers between generations in the family and society at large, and fair resource allocation in aging populations. However, the relevance of these age-related categories and criteria is rarely considered and therefore less than clear in both empirical research and ethical theory.

Research on the roles and perceptions of older people in different eras and cultures makes clear that (old) age is not just an objective chronological or biological fact but also a matter of historically variable social construction and cultural interpretation (Thane 2005). For example, old age was long envisioned as a phase of social disengagement and accommodation with biological finiteness; or as a stage of natural decline in opportunities and outlooks on life; or as a state of self-containment and relinquishment in favor of younger and future generations (ibid.). Conversely, old age may also be regarded as a state of undiminished individual and social standing that should be accompanied by a fair range of opportunities and an equitable quality of life; or as a status that deserves special respect, care and gratitude from younger generations; or even as a phase of life that opens new chances and perspectives (ibid.).

As a matter of fact, a number of recent studies indicate that many of the arguments in the public political and bioethical debate on age as a factor in biomedical and health policy decision making seem to be based upon such cultural conceptions of aging and old age, especially when it comes to treatment decisions or resource allocation (Schweda et al. 2015; Ubachs-Moust et al. 2008). However, rather than being explicitly addressed and discussed, such sociocultural images and conceptions of aging and old age are usually implicit in debates, taken for granted as a self-evident basis for bioethical reasoning. Especially in modern pluralistic societies and liberal democracies, it appears increasingly problematic to presume traditional understandings of aging and old age as a basis for moral arguments, political decisions, or even legal regulations, since these may reinforce stigmatization of and discrimination against particular groups of older people. As the baby boomers are growing old, it seems likely that the changes in values accompanying this generation's pathway through life are beginning to transform our perceptions of aging and old age, for example emphasizing aspects of individual flourishing and self-fulfillment. The underlying shifts in the conception of the individual life course and the fabric of intergenerational relations challenge the traditional coordinate system of many bioethical and public health debates. A "fresh map of life" (Laslett 1989) is emerging, which calls for a systematic empirical analysis and ethical reflection on the moral significance of the life course and intergenerational relations in bioethics and public health (Schweda 2017).

To date there has been little empirical research on public perspectives regarding the moral significance of aging and old age in the context of organ donation. A few studies explore attitudes towards age rationing in the distribution of organs and hint at a growing acceptance of age as a criterion for health care prioritization (Diederich et al. 2011). In a quantitative survey, Stahl and colleagues (2008) confronted participants with trade-offs between age and urgency and found that the older the patient was the more urgency was required to receive priority. The study indicates that clinical urgency is only one of many factors influencing attitudes to allocation decisions and that respondents apply different principles of fairness, including age, depending on the relative clinical status of patients. By contrast, several other quantitative and qualitative studies show a strong rejection of the idea that young patients should be given priority over older patients (Fattore et al. 1999). Schweda and Wöhlke (2016) found that lay people were against a general limitation of access to health care resources based solely on chronological age but nevertheless acknowledged that age can be a relevant factor in ethical decision-making processes, e.g., with regard to biographical concepts and viewpoints such as age roles, ideas of the course and prime of life, or responsibilities between generations.

Regarding living donation, the role of age and generational relations has been even less investigated. A few qualitative studies indicate how age and relationships between generations within the family can play an important role in this context (Wöhlke 2015; Lock/Crowley-Makota 2008). Thus, as mentioned above, traditional life models and gender roles can make organ donation by adult parents and especially mothers to their minor children a matter of course (Zeiler 2010; Schicktanz et al. 2010; Motakef/Wöhlke 2013). In this context, age difference is sometimes associated with the perception of an asymmetric relationship between parents and children that involves unilateral parental obligations of care, responsibility and sacrifice for the health of the family and especially the children (Schicktanz et al. 2010). By the same token, when a child offers to help a parent with an organ donation, limits on filial responsibilities in parent–child relationships can be brought to the fore (Schweda/Wöhlke 2013). However, we have already seen that an expanding range of medical possibilities, increasing life expectancies, and social value change seem to challenge traditional age norms and facilitate organ donations from adult children to their parents, or even grandparents, as a new expression of intergenerational familial care and solidarity (Kaufman et al. 2009). In this context, traditional ideas and expectations regarding advanced age are increasingly called into question. The medicalization of aging reframes age-associated ailments and impairments as medical conditions that require professional treatment (Kaufman et al. 2004). In addition, more ambitious standards of adequate functionality, wellbeing, possibilities, and prospects in later life promote intensified efforts and expanding expenses for the health care of older people (Kaufman et al 2009).

5.   Conclusions and Outlook

Population aging and medical progress promote new possibilities of organ transplantation at different stages of life and between different age groups. As a result, aspects of medical feasibility and ethical questions regarding the moral implications and consequences of age in the context of organ donation are gaining relevance. In everyday life, clinical practice, and public health contexts, such questions challenge traditional understandings of the individual life course as well as intergenerational relations, and they produce serious moral insecurities, perplexities, and conflicts. This is the case, for example, when adult children offer to donate a kidney to their parents; or when organ transplantations across considerable age differences are envisaged; or when decisions have to be made regarding old and very old persons' access to (and position on) waiting lists for post mortem donor organs.

In the academic discourse, there has been comparatively little systematic consideration regarding the significance of age and generational relations in transplantation medicine to date. While there have been at least a few studies on organ donation from and to neonates and very young children (Campbell et al. 2013; Sarnaik 2015), similar systematic research concerning old age is largely absent. On the one hand, biomedical studies increasingly examine the different medical chances and risks of organ transplantation from and to older people. On the other hand, however, the relevant medical possibilities are still not sufficiently investigated, and the underlying measures of medical efficacy and cost-efficiency involved in this context are still in need of clarification and justification. The relevant bioethical discussion is only just beginning and still seems to be informed by mostly traditional conceptions of aging, the individual life course, and intergenerational relations. Such conceptions frequently suggest premature and poorly reflected proposals, such as implicitly agist utilitarian calculations or even age-based rationing of donor organs.

Only recently have more informed and differentiated approaches towards these issues been brought forward. They suggest that questions related to aging and generational relations actually mark an emerging field of empirical research and ethical debate in the context of organ donation. Three aspects in particular deserve closer consideration: First, it is imperative to collect more comprehensive and systematic evidence about the medical chances and risks of transplantations from and to older people, but also about the health economic benefits and costs of 'old for old' schemes like the European Senior Program. This research especially has to take into account that medical possibilities of organ transplantation are still evolving, and the health of older people will also be different in more recent birth cohorts such as the baby boomer generation. Second, since the success of transplantation medicine largely depends on the social acceptance of the principles of organ donation and allocation, empirical research on public opinion must more systematically address aging and intergenerationality. We need to know more about how ideas of old age and generational roles and responsibilities factor into public moral attitudes towards organ donation and transplantation. Third, a more differentiated ethical debate on the moral significance of age in organ donation is necessary. In this context, the analysis and critical reflection on outdated notions of old age, the life course, and generational relations remains an important desideratum.

References

Alexander, Shana (1962): "They Decide Who Lives, Who Dies." In: Life Magazine 53, pp. 102–125.

Bentas, Wassilios/Jones, Jon/Karaogouz, Akay/Tilp, Ursula/Probst, Michael/Scheuermann, Ernst/Hauser, Ingeborg A./Jonas, Dietger/Gossman, Jan (2008): "Renal Transplantation in the Elderly: Surgical Complications and Outcome with Special Emphasis on the Eurotransplant Senior Programme." In: Nephrology Dialysis Transplantation 23/6, pp. 2043–2051.

Boesmueller, Claudia/Biebl, Matthias/Scheidl, Stefan/Oellinger, Robert/Margreiter, Christian/Pratschke, Johann/Margreiter, Raimund/Schneeberger, Stefan (2011): "Long-Term Outcome in Kidney Transplant Recipients Over 70 Years in the Eurotransplant Senior Kidney Transplant Program: A Single Center Experience." In: Transplantation, 92/2, pp. 210–216.

Caille-Brillet, Anne-Laure/Schmidt, Karolina/Watzke, Daniela/Stander, Volker (2015): Bericht zur Repräsentativstudie 2014 „Wissen, Einstellung und Verhalten der Allgemeinbevölkerung zur Organ- und Gewebespende", Köln: BZgA.

Caille-Brillet, Anne-Laure/Zimmering, Rebecca/Thaiss, Heidrun M. (2019): Bericht zur Repräsentativstudie 2018 „Wissen, Einstellung und Verhalten der Allgemeinbevölkerung zur Organ- und Gewebespende", Köln: BZgA.

Callahan, Daniel (1987): Setting Limits. Medical Goals in an Aging Society, New York: Simon & Schuster.

Callahan, Daniel (1992): "Limiting Health Care for the Old." In: Nancy Jecker (ed.), Aging and Ethics, Totowa: Humana, pp. 219–226.

Campbell, Michael/Wright, Linda/Greenberg, Rebecca A./Grant, David (2013): "How Young is too Young to be a Living Donor?" In: American Journal of Transplantation 13/7, pp. 1643–1649.

Cooper, Matthew/Forland, Cynthia L. (2011): "The Elderly as Recipient of Living Donor Kidneys, how Old is too Old?" In: Current Opinion in Organ Transplantation 16/2, pp. 250–255.

Crombie, Alison K./Franklin, Patricia M. (2006): "Family Issues Implicit in Living Donation." In: Mortality 11/2, pp. 196–210.

Crouch, Robert A./Elliott, Carl (1999): "Moral Agency and the Family. The Case of Living Related Organ Transplantation." In: Cambridge Quarterly of Healthcare Ethics 8/3, pp. 275–287.

Cuende, Natividad/Cuende, José I./Fajardo, José/Huet, Jesus/Alonso, Manuel (2007): "Effect of Population Aging on the International Organ Donation Rates and the Effectiveness of the Donation Process." In: American Journal of Transplantation 7/6, pp. 1526–1535.

Daniels, Norman (1988): Am I my Parents' Keeper? An Essay on Justice between the Young and the Old, New York: Oxford University Press.

De Fijter, Johann W. (2009): "An Old Virtue to Improve Senior Programs." In: Transplant International 22/3, pp. 259–268.

Diederich, Adele/Winkelhage, Jeanette/Wirsik, Norman (2011): "Age as a Criterion for Setting Priorities in Health Care? A Survey of the German Public View." In: PLoS ONE 6/8, e23930. DOI: 10.1371/journal.pone.0023930

Doxiadis, Ilias/Smits, Jacqueline/Persijn, Guido/Frei, Ulrich/Claas, Frans (2004): "It Takes Six to Boogie: Allocating Cadaver Kidneys in Eurotransplant." In: Transplantation 77/4, pp. 615–617.

Eurotransplant (2018): Annual Report 2017, Leiden: Eurotransplant.

Fattore, Giovanni (1999): "Clarifying the Scope of Italian NHS Coverage. Is it feasible? Is it desirable?" In: Health Policy 50/1–2, pp. 123–142

Feuerstein, Günter (1995): Das Transplantationssystem, Weinheim: Juvena.

Frei, Ulrich/Noeldeke, Jana/Machold-Fabrizii, Veronika/Arbogast, Helmut/Machold, Klaus/Fricke, Lutz/ Voiculescu, Adina/Kliem, Volker/Ebel, Horst/Albert, Ulla/Lopau, Kai/Schnuelle, Peter/Nonnast-Daniel, Barbara/Pietruck, Frank/Offermann, Ralf/Persijn, Guido/Bernasconi, Corrado (2008): "Prospective Age-Matching in Elderly Kidney Transplant Recipients – a 5-year Analysis of the Eurotransplant Senior Program." In: American Journal of Transplantation 8/1, pp. 50–57.

Fritsche, Lutz/Hörstrup, Jan Henrik/Budde, Klemens/Reinke, Petra/Giessing, Marcus/Tullius, Stefan G./Loening, Stefan/Neuhaus, Peter/Neumayer, Hans-Hellmut/Frei, Ulrich (2003): "Old-For-Old Kidney Allocation Allows Successful Expansion of the Donor and Recipient Pool." In: American Journal of Transplantation 3/11, pp. 1434–1439.

Goldstein, Daniel R. (2012): "The Graying of Organ Transplantation." In: American Journal of Transplantation 12/10, pp. 2569–2570.

Harris, John (1985): The Value of Life, London: Routledge and Kegan Paul.

Hebert, Sean. A./Ibrahim, Hasan. N. (2019): "Kidney Transplantation in Septuagenarians: 70 Is the New 60!" In: Kidney International Reports, 4/5, pp. 640–642.

Heemann, Uwe/Renders, Lutz (2018): „Nierenallokation in Deutschland. Gegenwärtiger Stand und mögliche Weiterentwicklungen." In: Der Nephrologe 13/5, pp. 355–365.

Heldal, Kristian/Leivestad, Torbjørn/Hartmann, Anders/Veel Svendson, Martin/Lien, Bjørn Herman/Midtvedt, Karsten (2008): "Kidney Transplantation in the Elderly – the Norwegian Experience." In: Nephrology Dialysis Transplantation 23/3, pp. 1026–1031.

Kaufman, Sharon R. (2007): "Fairness and the Tyranny of Potential in Kidney Transplantation." In: Current Anthropology 54/57, pp. 56–66.

Kaufman, Sharon R./Fjord, Lakshmi (2011): "Medicare, Ethics, and Reflexive Longevity: Governing Time and Treatment in an Aging Society." In: Medical Anthropology Quarterly 25/2, pp. 209–231.

Kaufman, Sharon R./Russ, Ann J./Shim, Janet K. (2009): "Aged Bodies and Kinship Matters: The Ethical Field of Kidney Transplant." In: Helen Lambert/Maryon McDonald (eds.), Social Bodies, New York: Berghahn, pp. 17–46.

Kaufman, Sharon R./Shim, Janet K./Russ, Ann J. (2004): "Revisiting the Biomedicalization of Aging: Clinical Trends and Ethical Challenges." In: The Gerontologist 44/6, pp. 731–738.

Kilner, John F. (1988): "The Ethical Legitimacy of Excluding the Elderly when Medical Resources are Limited." In: The Annual of the Society of Christian Ethics, pp. 179–203.

Ladin, Keren/Hanto, Douglas W. (2011): "Rational Rationing or Discrimination: Balancing Equity and Efficiency Considerations in Kidney Allocation." In: American Journal of Transplantation 11/11, pp. 2317–2321.

Laslett, Peter (1989): A Fresh Map of Life: The Emergence of the Third Age, London: Weidenfeld and Nicolson.

Lee, Shui Chuen (2015): "Intimacy and Family Consent: a Confucian Ideal." In: Journal of Medicine and Philosophy 40/4, pp. 418–436.

Lindemann Nelson, Hilde/Lindemann Nelson, James (1995): The Patient in the Family: An Ethics of Medicine and Families, New York: Routledge.

Lock, Margaret/Crowley-Makota, Megan (2008): "Situating the Practice of Organ Donation in Familial, cultural, and Political Context." In: Transplantation Reviews 22/3, pp. 154–157.

Lopp, Leonie (2013): Regulations Regarding Living Organ Donation in Europe. Possibilities in Harmonisation, Heidelberg: Springer.

Macrae, Jeanne/Friedman, Amy L./Friedman, Eli A./Eggers, Paul (2005): "Live and Deceased Donor Kidney Transplantation in Patients Aged 75 Years and Older in the United States." In: International Urology and Nephrology 37/3, pp. 641–648.

McAdams-DeMarco, Mara A./Ying, Hao/Olorundare, Israel/King, Elizabeth A./Haugen, Christine/Buta, Brian/Gross, Alden L./Kalyani, Rita/Desai, Niraj/Dagher, Nabil N./Lonze, Bonnie E./Montgomery, Robert A./Bandeen-Roche, Karen/Walston, Jeremy D./Segev, Dory L. (2017): "Individual Frailty Components and

Mortality in Kidney Transplant Recipients." In: Transplantation 101/9, pp. 2126–2132.

Meier-Kriesche, Herwig Ulf/Schold, Jesse D./Gaston, Robert S./Wadstrom, Jonas/Kaplan, Bruce (2005): "Kidneys from Deceased Donors: Maximizing the Value of a Scarce Resource." In: American Journal of Transplantation 5/7, pp. 1725–1730.

Mistry, Bhargav/McKeever, Brian/Phadke, Gautam/Mahale, Adit (2010): "World's Oldest Donor-Recipient Solid Organ Transplantation?" In: Dialysis & Transplantation 39/12, pp. 534–535.

Montgomery, Robert A./Gentry, Sommer E./Marks, William H./Warren, Daniel S./Hiller, Janet/Houp, Julie/Zachary, Andrea A./Melancon, J. Keith/Maley, Warren R./Rabb, Hamid /Simpkins, Christopher/Segev, Dorry L. (2006): "Domino Paired Kidney Donation: A Strategy to Make Best Use of Live Non-Directed Donation." In: Lancet 368/9533, pp. 419–21.

Motakef, Mona/Wöhlke, Sabine (2013): "Ambivalente Praxen der (Re)Produktion: Fürsorge, Bioökonomie und Geschlecht in der Lebendorganspende" In: Gender 5/3, pp. 94–113.

Oniscu, Gabriel C./Brown, Helen/Forsythe, John L. (2004): "How Old is Old for Transplantation?" In: American Journal of Transplantation 4/12, pp. 2067–2074.

Oniscu, Gabriel C./Brown, Helen/Forsythe, John L. (2005): "Impact of Cadaveric Renal Transplantation on Survival in Patients Listed for Transplantation." In: Journal of the American Society of Nephrology 16/6, pp. 1859–1865.

Persad, Govind/Wertheimer, Alan/Emanuel, Ezekiel J. (2009): "Principles for Allocation of Scarce Medical Interventions." In: The Lancet 373/9661, pp. 423–431.

Rao, Panduranga/Merion, Robert/Ashby, Valarie/Port, Friedrich/Wolfe, Robert A./Kayler Liise (2007): "Renal Transplantation in Elderly Patients Older than 70 Years of Age: Results from the Scientific Registry of Transplant Recipients." In: Transplantation 83, pp. 1069–1074.

Reese, Peter P./Bloom, Roy D./Feldman, Herold/Rosenbaum, Paul/Wang, Wei/Saynisch, Philip/Mukherjee, Nabanita/Garg, Amit X./Mussell, Adam/Shults, Justine/Even-Shoshan, Orit/Townsend, Raymond R./Silber, Jeffrey H. (2014): "Mortality and Cardiovascular Disease Among Older Live Kidney Donors." In: American Journal of Transplantation 14/8, pp. 1853–1861.

Reese, Peter P./Caplan, Arthur L./Bloom, Roy D./Abt, Peter/Karlawish, Jason H. (2010): "How Should we Use Age to Ration Health Care? Lessons from the Case of Kidney Transplantation." In: Journal of the American Geriatrics Society 58/10, pp. 1980–1986.

Rickert, Charles G./Markmann, James F. (2018): "Aging, Immunosenescence, and Transplantation Tolerance." In: Tamas Fulop/Claudio Franceschi/Katsuiku Hirokawa/Graham Pawelec (eds), Handbook of Immunosenescence: Basic Understanding and Clinical Implications, Cham: Springer, pp. 1–17.

Sarnaik, Ajit A. (2015): "Neonatal and Pediatric Organ Donation: Ethical Perspectives and Implications for Policy." In: Frontiers in Pediatrics 3/100, pp. 1–7.

Schamberger, Beate/Lohmann, Dario/Sollinger, Daniel/Stein, Reimund/Lutz, Jens (2018): "Association of Kidney Donor Risk Index with the Outcome after Kidney Transplantation in the Eurotransplant Senior Program." In: Annals of Transplantation 23, pp. 775–781.

Schicktanz, Silke/Pfaller, Larissa/Hansen, Solveig Lena/Boos, Moritz (2017): "Attitudes towards Brain Death and Conceptions of the Body in Relation to Willingness or Reluctance to Donate: Results of a Student Survey before and after the German Transplantation Scandals and Legal Changes." In: Journal of Public Health 25/3, pp. 249–256.

Schicktanz, Silke/Schweda, Mark/Wöhlke, Sabine (2010): "Gender Issues in Living Organ Donation: Medical, Social and Ethical Aspects." In: Ineke Klinge/Claudia Wiesemann (eds.), Gender and Medicine, Göttingen: Universitätsverlag Göttingen, pp. 33–55.

Schlieper, Georg/Ivens, Katrin/Voiculescu, Adina/Luther, Bernd/Sandman, Wilhelm/Grabensee, Bernd (2001): "Eurotransplant Senior Program 'Old for Old': Results from Ten Patients." In: Clinical Transplantation 15/2, pp. 100–105.

Schulte, Kevin/Klasen, Vera/Vollmer, Clara/Borzikowsky, Christoph/Kunzendorf, Ulrich/Feldkamp, Thorsten (2018): "Analysis of the Eurotransplant Kidney Allocation Algorithm: How Should We Balance Utility and Equity?" In: Transplantation Proceedings 50/10, pp. 3010–3016.

Schweda, Mark (2017): "'A Season to Everything'?: Considering Life-course Perspectives in Bioethical and Public Health Discussions on Aging." In: Mark Schweda/Larissa Pfaller/Kai Brauer/Frank Adloff/Silke Schicktanz (eds.), Planning Later Life. Bioethics and Public Health in Aging Societies, Abingdon: Routledge, pp. 11–30.

Schweda, Mark/Inthorn, Julia/Wöhlke, Sabine (2015): "'Not the Years in Themselves Count': The Role of Age for European Citizens' Moral Attitudes towards Resource Allocation in Modern Biomedicine." In: Journal of Public Health 23/3, pp. 117–126.

Schweda, Mark/Wöhlke, Sabine (2013): "Lasting Bonds and New Connections: Public Views on the Donor-Recipient-Relation and their Implications for the Ethics of Organ Transplantation." In: Mary Anne Lauri (ed.), Organ Donation and Transplantation: An Interdisciplinary Approach, New York: Nova, pp. 171–188

Schweda, Mark/Wöhlke, Sabine (2016): "Age and Generational Relations in Organ Donation: An Emerging Field of Empirical Research and Ethical Controversy." In: Willem Weimar/Emma Massay (eds.), Globale Challenges, Lengerich: Pabst, pp. 44–52.

Smith, George P. (1996): "Our Hearts Were Once Young and Gay: Health Care Rationing and the Elderly." In: University of Florida Journal of Law and Public Policy 8/1, pp. 1–23.

Smits, Jacqueline/Persijn, Guido/Van Houwelingen, Hans C./Claas, Frans/Frei, Ulrich (2002): "Evaluation of the Eurotransplant Senior Program. The Results of the First year." In: American Journal of Transplantation 2/7, pp. 664–670.

Smits, Jacqueline/ Van Houwelingen, Hans C./De Meester, Johann/Persijn, Guido/Claas, Frans (1998): "Analysis of the Renal Transplant Waiting List. Application of a Parametric Competing Risk Method." In: Transplantation 66, pp. 1146–1153.

Stahl, James E./Tramontano, Angela C./Swan, John S./Cohen, Brian J. (2008): "Balancing Urgency, Age and Quality of Life in Organ Allocation Decisions—What Would you Do? A Survey." In: Journal of Medical Ethics 34/2, pp. 109–115.

Süsal, Caner/Kumru, Gizem/Döhler, Bernd/Morath, Christian/Baas, Marije/Lutz, Jens/Unterrainer, Christian/Arns, Wolfgang/Aubert, Olivier/Bara, Christoph/Beiras-Fernandez, Andres/Böhmig, Georg A./Bösmüller, Claudia/Diekmann, Fritz/Dutkowski, Philipp/Hauser, Ingeborg/Legendre, Christophe/Lozanovski, Vladimir J./Mehrabi, Arianeb/Melk, Anette/Minor, Thomas/Mueller, Thomas F./Pisarski, Przemyslaw/Rostaing, Lionel/Schemmer, Peter/Schneeberger, Stefan/Schwenger, Vedat/Sommerer, Claudia/Tönshoff, Burkhard/Viebahn, Richard/Viklicky, Ondrej/Weimer, Rolf/Weiss, Karl-Heinz/Zeier, Martin/Živčić-Ćosić, Stela/Heemann, Uwe (2020): "Should kidney allografts from old donors be allocated only to old recipients?" In: Transplant International 33/8, pp. 849-857.

Tsuchiya, Aki (2000): "QALYs and Ageism: Philosophical Theories and Age Weighting." In: Health Economics 9/1, pp. 57–68.

Ubachs-Moust, Josy/Houtepen, Rob/Vos, Rein/Ter Meulen, Ruud (2008): "Value Judgements in the Decision-Making Process for the Elderly Patient." In: Journal of Medical Ethics 34/12, pp. 863–868.

U.S. Department of Health and Human Services, Health Resources and Services Administration (2012): "If you were there then, we Need you Now. Organ, Eye, and Tissue Donation for People 50 and Over", Washington, DC: U.S. Department of Health and Human Services.

Veatch, Robert (2002): Transplantation Ethics, Washington: Georgetown University Press.

Veatch, Robert/Ross, Lainie (2015): Transplantation Ethics, 2nd Edition, Washington: Georgetown University Press.

Wöhlke, Sabine (2015): Geschenkte Organe? Ethische und kulturelle Herausforderungen bei der familiären Lebendorganspende. Frankfurt a.M.: Campus.

Wu, Christine/Shapiro, Ron/Tan, Henkie/Basu, Amit/Smetanka, Cynthia/Morgan, Claire/Nirav, Shah/McCauley, Jerry/Unruh, Mark. (2008): "Kidney Transplantation in Elderly People: The Influence of Recipient Comorbidity and Living Kidney Donors." In: Journal of the American Geriatrics Society 56/2, pp. 231–238.

Zeiler, Kristin/Guntram, Lisa/Lennerling, Anette (2010): "Moral Tales of Parental Living Kidney Donation: a Parenthood Moral Imperative and its Relevance for Decision Making." In: Medicine, Health Care and Philosophy 13/3, pp. 225–236.

Zhou, Xin. J/Rakheja, Dinesh/Yu, Xueging/Saxena, Ramesh/Vaziri, Nosratola D./Silva, Fred G. (2008): "The Aging Kidney." In: Kidney International 74/6, pp. 710–720.

IV. ORGAN RECIPIENTS

13. Living with a Transplant
Identity and a Good Life[1]

Paweł Łuków

1. Introduction

The intuitive rationale behind transplants is that they save life and improve its quality. While obviously sound, these reasons can only be elements of any plausible answer to the more fundamental question about a good post-transplant life. 'Good life' does not reduce to survival or quality of life, or the two combined. A good life is a life that is good all things considered, taking account of all the values, circumstances, and considerations that matter in a particular person's life or make their life worthy for them. It can include balance of pleasure and pain, satisfaction of desires or fulfillment of expectations, achievement of objective goods, pursuit of personal goals, discharge of obligations, and various other elements and circumstances, as judged from the objectivizing perspective human beings take when they reflect on their own lives.

Human beings are planning and decision-making beings. When they plan their actions or make decisions they ask the ethical question: 'How should one live?' (Williams 1985). An answer to that question, which relies on the person's self-knowledge and self-understanding, entails a conception of a good life. To judge how well one's life is going, all things considered, and to choose how to act, one must appeal to such an objectivizing view of a good life; to provide guidance to planning and action, the conception must be sufficiently stable and instructive and relate to the actual circumstances of the individual's embodied existence. To *have* a good life, the human being needs a sufficiently stable and instructive conception *of* a good life.

This chapter will discuss the difficulties that transplant patients can encounter in their efforts to arrive at a conception of a good life as applying to their own life after surgery. While most authors discuss the social and psychological aspects of the transplant patient's life, as well as its quality, they generally remain silent about the interaction between the transplant patient's identity and their sense of how well their life is going. This is a serious omission. The decision to undergo transplant treatment and the process of recovery necessarily involve the most fundamental values and commitments (e.g. life itself, social bonds and relations, life goals). Those values and their

1 Research for this chapter was funded by the National Science Centre, Poland; Project No. 2015/17/B/ HS1/02390.

interrelations contribute to the identity of the patient. The removal of a diseased body part and its replacement with one that comes from another person shapes that identity in the most basic, physical way, and thus, together with the demands of a post-transplant treatment regime, it often demands rethinking or rearrangement of one's own conception of a good life. Thus, the focus on a good life and identity is of central importance to the perception of transplant patients as persons or agents. It can also help medical professionals to achieve a rich, comprehensive and integrated understanding of the existential situation of transplant patients, and therefore to respond adequately to their needs.

In this chapter it will be argued that due to the embodied nature of a human being and the central place embodied identity must occupy in every conception of a good life, and in every judgment of the worth of an individual life all things considered, transplants, by modifying the patient's bodily make-up, challenge their prospects for arriving at a sufficiently stable and instructive view of a good post-transplant life, and thus a reliable judgment about how well their life is going. The instabilities and indeterminacies of that conception may in turn result in problems with the patient's future identity. The instabilities in the patient's present identity, and in their conception of a good life, can prevent them from developing a sufficiently stable and instructive future identity, and so from having a good post-transplant life. An adequate response to such challenges may involve not only reciprocal adaptation of the patient's post-transplant identity and their conception of a good life but also a reframing of the very concept of the good life when applied to life after transplant surgery.

The discussion that follows will not investigate the components of conceptions of a good life. Such conceptions can differ vastly from theory to theory and from person to person. There thus seems to be insufficient grounds for adopting an overarching framework that relates those conceptions to post-transplant life. Additionally, since well-being seems to be a necessary component of every conception of a good life, and well-being during illness is not necessarily significantly lower than when healthy (Angner et al. 2009; Chwalisz et al. 1988; de Haes & van Knippenberg 1985; Riis et al. 2005), one should not assume that post-transplant life is necessarily worse, all things considered, than life in health. An attempt to judge whether a post-transplant life is necessarily good or not would presuppose a particular view of a good life, and so it would risk an imposition of such a view on post-transplant patients, effectively foreclosing some intuitively plausible alternative views of a good life.

The discussion will focus on post-transplant identity as a prerequisite of the process of arriving at, and sustaining, a conception of a good life and judging one's own life to be good, independently of the particular contents or structure of such a conception. These processes can be explicit, involving cognitively and affectively committed reflection on various aspects of one's own life; but they can also be tacit and result in cognitive and affective engagement with life events; and they can be a combination of the two. The identity to be discussed will not be understood as an individual's or object's sameness over time, or a person's sense or feeling of being one and the same at different points in time, although some aspects of this will transpire in the discussion. The identity considered in this chapter refers to the embodied experiences that collectively constitute one biography of a human being, and in this way define a particular human being as having a personality composed of, among other things, beliefs, habits, preferences, skills, and traits of character (Goldie 2004; Rorty/Wong 1990). A human being's biography is necessarily extended over time and susceptible to change. Thus, the identity of a human being is temporal, changeable, and therefore incomplete. To be a whole, a human being's life and identity need a significant degree of consistency between their events and phases. Although they may include significant disruptions, they can remain one biography and one identity.

This chapter begins with a phenomenological perspective on the embodied identity of the human being and illness. The insights deriving from this perspective will be then applied to the situation of the transplant patient. Such an outlook draws attention to the subjectivity of patients, thereby revealing the interrelations between patient identity and a good life, and moving beyond a focus on the physiological and socio-psychological aspects of medical care.

The theses that will be presented in this chapter regarding the possibility of arriving at a sufficiently stable and instructive conception of a good post-transplant life should not be understood as reports from empirical research or universal truths. Collectively, empirical data on the lived experiences of transplant patients form a repertoire of the various experiences that constitute illness and identity, and post-transplant identity. This repertoire will serve as the basis for an exploration of the interrelations between post-transplant identity, conception of a good life, and the potential difficulties in achieving such a life after transplant surgery. The elements of that repertoire form a range of experiences which can come in various combinations, depending, among other things, on the patient's biography, health status and history, social context, medical and lay ideologies, or the organ involved. Accordingly, the discussion of the possibility of achieving a sufficiently stable and instructive view of a good post-transplant life is not about universal phenomena. Rather, it is to be read as an exploration of the various challenges that transplant patients can face in their attempts to form a conception of a good post-transplant life.

The first section sketches the lived bodily experience of illness. It relies on the idea that a human body is not a mere Cartesian vehicle for a soul but a constituent of a specifically human identity, both species identity and identity as a particular member of that species. This section provides background for the discussion of post-transplant identity in the second section. As the available anthropological studies show, post-transplant identity is in many, often unique, ways fragile and unstable; it is frequently disrupted and in need of restructuring. In many respects this identity eludes the patient's control by subordinating their daily affairs to medical surveillance, and it is repeatedly challenged by the risk of organ rejection, the demands of immunosuppressive therapy, and medical complications. Building on these insights, the third section offers a philosophical investigation into the potential impact of post-transplant identity on the process of arriving at a sufficiently stable and instructive view of a good post-transplant life.

Due to the diversity and uniqueness of post-transplant experiences as they relate to the question of a good post-transplant life, this section cannot and will not report empirical data, although such data are appealed to. It is an exploration of the difficulties that transplant patients can encounter in their attempts to arrive at a stable and instructive conception of a good life. This exploration reveals that patients may need to reframe their conceptions of a good post-transplant life rather than merely rearrange or reconstruct them. A reframed conception of a good post-transplant life will often need to be open-ended to make room for the creative process of assimilation of the conflicts, uncertainties and instabilities of the post-transplant identity. In this way the conflicts, uncertainties and instabilities of the post-transplant identity can become a whole which makes the patient's life undoubtedly theirs.

2.   The Experience of Illness

The human body is the essential constituent of a human biological and biographical life. It is the basis both of an individual's membership in the human species and of their particular identity. An individual human body sustains the existence and identity of a particular human being over time and is the central instrument of their interactions with their natural and social environments. Embodiment makes human beings capable of good and evil, of having a conception of a good life, and of being susceptible to diverse benefits and harms. Additionally, human beings can form views of a good life because they are aware of the fragilities of their existence, which are brought about in a profound way by their embodiment.

The body is not only the physical substratum of a human being's existence (*Körper*); it is also the lived body (*Leib*) (Husserl 1989: §36) or embodiment, which is the conscious presence in, and involvement with, an environment. A person[2] as a particular lived body relates to the objects in their environment (which are perceived as really there) through their sensory experiences (Merleau-Ponty 1962), feelings, and emotions (Buytendijk 1987). In contrast to the physical body, the lived body is not simply the site of experiences, feelings and emotions. Experiences, feelings and emotions locate a human being as an entity in the world rather than as a sovereign Cartesian mind or mode of reference to things or to oneself. The lived body makes it possible to conceive of the objects and oneself as belonging to the same world. This double relationship to the things out there and to oneself establishes a particular person's sense of identity and individuality as a unique and separate entity (Merleau-Ponty 1962), and includes, among other things, their beliefs, habits, preferences, skills, and traits of character.

Despite its obvious centrality for human life, filled with thinking, planning, deciding, feeling, etc., the lived body usually remains transparent to human beings because life in health involves relating oneself as a whole, rather than as an aggregate of parts, to the objects in the environment rather than relating to oneself (Gadamer 1996; Leder 1990; Merleau-Ponty 1962; Sartre 1978 [1956]: 324–326; Zaner 1981). The absence of discomfort or pain makes one's own embodiment and the arrangement of one's own body parts imperceptible (Leder 1990; Zeiler 2010) and so unproblematic. One's own embodiment is brought to one's attention in health only occasionally, as a result of effort or fatigue (Van Den Berg 1987) or during pregnancy (Young 2005: 46–61). Unlike most instances of discomfort or pain, the absence of unpleasantness and pleasure does not have a specific place in the body. The lived body, which in various ways founds the person's being and presence in the world and mostly remains a transparent whole in times of health, can become an experienced sum of its parts in times of illness.

Illness, which is a fundamentally subjective experience, brings one's own body to one's attention, initially through a general and indeterminate discomfort (Zeiler 2010).

---

2 "Human being" and "person" will be used interchangeably. No substantive ethical assumptions typically associated with "person" are made in this chapter.

An attempt to make illness objective, or to develop an objective account of it, would presuppose its separation from the ill person. The resulting account would be alienated from the things which make the experience of illness possible and actual; it would also be limited to what is intersubjectively available (Agazzi 2001). Illness may begin with an unspecified and often pre-reflective experience that "something is the matter", that "one somehow does not feel quite right" (Gadamer 1996: 111), or that something is wrong with the person (Gert et al. 2006: 136). At more advanced stages of illness, the experience can be conceptualized as biographical disruption (Bury 1982), disruption of the lived body (Toombs 1988), otherness or alienation of the body from the ill person (Cassell 1985; Svenaeus 2000a, 2000b; Zaner 1981), disconnection of the body from the self of the ill person (Leder 1990), objectification of the body (Toombs 1988, 1992: 201–226), uncanniness and unhomelikeness (*Unheimlichkeit*) of the body (Svenaeus 2000b, 2011), or doubt in one's own body (Carel 2016: 86–105).

Illness drives a wedge between a person's sense of the integrity of their self and their body, making the body perceptible to that person (Kass 1985: 220; Merleau-Ponty 1962; Sartre 1978 [1956]: 337–338) and problematic (Frank 1995). Illness is defined by dualities which are usually absent in life in health. The first, most prominent duality is that of the body and the self (Cassell 1985: 55–65; Toombs 1988). The pains and discomforts caused by a disease and the limited capabilities of the diseased body shift the person's focus from the surrounding objects to the body, revealing it as an entity somewhat separated or distanced from the self. Bodily movements, whose technicalities usually escape the person's awareness, as well as the wholeness of the body in health, are now analyzed into their parts and processes, which must be controlled individually. Pain in the knee, for example, usually requires planning of how to position the foot or balance the body's weight while walking. The lived body in illness is no longer a unitary and harmonious whole, but a precarious structure made of processes and parts, which, due to the discord brought about by illness, need individual attention and corrections. The second duality in illness is a dissonance between the individual's self-image and their actual presence in the world. By depriving the lived body of some of its experiences, as well as affording new ones, illness confronts the person with change at the most intimate level; it surprises them and calls for self-reflection and sometimes re-construction of the self-image.

The dualities of illness make the human being realize that their body is the only form of existence available to them; experientially there is no alternative to their embodied existence, which determines who they are. The dualities of illness show that the human body is not an instrument that occasionally works badly, has defects, ceases to work as usual, or lets the person down. They reveal that illness is a total experience. It is the whole human being who is ill, not just their body or its part. This suggests that the ill person *is* the ailing lived body in a way similar to that in which a healthy human being is a healthy lived body.

The weaknesses, limitations, and dualities of the ill human being's diseased body can be experienced as chronic sorrow, frustration, anger and a sense of futility in making long term plans (Kierans 2005; Michael 1996), loss of self, diminished sense of self-identity, or as grieving for one's former identity (Charmaz 1983, 1995; Matson/ Brooks 1977). This is not to say that the weaknesses, limitations and dualities of illness have only negative impact on the ill person. They can also prompt adaptation and desirable changes, giving rise to the need to regain control over one's own affairs, promote personal growth and change (Michael 1996; Moch 1989), or struggle for normalcy (Öhman et al. 2003). Whether judged negatively or positively, the bodily changes brought about by illness affect the physical and perceptual abilities of the human being and their very subjectivity(Merleau-Ponty 1962).

3.   The Fragility of Post-transplant Identity

While in illness identity disruption is likely, organ transplants, much like chronic illness, necessarily affect the person's identity due to the bodily discontinuity brought about by removal of the diseased organ, and the bodily re-constitution prompted by implantation of someone else's body part. Due to the temporal dimension of transplant treatment, the impact of a transplant on a person's identity must be seen as a process which starts at the latest at the moment of removal of the diseased organ and continues during recovery and, potentially, the rest of the patient's life. Not infrequently, this "identity process" begins before the surgery, with the illness reaching the stage at which a transplant is considered (e.g. burdens of the treatment of the underlying disease, dependence on health care services, waiting for the organ) (Ådahl 2013; Kierans 2005), and lasts through the surgery into the remainder of the patient's life (Cormier et al. 2017; Varela 2001). The gravity of the impact of the transplant process on the patient's identity will vary not only depending on the characteristics of the recipient but also on the experiential identity significance of the body part to be removed and replaced (Svenaeus 2012, 2016: 28). The identity significance of a body part can be related to its visibility (e.g. a hand), indispensability for the human being's survival (e.g. the lungs), potential for spontaneous regeneration (e.g. the liver), cultural meaning related to traits of character, and association with expression of the individual's perceived personality (e.g. the heart).

The identity-related experiences of transplant patients will typically have two stages, often overlapping and varying, depending on the identity significance of the body part to be replaced. One is the experience of the anticipated and actual loss of the body part to be removed, the resulting fear of a loss of one's self (Belk 1992), and the subsequent loss of the imagined past "(compiled of experiences, sensations and achievements) that transplant patients consider that they might have had" (Baines/Jindal 2003: 124) if they had not suffered from the disease that had led to the loss of this organ. Depending on the identity significance of the diseased organ or the life stage at which the loss happens, the occurrence, forms and intensity of grieving for the loss of the organ can differ. For example, adolescents who – due to the burdens of the underlying condition – may miss out on some developmental stages may not grieve after the organ is removed because they have not had an opportunity to assimilate it in forming that identity, a process still underway (Anderson et al. 2017).

The second stage of the identity-related experiences of transplant patients is connected with the acquisition of a new body part and the need to incorporate it into the patient's identity. Again, the form and dynamics of this stage will vary depending on the identity significance of the body part replaced and the stage of life of the patient. It will also be shaped by the patient's health status (urgent or planned) and prognosis, the type of donor (deceased or living), the information about the donor that is available to the patient (ranging from anonymity to personal knowledge), and by the emotional links between the recipient and the donor (non-related versus related donation).

The following discussion of post-transplant identity covers both stages of the post-transplant identity process in its sequential dynamics of a living experience, whose elements – depending on the patient and their social circumstances – can be variously arranged and can differ in their prominence. Special attention will be paid to the post-transplant stage.

As noted in the section above, a person's own identity usually escapes their awareness, the body being taken for granted. The sequence of organ failure, removal, and replacement brings the individual's body to their attention. This sequence both questions their identity and reveals its importance, calling for its reconstruction. Clearly, the key element of the identity process in transplant recipients is the presence and functioning of a 'foreign' body part which, when combined with the patient's dependence on that organ for survival, can result in a conflicted or problematic identity. The foreign body part challenges the patient's identity by its presence in their body, but in most cases it simultaneously sustains that identity by making continued life possible (Nancy 2008). The patient must therefore incorporate the transplanted body part into their new or modified identity (Mauthner et al. 2015).

This conflict may be intensified by the patient's sense of connectedness to the organ donor as well as the contradictory messages medical staff communicate about the implanted body part. On the one hand, to motivate patients to comply with the demands of the immunosuppressive therapy, medical professionals often refer to the precious "gift of life", which imaginatively and affectively links the transplanted organ to its donor. Depending on the identity significance of the transplanted body part, such linking can initiate imaginative bonding of the patient with the donor, and in this way modification of the patient's identity. Not infrequently, patients contemplate the possibility of inheriting their donor's traits (Ådahl 2013; Bunzel et al. 1992; Inspector et al. 2004; Kaba et al. 2005; Neukom et al. 2012; Sanner 2001, 2003). Additionally, the stress on the value of the transplanted body part may trigger guilt over the fact that someone had to die to allow the patient to survive (Anthony et al. 2019; Forsberg et al. 2000; Inspector et al. 2004; Kaba et al. 2005; Mai 1986; Neukom et al. 2012; Sanner 2003; Schmid-Mohler et al. 2014). On the other hand, medical professionals routinely objectify transplanted organs as spare parts (e.g. the heart as "just a pump"), thus depersonalizing the sources of the body parts (Bunzel et al. 1992; Mai 1986; Sanner 2003; Sharp 1995). In combination with the gift-of-life imagery and corresponding to the identity significance of the transplanted organ, depersonalization can make it difficult for the transplant patient to perceive the organ as an integral part of their own body and identity (Nancy 2008), which can prompt confusion about their own identity (Forsberg et al. 2000; Tong et al. 2011). Accordingly, patients need to take steps to rebuild their identities and regain a sense of personal consistency and continuity.

As in life in health (Carr 1986; Ricoeur 1986), attempts to reconstruct one's own identity during serious illness often take the form of identity-shaping narratives (Bury 2001; Frank 1995; Williams 1984). The stories draw on the patient's biography as well as the (imagined or actual) biography of the donor and the implanted body part and reflexively shape the patient's biography. Since the transplanted body part belongs to the donor's biography, the recipient may view it as having its own story (Sharp 1995), which needs to be integrated, sometimes in combination with the donor's biography, into the patient's life story. Thus, recipients sometimes personalize transplanted organs, internalize images of their donors, or integrate those images into their newly constructed identities (Forsberg et al. 2000; Sharp 1995).

The consistency and continuity of the post-transplant identity can be extremely difficult to achieve and maintain. The popular rhetoric (intended to encourage post-humous donation) of the cadaveric donors "living on" in recipients imposes the donor's (actual or imagined) biography on the patient's construal of their identity, which is thus modified or perhaps even compromised. Thus, as suggested by frequent retro-spective conceptualizations of the surgery as renewal, rebirth, or becoming a new per-son (Ådahl 2013; Inspector et al. 2004; Kierans 2011; Neukom et al. 2012; Sharp 1995), post-transplant identity is not simply a modified pre-transplant identity; it can be a new identity which calls for its own narrative. The transplant patient may have to re-invent themselves as a unique individual who is both continuous with their pre-transplant self and transformed after the surgery. This process can be disturbed by the immunosup-pressive treatment, which requires commitment to continued medical surveillance of their life (Cormier et al. 2017), and so it removes from the patient's control a significant part of their future life story and their new identity. Additionally, since the demands of immunosuppression regularly remind the recipient of the presence of a body part that comes from another individual, which, together with the fear of rejection (Baines/Jin-dal 2003: 133–136; Forsberg et al. 2000; Juneau 1995; Schmid-Mohler et al. 2014; Sharp 1995), becomes the recipient's lifetime companion, the transplant patient's identity is repeatedly questioned, frequently uncertain, dependent, and leaves the patient in the precarious space between a world of abnormality, illness, limited productivity and dependence, and a world of normalcy, health, productivity and independence (Juneau 1995; Schmid-Mohler et al. 2014).

The varieties of post-transplant experiences and their impact on post-trans-plant identity are akin to the experience of chronic illness. The need to incorporate a transplanted organ into one's body and identity, as well as to adjust one's affairs to the demands of immunosuppression, can alternatively lead to rejection, engulfment, acceptance, or enrichment (Oris et al. 2018). One may reject the fact of being a trans-plant patient by disregarding various aspects of the post-transplant regimen. Or hav-ing a transplanted body part may engulf the patient to the extent that it will dominate all spheres, activities and efforts in their life. Alternatively, the patient may accept the fact of having an implanted organ without being overwhelmed by it or by the require-ments of the post-transplant regimen. Finally, the patient may be enriched by their new bodily make-up, seeing it as an opportunity for growth and personal development.

These beliefs and attitudes are responses to the lasting instability of the post-trans-plant identity, which is questioned, compromised, restructured, difficult to control, and uncertain – repeatedly and on many different levels. Such identity instability can have profound implications for the patient's ability to design their conception of a good life, and to live a good life at all. But it also harbors the promise of a good post-trans-plant life.

4.   The Continuing Challenge of Good Post-transplant Life

Human beings are not only cognizant of, and respond to, the environment. They are also aware of themselves, notably while thinking about their future (Klinger 1994). Future-oriented activities like planning and making decisions involve both self-aware-ness and awareness of the surrounding environment, which includes knowledge of its current and past states and causal links between its elements. These activities also include beliefs about agreement or disagreement between the objects of awareness and the self-awareness, and positive or negative attitudes towards these relations. These attitudes are not exclusively unreflective or instinctual. To a significant extent they rely on fundamental normative beliefs, which, when combined into sufficiently consistent wholes that include a person's 'ground projects' (Williams 1981), form that person's conception of a good life. Such a conception includes moral beliefs – such as those about obligations, values, rights, virtues etc. – but need not be limited or reducible to them (Nagel 1986; Williams 1981). Regardless of its contents, this concep-tion offers the person an impersonal or objectivizing perspective on their life affairs that allows them to make judgments about their life as good or worth pursuing (Annas 2004).

Within such an objectivizing perspective, a conception of a good life mediates between the person's past and present identity and their future identity according to the normative beliefs that comprise that conception. A person's view of a good life makes it possible for them to care about their future identity as specifically *theirs* (Williams 1981) – that is, to combine their past, present and future into a consistent personal narrative (Ricoeur 1986). This process is a two-way interaction between the person's conception of a good life with a focus on the future, and their unique present identity as it has been shaped by the preceding events in their life. Accordingly, the fundamental normative beliefs that make up a person's conception of a good life nec-essarily belong to their present identity (Williams 1981). Making (far-reaching) deci-sions and taking an impersonal or objectivizing perspective on their present identities afforded by the conception of a good life, the human being shapes a future identity, conceived of as continuation of the present one. Thus, the mutual interaction of a per-son's identity with their conception of a good life leads to an interdependence between their identity's present and its future. A major change in a person's present identity is thus likely to affect their conception of a good life; modifications to their view of a good life can shape their future identity.

The interaction between a person's identity and their conception of a good life indi-cates that if a conception of a good life is to provide the required guidance for thinking and action, and if it is to successfully link their past, present and future, the present identity must be sufficiently stable and consistent. Significant instability or incon-sistency of the present identity may prevent a person from successful formation of a sufficiently stable future identity, or even from making any attempts to shape that identity. Instabilities and inconsistencies in the person's present identity can result in their failure to implement their conception of a good life and may prevent their life from being good.

The conception of a good life involved in thinking, planning, and deciding is often explicit, but it need not be so. Judgments about how well one's own life is going can be overt, taking the form of cognitively and affectively committed considerations of various components and aspects of human life, one's own biography, and relations between the two. Alternatively, a person's view of a good life and their judgment about how well their life is going can remain unarticulated; however, it can be reconstructed from their statements, decisions, actions, and commitments. Such a reconstruction can take various forms. It can be a list of priorities or goals and judgments; or it can, particularly in the face of such life-changing events as the onset of a serious illness or a demanding therapy, take the form of a patient's life narrative (Bury 2001; Frank 1995; Williams 1984).

There are at least three possible types of conception of a good life. The conception can be organized around the hedonistic idea of a life characterized by a suitable balance of pleasures and pains experienced by a person or, less subjectively, around the concept of a life of fulfillment of that person's desires; alternatively, a good life can be conceived of in a perfectionist way as offering the person access to the goods on a list of goods required for a human being (Parfit 1984). A conception of a good life can play its role of the standard of the worth of the life of a human being all things considered exactly because it relates to that person's identity. Since post-transplant identity is usually different from that of life in health, the transplant patient's thinking, planning and deciding on the ground of their conception of a good life can face challenges unknown to healthy persons or to those living with a serious or chronic illness.

As explained in the first section, being ontologically and experientially constitutive for an individual identity, the body in health is for the most part experientially transparent to the healthy person, leaving questions of their identity and a good life mute for the majority of the time. This fragility of identity, which belongs to the human condition, remains invisible in a way akin to the invisibility of the body in health. It is noticed at times of illness and 'forgotten' again after recovery. The fragility of the patient's identity becomes visible during (serious) illness, when the body becomes perceptible to them due to the changes, discomforts, and difficulties in controlling their affairs. By revealing these fragilities, such disruptive phenomena can prompt re-examination of how well one's own life has been going so far, and so they can encourage a critical reflection on one's own identity and one's conception of a good life. Except where illness is chronic or associated with extremely traumatic experiences, such concerns are likely to cease after recovery.

Post-transplant life is different because post-transplant identity is different. As the data on transplant patients' experiences suggest, the fragility of a transplant patient's identity is brought to their awareness by the fragility of their changed body. Additionally, the degree of fragility of the post-transplant patient's body and identity fluctuates together with crises that occur in the recovery process and the demands of the post-transplant therapy. As a result, the patient's body and identity will often be significantly more unstable than in passing illness, and identity persistently fragmented. The patient might need to reconstruct their identity because the replacement of their organ with someone else's brings their present identity into question. Their present identity can no longer be a fixed point of reference to which their conception of a good life can be readily applied in their planning, deciding and acting.

The instability of the patient's present identity in planning and decision making can be exacerbated by the demands of immunosuppression, which bring the fragility of the patient's body and identity to their attention. The repeated challenges to post-transplant identity, caused by the fragile reconstitution of the patient's body, give rise to *recurring* explorations of their identity. Such explorations can impact deeply the patient's potential to arrive at a conception of a good life and make credible judgments of the worth of their present life. First, due to its fragility, the patient's present identity is likely to be less stable than their identity in health, and so it will be more difficult to design a conception of a good life which would be adjusted to a fixed identity. Although the identity of a human being is never complete, it usually remains sufficiently stable in the present and linked to the past to provide a basis for a conception of a good life. By contrast, a transplant patient's present identity is lastingly and profoundly 'unfinished' – due to the presence of a foreign body part, the responses of their immune system to it, and the regimen of immunosuppression – to a much higher degree than in health. Accordingly, post-transplant identity may require more frequent and perhaps deeper and more comprehensive redesign of the patient's conception of a good life as compared to responses to typical events of life in health.

Secondly, the patient's evaluations of their own post-transplant life may fluctuate more relative to their repeatedly rebuilt identity. The aspects of their identity to which the patient has adjusted their new conception of a good life may undergo changes caused by clinical events (e.g. onset of diabetes or high blood pressure) and the demands of immunosuppression (e.g. the regime of immunosuppressant therapy or effects of compromised resistance to infections). Such changes can be incompatible with the patient's recently developed conception of a good life. To the extent to which the new identity is beyond the patient's control (e.g. changes in the bodily composition or the limits placed on the patient's lifestyle), the conception of a good life will need more frequent adaptation and *redesign*. Thus, changes in the patient's identity and of their conception of a good life will be mutually dependent: changes of the patient's clinical status will require modifications to their conception of a good life, which will become part of their present identity, which, in turn, may necessitate changes in the conception of a good life, which, again, potentially will change the patient's future identity. The patient's thinking about a good life and identity cannot therefore be focused on their future to the same extent as in a life in health. The patient's preferred identity, that is what they, explicitly or not, intend, plan or wish to be (Charmaz 1987), cannot play the organizing role it usually plays in life in health because, potentially, the preferred identity is significantly less determinate and complete. While past events may still pertain to their identity, the events relating to the preferred identity are undefined.

Since, as already noted, the conception of a good life necessarily belongs to the person's identity, the fragility of post-transplant identity, rooted in the fragility of the transplant patient's body, can result in instability of their conception of a good life. These fragilities cumulatively affect the patient's life, and so they may affect its worth all things considered, in that they will make the central components of that life, whatever its constituents, uncertain and unpredictable (Inspector et al. 2004). The strategies of coping with uncertainty, such as resolve, benefiting from the support of others, or compliance with the demands of immunosuppression or lifestyle (Cormier et al. 2017), are likely to be insufficient due to the instability of the very conceptual framework of a good life brought about, sustained by, and nourishing the sequence of fragilities. The instability of that framework, intended to organize the patient's planning, deciding, and acting is likely to make a good life relatively elusive as an idea and problematic as a fact.

Transplant patients may respond to the conflicts, uncertainties and instabilities of their post-transplant identity and their conception of a good life in two ways. One is resignation and acquiescence to the limited, elusive, or in extreme cases, non-existent prospects for a good life, which might take the form of an express or tacit decision to live in the present and refrain from setting goals or planning for the future (Michael 1996). Attempts to design their own conception of a good life can then be seen as pointless or futile. This, however, would deprive the transplant patient of a good life. To the extent that human beings need a view of a good life, which is directed to the future to structure their current affairs, to have a good life, such a resignation can question the very decision to undergo the transplant treatment. Why save life or improve its quality if that life cannot be good, as measured by the standard of the person saved?

An alternative response to the post-transplant conflicts, uncertainties and instabilities of identity and the conception of a good life is to see those conflicts, uncertainties and instabilities as opportunities for enrichment, growth, and personal development (Oris et al. 2018). For this to be effective, it is not enough to rely on conceptualizations of a good life that presuppose a stable present identity rooted in a past identity. Whether in the form of a list of statements about what matters in life or as a narrative, the conception of a good life would need to be based on a re-conceptualized or reframed idea of a good life. Such an idea should assimilate or incorporate post-transplant conflicts, uncertainties, and instabilities. As a result of their heightened bodily awareness and (actual or imagined) connection to the donor, their family members, and perhaps (for example, through the feelings of gratitude) to society at large, the patient could make the conflicts, uncertainties and instabilities important parts of their conception of a good life. This conception could respond to the needs and experiences of the transplant patient based on their particular identity.

It is impossible to discuss the details of the reframed idea of a good post-transplant life here. These will depend on personal characteristics and the situation of a given patient. Some general points, however, can be made. First, a reframed view of a good post-transplant life would need to respond to the conflicts, uncertainties, and instabilities of post-transplant identity in its relationship to the patient's past. Seeking continuity with their pre-transplant lives, patients need to incorporate into their thinking both their own past as well as the (imagined) biography of the transplanted organ or, perhaps, of the donor. In such cases, a patient's conception of a good life would have to combine two pasts with one present and a future in order to reconstitute their identity and biography as undoubtedly *theirs*. Accordingly, their view of a good life would not only connect their own body with the received organ and the two biographies that precede the failure of their own organ into a sufficiently unified whole; it would also have to contain conceptual, imaginative and affective resources that allow the patient to 'domesticate' the implanted body part and its biography, that is, to make their presence in the patient's life a legitimate basis of the worth of their life all things considered.

One of the more specific and socially important aspects of the 'domestication' of the new body part and the biographies linked to it could be negotiation of the conflict between the idea of the gift of life and that of 'just a body part'. Since embodiment is central to identity and identity is the basis of a good life, a conception of a good post-transplant life will need to include appreciation of the organ without making the patient victim to the feelings of unrepayable debt or guilt. This may be difficult in view of the recipient's possibly unstable health status and the demands of the recovery process, which makes reappearance of the conflicts, uncertainties and instabilities of the post-transplant identity more likely.

Secondly, as explained above, the conflicts and tensions inherent to the post-transplant identity do not allow the patient to take their body and their bodily identity for granted as while living in health. By being repeatedly questioned, they prompt re-examination of the patient's perspective on their own life, and so of their conception of a good life. In this way the identity of the transplant patient is likely to be a process rather than a relative constant, and development of the conception of a good life a continuing task to be accomplished with relatively high awareness. Although the identity of every human being changes over time, the transformations are stretched over periods which are sufficiently long for identity to be taken as a given and a constant. In transplants, the changing nature of the patient's identity is perceptible, becoming more prominent in periods of medical crisis, in proportion to the identity significance of the transplanted body part. This processual aspect of post-transplant identity calls for an analogously processual conception of a good life whose components are dynamically related to the patient's life events. In such a conception of a good life the patient's bodily fragility and uncertainty about their future are essential. Thus, plans will often need to be open-ended and responsive to unexpected changes. They will have to result from a creative and learning approach to new events in order to maintain a sufficient level of consistency and continuity of the post-transplant life.

5.   Conclusion

Good post-transplant life is not limited to quality of life. It encompasses medical and psychological as well as existential and moral aspects of life, which are intimately related to the patient's goals and priorities. A transplant patient's identity can be seriously disturbed due to the embodied nature of human existence. The taken-for-grantedness and transparency of the lived healthy body, which is normally underappreciated as the basis for both identity and a conception of a good life, tends to disappear after transplant. The conflicts, uncertainties and instabilities of the post-transplant identity call for the reconstitution of identity as well as the reconstruction and, more fundamentally, reframing of the conception of a good life. Since after transplant surgery the patient's embodiment is acutely perceptible and their identity prone to contestation, their conception of a good life may need to include the conflicts, uncertainties and instabilities associated with the transplant identity process and the processual nature of the conception of a good post-transplant life. The patient's bodily and experiential identity will have to be negotiated to be included in their view of a good life. Since these negotiations are ostensibly inconclusive and may recur due to the demands of immunosuppression and the fragile status of the patient's bodily integrity, a patient's view of a good life must include resources necessary for adequate responses to their potentially changing identity.

Thus, not only is it the worth of a person's own life, all things considered, that is repeatedly re-examined in the face of the fragility and instability of the post-transplant identity, it is also their very view of a good life. Thrown into question by the uncertain status of the implanted body part, a patient's limited control of their affairs brought about by the demands of immunosuppression and medical surveillance, as well as by the chronic uncertainty of the future, post-transplant identity not only calls for a new perspective on the worth of the patient's life; it also calls for reframing of the very idea of a good life.

The reframed conception of a good post-transplant life needs to respond to the recurring episodes of questioning of the patient's identity by becoming an explicitly unfinished and open-ended process in which the patient's bodily fragility and the relatively high instability of their future are an inherent part of that conception. Because consistency and continuity in the patient's life are necessary preconditions of its worth for the patient, all things considered, the patient needs a health care environment that provides a more creative and adaptive approach to their future as well as personal skills to help them design the best possible conception of a good post-transplant life.

References

Ådahl, Susanne (2013): "When Death Enables Life: Incorporation of Organs from Deceased Donors in Finnish Kidney Recipients." In: Mortality, 18/2, pp. 130–150.

Agazzi, Evandro (2001): "Illness as Lived Experience and as the Object of Medicine." In: Anna-Teresa Tymieniecka/Evandro Agazzi (eds.), Life Interpretation and the Sense of Illness within the Human Condition: Medicine and Philosophy in a Dialogue, Dordrecht: Springer, pp. 3–15

Anderson, Sara M./Wray, Jo/Ralph, Andrea/Spencer, Helen/Lunnon-Wood, Tracey/Gannon, Kenneth (2017): "Experiences of Adolescent Lung Transplant Recipients: A Qualitative Study." In: Pediatric Transplantation 21/3. DOI: 10.1111/petr.12878

Angner, Erik/Ray, Midge N./Saag, Kenneth G./Allison, Jeroan J. (2009): "Health and Happiness among Older Adults: a Community-Based Study." In: Journal of Health Psychology, 14/4, pp. 503–512.

Annas, Julia (2004): "Happiness as Achievement." In: Daedalus, 133/2, pp. 44–51.

Anthony, Samantha J./Nicholas, David B./Regehr, Cheryl/West, Lori J. (2019): "The Heart as a Transplanted Organ: Unspoken Struggles of Personal Identity Among Adolescent Recipients." Canadian Journal of Cardiology 35/1, pp. 96–99.

Baines, Lyndsay S./Jindal, Rahul M. (2003): The Struggle for Life: a Psychological Pperspective of Kidney Disease and Transplantation.,Westport: Praeger.

Belk, Russell W. (1992): "Me and Thee versus Mine and Thine: How Perceptions of the Body Influence Organ Donation and Transplantation." In: James Shanteau/Richard J. Harris (eds.), Organ Donation and Transplantation: Psychological and Behavioral Factors, Washington: American Psychological Association, pp. 139–149.

Bunzel, Brigitta/Schmidl-Mohl, Brigitte/Grundböck, Alice/Wollenek, Gregor (1992): "Does Changing the Heart Mean Changing Personality? A Retrospective Inquiry on 47 Heart Transplant Patients." In: Quality of Life Research 1/4, pp. 251–256.

Bury, Mike (1982): "Chronic Illness as Biographical Disruption." In: Sociology of Health and Illness 4/2, pp. 167–182.

Bury, Mike (2001): "Illness Narratives: Fact or Fiction?" In: Sociology of Health and Illness 23/3, pp. 263–285.

Buytendijk, Frederik J. J. (1987): "The Phenomenological Approach to the Problem of Feelings and Emotions." In: Joseph J. Kockelmans (ed.), Phenomenological Psychology: The Dutch School, Dordrecht: Springer, pp. 119–132.

Carel, Havi (2016): Phenomenology of Illness, Oxford: Oxford University Press.

Carr, David (1986): Time, Narrative, and History, Bloomington: Indiana University Press.

Cassell, Eric J. (1985): Talking with Patients, Cambridge: MIT Press.

Charmaz, Kathy (1983): "Loss of Self: a Fundamental Form of Suffering in the Chronically Ill." In: Sociology of Health and Illness 5/2, pp. 168–195.

Charmaz, Kathy (1987): "Struggling for a Self: Identity Levels of the Chronically Ill." In: Research in the Sociology of Health Care 6, pp. 283–321.

Charmaz, Kathy (1995): "The Body, Identity and Self." In: The Sociological Quarterly 36/4, pp. 657–680.

Chwalisz, Kathleen/Diener, Ed/Gallagher, Dennis (1988): "Autonomic Arousal Feedback and Emotional Wxperience: Evidence from the Spinal Cord Injured." In: Journal of Personality and Social Psychology 54/5, pp. 820–828.

Cormier, Nicholas R./Gallo-Cruz, Selina R./Beard, Renee L. (2017): "Navigating the New, Transplanted Self: How Recipients Manage the Cognitive Risks of Organ Rransplantation." In: Sociology of Health and Illness 39/8, pp. 1496–1513.

De Haes, Johanna C. J. M./van Knippenberg, Ferdenand C. E. (1985): "The Quality of Life of Cancer Patients: a Review of the Literature." In: Social Science & Medicine 20/8, pp. 809–817.

Forsberg, Anna/Bäckman, Lars/Möller, Anders. (2000): "Experiencing Liver Transplantation: a Phenomenological Approach." In: Journal of Advanced Nursing 32/2, pp. 327–334.

Frank, Arthur W. (1995): The Wounded Storyteller: Body, Illness and Ethics, Chicago/London: University of Chicago Press.

Gadamer, Hans-Georg (1996): The Enigma of Health: the Art of Healing in a Scientific Age, Stanford: Stanford University Press.

Gert, Bernard/Culver, Charles M./Clouser, K. Danner (2006): Bioethics: a Systematic Approach, 2nd ed., New York: Oxford University Press.

Goldie, Peter (2004): On Personality, London: Routledge.

Husserl, Edmund (1989): Ideas Pertaining to a Pure Phenomenology and to a Phenenological Philosophy. Second book: Studies in the Phenomenology of constitution, Dordrecht/Boston/London: Kluwer.

Inspector, Yoram/Kutz, Ilan/David, Daniel (2004): "Another Person's Heart: Magical and Rational Thinking in the Psychological Adaptation to Heart Transplantation." In: Israel Journal of Psychiatry and Related Sciences 41/3, pp. 161–173.

Juneau, Bonnie (1995): "Psychologic and Psychosocial Aspects of Renal Transplantation." Critical Care Nursing Quarterly 17/4, pp. 62–66.

Kaba, Evridiki/Thompson, David R./Burnard, Philip/Edwards, Deborah/Theodosopoulou, Eleni (2005): "Somebody Else's Heart Inside Me: a Descriptive Study of Psychological Problems after a Heart Transplantation." In: Issues in Mental Health Nursing 26/6, pp. 611–625.

Kass, Leon (1985): Toward a More Natural Science: Biology and Human Affairs, New York: Free Press.

Kierans, Ciara (2005): "Narrating Kidney Disease: the Significance of Sensation and Time in the Emplotment of Patient Experience." In: Culture, Medicine and Psychiatry 29/3, pp. 341–359.

Kierans, Ciara (2011): "Anthropology, Organ Transplantation and the Immune System: Resituating Commodity and Gift Exchange." In: Social Science & Medicine 73/10, pp. 1469–1476.

Klinger, Eric (1994): "On Living Tomorrow Today: the Quality of Inner Life as a Function of Goal Expectations." In: Zbigniew Zaleski (ed.), Psychology of Future Orientation, Lublin: Towarzystwo Naukowe, pp. 97–106.

Leder, Drew (1990): The Absent Body, Chicago: University of Chicago Press.

Mai, Francois M. (1986): "Graft and Donor Denial in Heart Transplant Recipients." In: The American Journal of Psychiatry 143/9, pp. 1159–1161.

Matson, Ronald R./Brooks, Nancy A. (1977): "Adjusting to Multiple Sclerosis: an Exploratory Study." In: Social Science & Medicine 11/4, pp. 245–250.

Mauthner, Oliver E./De Luca, Enza/Poole, Jennifer M./Abbey, Susan E./Shildrick, Margrit/ Gewarges, Mena/Ross, Heather J. (2015): "Heart Transplants: Identity Disruption, Bodily Integrity and Interconnectedness." In: Health 19/6, pp. 578–594.

Merleau-Ponty, Maurice (1962): Phenomenology of Perception, London/New York: Routledge.

Michael, Susan R (1996): "Integrating Chronic Illness Into One's Life: a Phenomenological Inquiry." In: Journal of Holistic Nursing 14/3, pp. 251–267.

Moch, Susan Diemert (1989): "Health within Illness: Conceptual Evolution and Practice Possibilities." In: Advances in Nursing Science 11/4, pp. 23–31.

Nagel, Thomas (1986): The View from Nowhere, New York/Oxford: Oxford University Press.

Nancy, Jean-Luc (2008): The Intruder Corpus, New York: Fordham University Press.

Neukom, Marius/Corti, Valentina/Boothe, Brigitte/Boehler, Annette/Goetzmann, Lutz (2012): "Fantasized Recipient–Donor Relationships Following Lung Transplantations: A Qualitative Case Analysis Based on Patient Narratives." In: The International Journal of Psychoanalysis 93/1, pp. 117–137.

Öhman, Marja/Söderberg, Siv/Lundman, Berit (2003): "Hovering Between Suffering and Enduring: The Meaning of Living With Serious Chronic Illness." In: Qualitative Health Research, 13/4, pp. 528–542.

Oris, Leen/Luyckx, Koen/Rassart, Jessica/Goubert, Liesbet/Goossens, Eva/Apers, Silke/Arat, Seher/Vandenberghe, Joris/Westhovens, René/Moons, Philip (2018): "Illness Identity in Adults with a Chronic Illness." In: Journal of Clinical Psychology in Medical Settings 25/4, pp. 429–440.

Parfit, Derek (1984): Reasons and Persons, Oxford: Oxford University Press.

Ricoeur, Paul (1986): "Life. A Story in Search of a Narrator." In: Marinus C. Doeser/John N. Kraay (eds.), Facts and Values: Philosophical Reflections from Western and Non-Western Perspectives, Dordrecht/Lancaster: Nijhoff, pp. 121–132.

Riis, Jason/Loewenstein, George/Baron, Jonathan/Jepson, Christopher/Fagerlin, Angela/Ubel, Peter A. (2005): "Ignorance of Hedonic Adaptation to Hemodialysis: a Study Using Ecological Momentary Assessment." In: Journal of Experimental Psychology: General, 134/1, pp. 3–9.

Rorty, Amelie Oksenberg/Wong, David (1990): "Aspects of Identity and Agency." In: Owen J. Flanagan/Amelie Oksenberg Rorty (eds.), Identity, Character, and Morality: Essays in Moral Psychology, Cambridge: MIT Press, pp. 19–36.

Sanner, Margareta A. (2001): "Exchanging Spare Parts or Becoming a New Person? People's Attitudes toward Receiving and Donating Organs." In: Social Science & Medicine 52/10, pp. 1491–1499.

Sanner, Margareta A. (2003): "Transplant Recipients' Conceptions of Three Key Phenomena in Transplantation: the Organ Donation, the Organ Donor, and the Organ Transplant." In: Clinical Transplantation 17/4, pp. 391–400.

Sartre, Jean-Paul (1978 [1956]): Being and Nothingness. An Essay in Phenomenological Ontology, New York: Pocket Books.

Schmid-Mohler, Gabriela/Schäfer-Keller, Petra/Frei, Anja/Fehr, Thomas/Spirig, Rebecca. (2014): "A Mixed-Method Study to Explore Patients' Perspective of Self-Management Tasks in the Early Phase after Kidney Transplant." In: Progress in Transplantation 24/1, pp. 8–18.

Sharp, Lesley A. (1995): "Organ Transplantation as a Transformative Experience: Anthropological Insights into the Restructuring of the Self." In: Medical Anthropology Quarterly 9/3, pp. 357–389.

Svenaeus, Fredrik (2000a): "The Body Uncanny – Further Steps towards a Phenomenology of Illness." In: Medicine, Health Care and Philosophy, 3/2, pp. 125–137.

Svenaeus, Fredrik (2000b): "Das Unheimliche – Towards a Phenomenology of Illness." Medicine, Health Care and Philosophy, 3/1, pp. 3–16.

Svenaeus, Fredrik (2011): "Illness as Unhomelike Being-in-the-World: Heidegger and the Phenomenology of Medicine." In: Medicine, Health Care and Philosophy 14/3, pp. 333–343.

Svenaeus, Fredrik (2012): "Organ Transplantation and Personal Identity: How does Loss and Change of Organs Affect the Self?" In: The Journal of Medicine and Philosophy 37/2, pp. 139–158.

Svenaeus, Fredrik (2015): "The Lived Body and Personal Identity. The Ontology of Exiled Body Parts." In: Erik Malmqvist/Kristin Zeiler (eds.), Bodily Exchanges, Bioethics and Border Crossing: Perspectives on Giving, Selling and Sharing Bodies. Abingdon/Oxon/New York: Routledge, pp. 19–34.

Tong, Allison/Morton, Rachael/Howard, Kirsten/McTaggart, Steven/Craig, Jonathan C. (2011): "'When I Had My Transplant, I Became Normal.' Adolescent Perspectives on Life after Kidney Transplantation." In: Pediatric Transplantation 15/3, pp. 285–293.

Toombs, S. Kay (1988): "Illness and the Paradigm of Lived Body." In: Theoretical Medicine 9/2, 201–226.

Toombs, S. Kay (1992): The Meaning of Illness: a Phenomenological Account of the Different Perspectives of Physician and Patient, Dordrecht/Boston: Kluwer.

Van Den Berg, Jan H. (1987): "The Human Body and the Significance of Human Movement." In: Joseph J. Kockelmans (ed.), Phenomenological Psychology: The Dutch School, Dordrecht: Springer Netherlands, pp. 55–77.

Varela, Francisco J. (2001): "Intimate Distances. Fragments for a Phenomenology of Organ Transplantation." In: Journal of Consciousness Studies 8/5–7, pp. 259–271.

Williams, Bernard (1981): "Persons, Character and Morality." In: Bernard Williams: Moral Luck: Philosophical Papers 1973–1980, Cambridge: Cambridge University Press, pp. 1–19.

Williams, Bernard (1985): "Socrates' Question." In: Bernard Williams: Ethics and the Limits of Philosophy, Cambridge: Harvard University Press, pp. 1–21.

Williams, Gareth (1984): "The Genesis of Chronic Illness: Narrative Re-Construction." In: Sociology of Health & Illness 6/2, pp. 175–200.

Young, Iris M. (2005): On Female Body Experience: 'Throwing like a girl' and Other Essays, New York: Oxford University Press.

Zaner, Richard M. (1981): The Context of Self: a Phenomenological Inquiry Using Medicine as a Clue, Athens/Ohio: Ohio University Press.

Zeiler, Kristin (2010): "A Phenomenological Analysis of Bodily Self-Awareness in the Experience of Pain and Pleasure: on Dys-Appearance and Eu-Appearance." In: Medicine, Health Care and Philosophy 13/4, pp. 333–342.

14. Problematizing the Rhetoric of Gift-Giving in Transplantation Narratives
Epistemic Authorities

Rhonda Shaw

1. Introduction

Social scientists have long argued that reciprocity is a basic principle of social life and a social norm of gift-giving (Berking 1999; Gouldner 1996; Simmel 1996). According to Komter (2005), however, the reciprocity rule does not directly apply to substances of human origin that are deemed bodily gifts, such as blood or organs. This is not only due to the treatment of blood and organs as part of a global economy of tissue exchange in which human body parts and products are transformed into commodities with biovalue (Waldby/Mitchell 2006), but because the donation of bodily gifts is typically assumed to be altruistic; freely given, one-way, and disinterested. Komter's sociological observation does not simply describe current institutional and organisational arrangements, it is also a value promoted by stakeholders, professional groups, and policy makers. That is, the prevailing moral guideline in global north jurisdictions is that bodily organs should be treated as gifts and only ever voluntarily donated as an act of altruism (Berglund/Lundin 2012). In this rendering, altruistic donative acts should be intentional, voluntary, and seek to enhance the welfare of others without external influence, expectations of reciprocation or commercialization (Shaw 2019).

There are multiple ways to conceptualize gifts and gift-exchange in social life. While many scholars emphasize the polysemic and paradoxical nature of the gift as unilateral and reciprocal, self-interested and altruistic, voluntary and normative (e.g. Berking 1999; Godbout/Caillé 2000; Godelier 2002; Mauss 1990; Osteen 2002; Schrift 1997), the complexities of this understanding tend to be subsumed by the language used in health care information manuals and in biomedical policy guidelines and protocol. As Tutton (2002) points out, the gift is typically conceptualized by ethics committees, medical councils, and research institutes interested in fostering the donation of body parts and products as a one-way transaction (e.g. *UK Human Tissue Authority* guidelines). Drawing on the legacy of Titmuss' (1997) comparative research on commercial and voluntary blood donation systems in the UK and US in the late 1960s, the language that is used in these contexts to talk about donation is couched in terms of the 'gift relationship'. Typically, the gift relationship, which is underpinned by the notion of reciprocity, is conflated with altruism and the pure gift as unconditional.

The example Tutton gives that exemplifies this kind of thinking comes from the Medical Research Council (MRC) in the UK, which states that treating bodily donations as gifts is "preferable from a moral and ethical point of view, as it promotes the 'gift relationship' between participants and researchers, and underlines the altruistic motivation for participation in research" (in Tutton 2002: 523).

However, as international researchers have shown (Fox/Swazey 1992; Sharp 2007; Shaw et al. 2012; Shaw/Webb 2015; Siminoff/Chillag 1999), the multiple meanings of the term gift and its conflation with altruism can lead to problems when people have different ideas about what a gift is and how to give and receive it. For some people who donate and receive substances of human origin, the transfer of bodily material is not an altruistic act over which control is unilaterally relinquished or surrendered (Shaw 2008). Rather, bodily gifts establish on-going reciprocity relations between donors and recipients and failure to return a gift, or to show gratitude for a gift, symbolizes a refusal to cement the social and moral bond. Treating bodily donations as an altruistic act can therefore fail to account for the complex entanglement of psychosocial and intercorporeal processes occurring between participants involved in organ donation and transplantation (Shildrick 2012).

In keeping with legislation and policy elsewhere in the global north, the language of the gift is used in New Zealand to promote organ donation as an altruistic act. In this chapter, I examine the salience of this terminology to describe and understand the experiences of organ donors, donor families, and transplant recipients. To do so, I draw on the concept of epistemic injustice as described by the philosopher Miranda Fricker (2007, 2008) as a dysfunction in our knowledge practices. The rationale for applying Fricker's approach to this discussion is to show why the inclusion of perspectives from the standpoint of organ donors, donor families, and transplant recipients is ethically needed and justified, and to emphasize the importance of qualitative social science research in bringing these views to bear on our collective understanding of organ donation and transplantation processes.

2.   Theoretical Framework: Epistemic Injustice in Organ Donation

Epistemic injustice occurs when "particular powerful or dominant groups, can limit or occlude knowledge production and transmission by powerless or marginalized groups" (Mason 2011: 294), resulting in a partial knowledge base. According to Fricker epistemic injustice can occur in two ways. Hermeneutic injustices occur when a gap in collective understanding delimits a group or individual's ability to make sense of or articulate their experiences to others (or oneself). Testimonial injustices occur when the hearer, usually a member of a dominant group, assigns "a prejudicially deflated degree of credibility" (Fricker 2008: 69) to a speaker's words or utterance, thereby discounting or ignoring the speaker's perspective based on preconceptions of their social identity. The harms that result from these forms of unknowing prevent a speaker from being heard or silence a certain group or individual unfairly through processes of testimonial quieting and testimonial smothering (Dotson 2011), making it difficult for such groups and individuals to reclaim or assert their epistemic agency.

Against the theoretical background of Fricker's and Dotson's work, I will draw on qualitative data from a series of linked empirical studies conducted in New Zealand on organ donation and transplantation, which I will call the New Zealand study for the purposes of the chapter. I suggest that the dominant health care discourse in this domain, including the discouragement of communication and contact between organ donor and transplant recipient families and communities, can result in forms of epistemic injustice as identified by Dotson. Testimonial quieting occurs when a patient's knowledge is devalued because they are perceived as lacking credibility, and testimonial smothering is the failure to acknowledge the content value of a patient's viewpoint, because it is at odds with so-called expert-knowledge, thereby leading to self-silencing and communicative editing to conform to dominant discourses or scripts. Adopting Dotson's reading of epistemic injustice, the New Zealand study findings indicate that framing organ donation as an altruistic gift "marginalizes the voices of those who are anything less than straightforwardly grateful for their transplant" (O'Brien 2017: 294) and obscures the multi-faceted nature of indebtedness and gratitude to the donor. I suggest that privileging dominant ideals around anonymity protocol prevent some donors and transplant recipients from voicing alternatives or questioning the values embedded in this discourse, such as diverse ways of thinking about the interplay of embodiment, bodily integrity, and identity; thereby diminishing the total knowledge base and service delivery in this context. This may explain why some donor families and transplant recipients experience difficulties and resistance to accepting status quo attitudes around gratitude and reciprocity when giving and receiving organs.

3.   Cultural Background: Organ Donation in New Zealand

Although the past decade has seen an increase in organ donations globally, low donation rates in many high-income countries are rendering transplant waitlists lengthy and unpromising (Larijani/ Zahedi 2007). Many countries with transplant programs have endeavored to boost the rate of altruistic donation, yet progress is often slow moving, and, in some countries, the rates of donation have plateaued (Matas/Delmonico 2012). When compared internationally, New Zealand's donation rates remain among some of the lowest across high-income countries at 15.2 deceased donors per million population (ANZDATA 2018).

Where deceased donation is concerned, unmediated contact between organ donors, donor families, and recipients of organs and tissues is institutionally discouraged, as is unmediated contact between living non-directed donors and transplant recipients. Various reasons are given not to allow meetings between donors and recipients, including support for the concept of organ donation as an unconditional gift, as well as protecting the anonymity of the donor (Ministry of Health 2004). The Organ Donation New Zealand (ODNZ) website states that donor families are given brief details about the recipients of their family member's organs and tissues, should they wish to receive this information.[1] Moreover, letters can be forwarded by transplant coordinators between donor and recipient families with their consent.

Meetings between donor and recipient families can occur, but they are infrequent due to the careful mediation of social distance between respective individuals and families by health professionals, psychologists and counsellors. One possibility for connec-

---

1   https://www.donor.co.nz/facts-and-myths/faqs/ (accessed February 9, 2020).

tion between donors and recipients occurs in major New Zealand cities in cathedrals where Thanksgiving Services are held for donor families and organ recipients. At these services, transplant recipients are invited to light a candle as a symbol of gratitude to those who have given them renewed life and members of donor families are invited to receive a variety of Camellia plant called 'Donation' in recognition of their 'gift'. The service is followed by Lunch at which it is possible for donor families and recipients to serendipitously meet, thereby collapsing the social distance required of anonymous donation to a stranger. Despite media anecdotes suggesting otherwise, professionals working in the donation area maintain that matching donors with recipients at these services is not common practice. It is nonetheless difficult to say categorically that people do not try to meet up at Thanksgiving Services and that the purpose of the ceremony, for people to recognize and share a view of the ceremonial significance of the ritual as a social good is paramount, as the ends of individuals attending these such services may be very different. Some people are keen to objectify the symbolic act of donation via more tangible social relationships and believe that prohibiting meetings is "the ultimate in paternalism" (Ministry of Health 2004: 95), preventing closure for families who may then go to lengths to circumvent so-called anonymity protocol.

4.   Methods

In this chapter I provide a general overview from previously published work of the perspectives of Transplantation specialists and Intensive Care specialists (Intensivists), deceased donor family members, non-directed living kidney donors, and organ transplant (heart, kidney, lung) recipients from a series of linked qualitative studies based on face-to-face interviews and fieldwork conducted in New Zealand between 2007 and 2013.[2] This includes data from studies with 15 Intensivists and Donor and Recipient Coordinators, 11 Transplantation specialists, nine members of deceased donor families, six non-directed live kidney donors, 27 transplant recipients, and 15 Māori donors, recipients and whānau (Māori are indigenous inhabitants of New Zealand; whānau is a term meaning extended family). Data from the health care professionals is included in this discussion because these practitioners are on the front-line of providing services and advice to those seeking organ transplantation and have an overview of issues that affect access and experiences supporting a range of different patients from various cultural backgrounds.

The Intensivists and Transplantation professionals, recruited by convenience and snowball sampling, were interviewed at their place of work. Advertisements in national media and websites were used to recruit organ donor family members and transplant recipients, who were interviewed in their homes or at a location convenient to participants. All participants were self-selected and written informed consent was obtained for interviews. The interviews took between 60 and 150 minutes. All the interviews were transcribed verbatim, and then sent to participants for review and editing upon request. The participants were asked open-ended questions structured around guid-

---

2 The studies all received research ethics clearance (Victoria University of Wellington 2-2007-SACS; Multi-Region Ethics Committee MEC/08/03/027; Victoria University of Wellington HEC 16628/4/06/09; Multi-Region Ethics Committee MEC/11/EXP/089).

ing interview themes relevant to each participant group. The natural pattern for organ recipients was to begin with explanations of illness onset and then discuss physical symptoms, mishaps and problems before broaching explicitly moral questions. Donor family members also began by discussing illness onset associated with their loved one, and the living non-directed donors began their conversation by recalling the event or occasion that gave rise to their decision to donate a kidney. Pseudonyms have been used to protect confidentiality.

The interview transcripts were read and re-read, and the data were coded manually and checked by the author before being analyzed thematically (Braun/Clarke 2006). The themes were then linked back to phenomenological theory about embodiment and perceptions of moral identity in relation to organ transfer (Haddow 2005, Shildrick 2008). Collectively, the data sets document how the respective roles, beliefs, and understandings of different groups of interviewees toward human embodiment, identity, and wellbeing shape and frame their attitudes and moral experience of organ donation and transplantation.

5.   Interpreting Results of the New Zealand Study

5.1   The Language of Gratitude

Although deceased donation has increased dramatically over the last four to five years in New Zealand, numbers remain comparatively low, despite concerted education programs and media publicity to increase awareness of donation rates. Such programs frame organ donation as unambiguously life-giving, emphasizing themes in the personal stories of transplant recipients around living one's life well to honor the donor and their gift. For example, ODNZ, which is currently the national coordinating agency for deceased donation in New Zealand, uses the tag line 'Organ Donation – the gift of life' to accompany its logo on the official website. In November 2019, a word search for the term 'gift' on the website produced 136 hits, mainly in reference to stories about people's transplantation journeys. Likewise, the opening statement of the Increasing Deceased Organ Donation and Transplantation national strategy summary reads: 'Organ donation is a very special gift'.[3]

Because organ donation is supposed to be a selfless act of giving and generosity that grants new life to the recipient, many of its rituals promote and memorialize its life-giving aspects. In the New Zealand study, for example, several transplant recipients talked about their 'second birthdays'. Helen, a mother of a transplant recipient, whose husband was also a deceased donor, spoke explicitly about the ritual of the 'second birthday', stating: "In our family we still celebrate [son's name] transplant birthday." Such comments follow a sanctioned script, heavily reliant on interlocutors to master certain phrases and expressions to describe their experiences. The following statement is typical: "I mean it really is like a rebirth. You just feel a sense of gratitude that you can never possibly feel... I mean, um, having a second chance of life is better than winning, being a billionaire."

---

3 https://www.health.govt.nz/publication/increasing-deceased-organ-donation-and-transplantation-national-strategy (accessed February 9, 2020).

The language of gratitude embedded in this discourse links the moral agency of the patient to expectations around self-care, including 'compliance' or 'adherence' to healthy diet and drug-taking regimens, as well as regular exercise. For those on kidney dialysis waiting for transplantation, and for transplant recipients who are required to take a cocktail of drugs each day at specified intervals their own and others' worthiness to receive an organ is a key concern. The following comment by a transplantation specialist emphasizes the magnitude of the gift that is conveyed to organ recipients. In the specialist's view, this requires acceptance of the sick role; that is, valuing the donated organ means seeking professional help, taking medication, getting better, and moving on with their life.

> It is vital that the recipient of a transplanted organ takes ownership, if you like, of that organ, and I think it's very appropriate that they are mindful that this is given from a family at a very difficult time. [...] Not that you'd want them to wander around and start saying 'thank you, thank you, thank you', but you want them to take their tablets, you want them to keep fit and you want them to attend appointments; that's all we ask.

Related to the specialist's characterization of the transplant recipient as a 'good patient' who takes personal responsibility for managing their health by avoiding risky, deviant, or resistant behaviors around dialysis, diet, and self-care, transplant recipients also speak about coming up against other interpersonal and organizational impediments that constrain their ability to express moral agency freely.

One concern for recipients in their efforts to connect with donors and donor families is related to the ability to convey gratitude and reciprocity. Some transplant recipients experience so much guilt associated with reciprocation that it produces anxiety around the process involved in thanking donor families. Consequently, transplant recipients are mindful of respecting the privacy of donor families and their rights to confidentiality, taking special care to avoid approaching them at public Thanksgiving services (held annually at city cathedrals) without warrant. For instance, Daphne, a kidney recipient who had two failed transplants, said she did the 'right thing' by not writing to her donor family, as she did not want them to think their donative act was in vain.

However, for many transplant recipients whose operations are successful, the desire to say thank you is a paramount concern. For some, making direct contact with non-related donors and donor families is an expressed desire, despite sometimes feeling overwhelmed by the prospect. Eryx, one kidney recipient, was actively interested in meeting his donor family until he heard the mother of a deceased donor unexpectedly share her grief over her daughter's death at a Thanksgiving service. The mother's distress at the distribution and re-location of her daughter's seven organs in strangers' bodies across Australia and New Zealand (there is a reciprocal organ sharing arrangement between these countries) was too much for this recipient to bear.

5.2   The Anonymity Imperative

To preserve the privacy of those involved from making direct contact, a so-called anonymity imperative protects donors and recipients in deceased organ donation and is carefully managed by those who work in this domain. There are various reasons given for ensuring anonymity between organ donor families, and transplant recipients and their families. The current practice in New Zealand is to support the sharing of general information about transplant outcomes, but withhold personal information about donors to transplant recipients and discourage meetings. Recipients do not know the name of their donor and they are not given contact details about their family. Many recipients know only their donor's age and occasionally their gender, although in one New Zealand District Health Board catchment the practice was strictly not to give out this information.

Sharp identifies the rationale health professionals in the USA have used for ensuring the anonymity mandate (which is similar elsewhere): to respect donors and donor families' privacy, free from intrusion in the grieving process; to prevent recipients identifying psychologically with donors; and to protect recipients from overwhelming feelings of guilt because "someone had to die so that they could live" (2006: 106). In Sharp's view, one of the problems associated with not naming donors to recipients is that the practice consigns deceased donors to a nameless and "generic category of dead" people (Sharp 2007: 35). Moreover, the inability of recipients to name donors obscures the identities of organ donors and not only silences recipients but also donor families. Anonymity protocol therefore denies people "the opportunity to tell their stories and speak of personal pain and loss" (ibid.). Data from the New Zealand study confirm Sharp's observation about the silent narrative of pain, loss, and guilt, especially in conjunction with attempts to establish moral connection with donors and donor families. A key question is how donors and recipients can give voice to these concerns within the constraints and parameters of public discourse around organ transfer.

The language available to participants to articulate themselves plays a key role in determining what one can say about the experience of organ donation and transplantation, whether one's testimony is likely to be heard, and how it is responded to by health care professionals and stakeholders. Recipients' stories told in the public arena in New Zealand, such as the ODNZ website, and at Thanksgiving services at national cathedrals designed to thank donors and their families, contain certain taboos in the storytelling (e.g. donor family members are not supposed to publicly express distress about their loved ones' organs being 'scattered' around the country). While the language used communicates shared feeling it also delimits what can be said and felt. For Siminoff and Chillag (1999), gift-of-life rhetoric is a key culprit, constantly operating as form of 'social control' to remind recipients to comply with care regimens as gratitude for their second lease of life. In short, the emphasis on life and repeated references to rebirth, renewal and salvation denies painful "emotional outbursts, [and] graphic accounts of suffering or death" (Sharp 2006: 109–110).

The stories that people are permitted to publicly impart about their experiences of organ donation and transplantation require them to manage their emotions by following scripts or adopting a prescribed narrative form. This relates specifically to gift rhetoric; terminology some organ recipients are more inclined to use than donors and members of donor families. Although most participants in the New Zealand study did not interpret the gift-of-life anthropologically, many transplant recipients nonetheless understand gifts as signifying relationships based on giving, receiving *and* reciprocating (Shaw/Webb 2015). This kind of gift relationship is cut short when organ transfer policies and practices conceptualise gifts as one-way transactions, promoting generalised but non-specific forms of reciprocity. So, although donor and recipient anonymity operate to ensure the unidirectional gift as unconditional and disinterested, some transplant recipients never feel free of their moral responsibilities toward donors, donor families, and the transplant community.

5.3   Reciprocity: Saying Thank You

In New Zealand, transplant recipients are permitted to write thank you letters to their donors or to donor families, which are then passed through recipient and donor coordinators to ensure anonymity and privacy between the two parties. This is clearly important for both organ and tissue recipients and donor family members. Indeed, it bothers recipients' moral memory, as Simmel (1996) put it, when they are unable to say thank you to their donor families. Many recipients talk about the difficulties of writing the thank you letter given the magnanimity of organ donation, especially when it is couched as a gift. For example, Anteia, a lung recipient commented that:

> It took me a year to write that letter. I started after about six months to write it and I had it on my PC, and I'd start to look at it, and I'd sit there and cry and make a few adjustments to it. And then I'd think no, that's not right either. What do you say to somebody who saved your life basically? And they are going through their grieving process because their family member died. So, it was a really, really, hard letter to write. And it must have been over a year before I thought; well I can't say any more than I did.

While letter writing provides an opportunity for recipients to say thank you, letters do not always ease the burden of guilt for many recipients who are troubled for years after their transplantation operation about how to say thanks. O'Brien (2017), drawing on research conducted in Australia, suggests that heart recipients feel this more acutely than do liver and kidney recipients, due to the higher social value accorded to the heart than to other organs. Andreus, a male heart recipient from the New Zealand study, emphasizes the magnitude of his 'gifted' organ in the following quotation:

> Obviously, I'm thankful and I'm glad that that's what they considered [organ donation]. But I tried to write some letters... and I just couldn't, it was just garbage. Emotionally it wasn't garbage, it was just straight from my heart, but you just couldn't read it. You can't tell someone something like that after they'd given you; you know given away I guess a part of their self or their family... I mean you need to be articulate and considerate and thoughtful, and it's just, I couldn't do that. I tried and tried and tried, it's, and I, and I remember [name of Transplant coordinator] saying, 'Just write something to the point, you know, just be simple', but... I think I probably should just do that, but it just doesn't seem like reciprocity, it doesn't seem like giving anything significant.

Likewise, Elissa, a female heart recipient who never wrote to her donor family, said:

> I have absolutely no idea of what I would say. I just couldn't bring myself to... I tried to write a few things and when my words were entirely, entirely inadequate I gave up. Now I've regretted that a few times, because I thought that the donor families probably, I don't know any donor families, so I can't comment for certain, but I believe that the

donor families actually like getting that communication. I think they like that, by and large.

Interviews with eight of the donor family members in the New Zealand study indicated that this is generally the case. Several appreciated the letters and cards they received and found them 'inspiring'. All stated they felt good knowing other people benefitted by their decision. However, one donor family member (Dymas) remarked that he did not know he could receive communication, and Castalia, another donor family member, remarked that the letter she received gave her no solace whatsoever. For Castalia, the donative act was simply 'intellectual', and she felt no connection to the recipient. Alluding to the sacrificial element in organ donation that is often hidden by an emphasis on giving the gift-of-life, Castalia conveyed a deep sense of ambivalence about organ donation as a social good and her failure to protect the body of her mother, whose organs her family donated. The vulnerability of the donor is also conveyed in the following account by a prospective interviewee in the New Zealand study. After some deliberation, this person eventually decided not to be involved in the project after initially consenting to an interview. This person, who offered to talk about donating her son's body tissues after his suicide declined to participate saying, "my rational mind says 'yes' [to an interview], but my emotional mind is cautious." Because she was engaged in her own research project at the same time the study was being conducted the woman conjectured that she would be too "emotionally depleted" to participate.

Given the global shortage of donor organs to save human life it is not surprising that discussion of sacrifice to which these donor family members allude is missing from the terms of reference in public debate. In short, the language of sacrifice speaks plainly of death and the literal disassembling of human bodily integrity. Reflecting on the difficult decision-making involved in deceased donation, several Intensivists spoke of it as a 'trade off' between viewing organ donation as altruistic and sacrificial. Their view was that organ donation is a painful event for donor families and not to be treated lightly (Shaw 2010). For this reason, Sque et al. (2007) maintain that understanding the sacrifices involved in organ donation may go some way to explain the reticence of some donor families to donate – especially in cases where these sacrifices are inadequately memorialized. While gift terminology partly captures the motivations and emotions of some participants involved in donation and transplantation processes, Sque et al. (2007) suggest that the dominant visibility of this theme in fact effaces a "darker side" to donative practices, articulated in terms of sacrifice.

5.4   Intercorporeality and Narratives of Solidarity

In contrast to narratives of sacrifice, grief, and loss, are accounts that foreground the intense identification some recipients feel for their donor and the importance they attach to being able to establish meaningful ties with donor families. From a phenomenological perspective, the notion of intercorporeality encapsulates the perception of ideas and feelings about donor-recipient connection – or the lack thereof – in a bodily, subjective, and social sense.

For some people, the incorporation of body parts is thought to reconstitute embodied identity in moral and spiritual ways (McKenny 1999; Sanner 2006), in that incorporating the body parts and tissues of others has implications for individual and social identity, culturally and subjectively. Because phenomenology holds that the body is inextricably interwoven with the self, relocating a donated organ into the body of a transplant recipient has the potential to produce anxiety for those who see the procedure as breaching norms about bodily integrity. If the organ is not only thought of as a spare part, but also has magical qualities, then the transplant recipient must integrate the new organ by becoming part of another individual.

As well as producing identifications at the level of recipients' embodied identity, the literal intercorporeality of organ transfer also produces dis-identifications, thus complicating the experience of tissue transfer for donors and recipients who regard body fragments as alienable. As transplantation research shows (Haddow 2005; Shildrick 2008), if donor families and transplant recipients think of the body as some 'thing' we 'have' and thus detachable from subjective identity after physical death then the problem of anonymity that this chapter raises may not be perceived as an issue. On the other hand, those who view the body as co-existent with personhood, and as something we 'are', may construe tissue exchange as intersubjective and corporeal, and interpret body part incorporation as permissible or impermissible for that reason.

For these individuals, organ donation is not viewed through the lens of pure altruism but as a gift relationship, bringing different groups of people together who would not otherwise be connected but for biomedical and technological innovation. For instance, several of the New Zealand study interviewees considered the donated organ alienable in terms of use but not in terms of ultimate possession, and created inexplicable kinship ties between the donor, the donor family, and the recipient that had cultural and social implications.

Some transplant recipients, for instance, did not regard the organ as property to be alienated from one body and relocated in another; rather, they treated the organ as would a custodian, with the view that it may be eventually returned (Shaw/Webb 2015). For several Māori research participants in the study, the origin of the gifted organ and the identity of the giver do not dissipate or erode when body parts or organs are exchanged, upon death, or when a body is buried (Webb/Shaw 2011). In Māori philosophy, body parts which live on outside the body can tamper with the ancestral line, if people have not followed the correct protocol or safeguards designed to recognize customary rules and observances. Knowing where donated organs come from and being able to return them, in the appropriate way, is thus important (Te Puni Kokiri 1999). In fact, for Māori who subscribe to a traditional cultural and spiritual worldview, living donation may be more acceptable under some circumstances than deceased donation. This perspective may reflect a hermeneutic gap for some health care professionals, especially as it is not aligned with the 'dead donor rule' of transplantation medicine and puts the living donor at risk.

While some study participants envisaged the idea of an imagined community of donors, recipients, and their families, for other participants in the study organ transplantation caused ontological anxiety. They reflected on incorporating the personal and embodied qualities of the donor through the organ transfer process and said they needed to know more about their donor to allay anxieties about the strangeness of the organ transfer experience. A woman lung recipient initially felt uncomfortable about the lung she received because she thought it was from a man. She subsequently "found out my donor was female, a lady in her forties, and I immediately felt happier."

Unlike recipients who had an intercorporeal view of embodiment through organ transfer, some interviewees thought the notion that one takes on personal attributes and qualities of the donor through tissue exchange was far-fetched. In contrast to what other researchers say about the symbolic weight of the heart for transplant recipients (cf. Svenaeus 2012), Elissa said the idea of psychic and social communion with her donor was "irrelevant". She remarked, "It's only about how the heart feels in a physical sense, like how it's functioning, that's all that matters." Likewise, Maia, a lung recipient who had received a transplanted lung did not invest her organs with personhood, stating that her old lung "was a hunk of meat" and that her body was simply a vessel for her soul or spirit.

It is significant, given these quotations, that researchers point to evidence indicating that people who view donated organs as spare parts do better post-transplant clinically and psychologically (at least initially) in terms of integrating the organ as part of their new sense of self (Siminoff/Chillag 1999; Shildrick 2008). These recipients are grateful, but they do not construct fantasies of establishing relationships with their donor and donor families. Their perspectives, furthermore, tend to be accepted by health care professionals as compatible with altruism as a one-way transaction and organ donation as a gift-of-life.

6.   Testimonial Quieting and Smothering in the Field of Organ Donation

Several scholars have argued that ill persons are vulnerable to epistemic injustice because they may be regarded by health care practitioners as cognitively unreliable, emotionally compromised, and existentially unstable in ways that render their own testimonies of their health and illness experiences suspect (Carel 2016; Schicktanz 2015). This situation arises because practitioners and health care services privilege certain forms of evidence and ways of knowing and sharing knowledge that patients are said to lack. For patients to be heard, Carel maintains that their testimonies need to be expressed in the "accepted language of medical discourse to be assigned epistemic authority" (2016: 3).

In tissue economies involving organ donation, educational and recruitment organizations incorporate altruistic ideals into promotional discourse to encourage donation awareness and engagement. Although the values of organ donors and tissue providers are not necessarily aligned with the interests of educational and recruitment organizations, individuals are obliged to make sense of their actions in institutional contexts by strategically drawing on the resources that these institutions and organizations provide. These institutionally constructed discourses become cultural scripts that provide people with tools to communicate linguistic competencies, and, as justifications for their actions, legitimize entitlement to inclusion as moral subjects and members of certain groups. Accessing and using a recognizable vocabulary is thus an important step in determining the credibility of transplant recipients, donor families, and donors (Shaw 2019).

While learning new terms can be hermeneutically empowering it can also result in ways of talking that enact testimonial smothering and silencing. For some donors, donor families, and transplant recipients, for example, the accepted vocabulary of gift terminology is regarded as hackneyed, trivial, and lacking in communicative nuance.

Individuals who are critical of gift terminology report that it sentimentalizes what could be emotionally and psychologically easier to deal with if the language used was more neutral. Several interviewees in the New Zealand study for instance regarded the descriptors 'health intervention' and 'donation' as preferable, although they felt that the appropriateness of these terms depends very much on what is being donated, to whom, and for what purposes. These participants contended that talking about organ donation as a gift of life overshadows how ill people with organ failure become, and conceals the difficulties of accommodating an alien body part and living day-to-day with the impact of immunosuppressant medication (Shildrick 2012, Sothern/Dickinson 2011). Aside from the experience of post-transplant health as a state of 'persistent liminality' (Crowley-Matoka 2005), permanently vacillating 'betwixt and between' life as sick and healthy, gift language fails to convey the impossibility of reciprocation, especially in the case of anonymous donation (Fox/Swazey 2009). It thus orchestrates what Hochschild has referred to as feeling rules around obligations to give and receive; scripting what is possible for recipients to say by framing accounts of the transplantation experiences in a language of indebtedness (Shaw 2015).

Like transplant recipients who self-silence their experience of organ transplantation as a state of 'persistent liminality' in order to become 'good patients' and present a positive public face, organ donors also self-edit to convince health care professionals that their offer to donate is free from coercion and that they are not seeking payment (Shaw 2019). One non-directed donor I spoke with recounted an experience of testimonial smothering as she talked about the difficulty of convincing people that her intention to become an anonymous donor was valid. She surmised that her initial appointment with a hospital renal department was double-booked because she was not expected to turn up, and then, after all the tests were done, which took "a very long time", she was told that the operation was not carried out at that particular hospital. Having gone through the entire process to determine donor suitability, the woman began inquiring at hospitals around New Zealand to see if any were willing to do the operation. She, "wrote a letter to [New Zealand city] Hospital and explained what I had done, and I got a very nasty letter back telling me that I was just after money for my kidney" (Shaw 2019). The string of micro-aggressions and invalidation this woman recalled, as evidenced by the quotation above, did not deter her. She did eventually donate a kidney as a non-directed donor, with another service provider at another New Zealand city.

Several of the non-directed donors in the study explained that passing as a genuine donor not only required 'persistence' but also meant saying the right thing to health care professionals and psychologists. To avoid appearing emotionally compromised, they explained that it was important to downplay emotion when communicating their donative intent to health care practitioners. This is not to say that they lacked reasons for wanting to become non-directed donors, but that their testimonial credibility largely rested on their ability to mobilize institutionally derived scripts to show that they fully comprehended the risks and benefits of their donative decision-making to medical professionals. Because of the longstanding perceived suspicion among the medical community regarding the existence of genuine altruism, living non-directed kidney donors go to great lengths to phrase their motivations using institutionally acceptable language, such as talking about their second kidney as a vital spare part that would go to waste if not donated (a perspective shared by many living directed donors), or by expressing their awareness of the physical impact of renal failure and dialysis on others' suffering (Shaw 2019). Consequently, non-directed kidney donors describe their donative decision-making in rational terms as non-emotional and carefully deliberated, having more to do with outcome than objectifying their moral identity as a good citizen.

For instance, one participant claimed that although she had "four or five different reasons" to donate, she could, for the purpose of convincing people it was the right thing to do, sum up her decision as a "simple, basic, logical equation" about functioning on one kidney and helping out if you can. Likewise, another participant stated, "I'm fairly clinical in my approach. [...] I know what good it will do. I know I can live with one kidney, and I didn't need to ask anybody that, to make up my own mind." This reasoning works as a useful, expedient rhetoric to fit the dominant view of the human body as an assemblage of interchangeable parts, able to be exchanged with little or no psychosocial, emotional or existential impact. Prospective donors are guarded about saying they view their acts as symbolizing human connection during the psychological assessment process, for fear of jeopardizing their donative plans. While beliefs about metaphysical communion with other human beings may be salient, these ideals are not typically articulated as the key driver for donative intent. Their accounts suggest that they find an event to identify as a precipitant for their acts (for example, saying they once knew an acquaintance with end-stage renal failure or being able to live a full life with one kidney) because they are compelled to rationalize their motivations to fit dominant institutional logic.

7.   Conclusion

This chapter discusses the significance of altruism and gift-of-life language as a cultural and institutional value motivating ethical practices of organ donation and transplantation in relation to gratitude as a moral imperative. As suggested, however, not all organ recipients tell the same story about their illness and transplantation experience, "with morally expected (appropriate) levels of gratitude" (O'Brien 2017: 293), nor do they frame their stories in uniform ways using gift-of-life terminology. How organ donors, donor families, and transplant recipients talk about their experiences of organ transfer in the context of patient-practitioner interactions and in public fora, and what they are permitted to say, is affected by the credibility they are afforded by health care professionals and the interpretative resources they have available, not only to articulate and make sense of their experiences, but also to be heard by those with epistemic authority. While the New Zealand study indicates that Intensivists and Transplantation specialists do not always resist epistemic humility with respect to patients' testimonies about gift-of-life terminology and expectations of gratitude (Shaw 2010, Shaw/Webb 2015), these understandings do not always translate to promotional and educational discourse or media discussion in the public domain. In order to create what Fricker calls "the positive space of epistemic justice" (2007: 7) and enhance the knowledge base and public understanding of organ donation and transplantation to assist the development of ethical guidelines and health policy discourse, we need to expand the conceptual toolkit explaining organ donation and transplantation (Shaw

2015) so voices that do not conform to sanctioned ways of encountering and speaking about transplantation can be heard and adequately addressed.

References

ANZDATA Registry (2018): 41st Annual Report, Australia and New Zealand Dialysis and Transplant Registry, Adelaide, Australia. Available at: http://www.anzdata.org.au (accessed June 29, 2020)

Berglund, Sara/Lundin, Susanne (2012): "'I Had to Leave': Making Sense of Buying a Kidney Abroad." In: Martin Gunnarson/Fredrik Svenaeus (eds), The Body as Gift, Resource, and Commodity: Exchanging Organs, Tissues and Cells in the 21st century, Huddinge, Stockholm: Södertörns Studies in Practical Knowledge, pp. 321–342.

Berking, Helmuth (1999): Sociology of Giving, London: Sage.

Braun, Virginia/Clarke, Victoria (2006): "Using Thematic Analysis in Psychology." In: Qualitative Research in Psychology 3, pp. 77–101.

Carel, Havi (2016): Epistemic Injustice in Healthcare. Oxford Scholarly Online. DOI:10.1093/acprof:oso/9780199669653.001.0001

Crowley-Matoka, Megan (2005): "Desperately Seeking 'Normal': The Promise and Perils of Living With Kidney Transplantation." In: Social Science & Medicine 61, pp. 821–831.

Dotson, Kristie (2011): "Tracking Epistemic Violence, Tracking Practices of Silencing." In: Hypatia 26/2, pp. 236–257.

Fox, Renee/Swazey, Judith (1992): Spare Parts, New York: Oxford University Press.

Fricker, Miranda (2007): Epistemic Injustice: Power and the Ethics of Knowing. Oxford: Oxford University Press.

Fricker, Miranda (2008): "Epistemic Injustice: Power and the Ethics of Knowing. Précis." In: Theoria: An International Journal for Theory, History and Foundations of Science 23/61, pp. 69–71.

Godbout, Jacques T./Caillé, Alain (2000): The World of the Gift. Montreal/Kingston: McGill-Queen's University Press.

Godelier, Maurice (2002): "Some Things You Give, Some Things You Sell, but Some Things You Must Keep for Yourselves: What Mauss Did Not Say about Sacred Objects." In: Edith Wyschogrod/Jean-Joseph Goux/Eric Boynton (eds), The Enigma of Gift and Sacrifice, New York: Fordham University Press.

Gouldner, Alvin (1996): "The Norm of Reciprocity: A Preliminary Statement." In: Aaafke E. Komter (ed.): The Gift: An Interdisciplinary Perspective, Amsterdam: Amsterdam University Press, pp. 49–66.

Haddow, Gillian (2005): "The Phenomenology of Death, Embodiment and Organ Transplantation." In: Sociology of Health & Illness 27/1, pp. 92–113.

Komter, Aaafke E. (2005): Social Solidarity and the Gift, Cambridge: Cambridge University Press.

Larijani, Bagher/Zahedi, Farzaneh (2007): "Ethical and Religious Aspects of Gamete and Embryo Donation and Legislation in Iran." In: Journal of Religion and Health 46/3, pp. 399–408.

Mason, Rebecca (2011): "Two Kinds of Unknowing." In: Hypatia 26/2, pp. 294–307.

Matas, Arthur J./Delmonico, Francis L. (2012): "Living Donation: The Global Perspective." In: Advances in Chronic Kidney Disease 19/4, pp. 269–275.

Mauss, Marcel (1990): The Gift: The Form and Reason for Exchange in Archaic Societies, New York: WW Norton.

McKenny, Gerald P. (1999) "The Integrity of the Body: Critical Remarks on a Persistent Theme in Bioethics." In: Mark J. Cherry (ed.), Persons and Their Bodies: Rights, Responsibilities, Relationships, Dordrecht: Kluwer, pp. 353–361.

Ministry of Health (2004): Review of the Regulation of Human Tissue and Tissue-based Therapies: Submissions Summary. Wellington.

O'Brien, Geraldine (2017): "Gift-of-life? The Psychosocial Experiences of Heart, Liver and Kidney Recipients." In: Rhonda M. Shaw (ed.) Bioethics beyond Altruism: Donating & Transforming Human Biological Materials, Cham: Palgrave Macmillan, pp. 215–237.

Osteen, Mark (2002) (ed.): The Question of the Gift: Essays Across Disciplines, London: Routledge.

Sanner, Margareta A. (2006): "People's Attitudes and Reactions to Organ Donation." In: Mortality 11/2, pp. 113–150.

Schicktanz, Silke (2015): "The Ethical Legitimacy of Patient Organizations' Involvement in Politics and Knowledge Production: Epistemic Justice as a Conceptual Basis." In: Peter Wehling/Willy Viehöver/Sophia Koenen (eds), The Public Shaping of Medical Research: Patient Associations, Health Movements and Biomedicine, London: Routledge, pp. 246–264.

Schrift, Alain D. (1997) (ed.): The Logic of the Gift: Toward an Ethic of Generosity, New York: Routledge.

Sharp, Lesley A. (2006): Strange Harvest: Organ Transplants, Denatured Bodies, and the Transformed Self, Berkeley: University of California Press.

Sharp, Lesley A. (2007): Bodies, Commodities, and Biotechnologies: Death, Mourning, & Scientific Desire in the Realm of Human Organ Transfer, New York: Columbia University Press.

Shaw, Rhonda M. (2008): "The Notion of the Gift in the Donation of Body Tissues." In: Sociological Research Online 13/6. DOI: 10.5153/sro.1832

Shaw, Rhonda M. (2010): "Perceptions of the Gift Relationship: Views of Intensivists and Donor and Recipient Coordinators." In: Social Science & Medicine 70/4, pp. 609–615

Shaw, Rhonda M. (2015): "Expanding the Conceptual Toolkit of Organ Gifting." In: Sociology of Health & Illness 37/6, pp. 952–966.

Shaw, Rhonda M. (2019): "Altruism, Solidarity and Affect in Live Kidney Donation and Breastmilk Sharing." In: Sociology of Health & Illness 41/3, pp. 553–566.

Shaw, Rhonda M./Bell, Lara/Webb, Robert (2012): "New Zealanders' Perceptions of Gift and Giving Back in Organ Transfer Procedures." In: Kotuitui 7/1, pp. 26–36

Shaw, Rhonda M./Webb, Robert (2015): "Multiple Meanings of 'Gift' and Its Value for Organ Donation." Qualitative Health Research 25/5, pp. 600–611.

Shildrick, Margrit (2008): "Contesting Normative Embodiment: Some Reflections on the Psycho-social Significance of Heart Transplant Surgery." In: Perspectives: International Postgraduate Journal of Philosophy 1, pp. 12–22.

Shildrick, Margrit (2012): Hospitality and the 'Gift of Life': Reconfiguring the Other in Heart Transplantation. In: Stella Gonzalez-Arnal/Gill Jagger/Kahtleen Lennon (eds), Embodied Selves. New York: Palgrave Macmillan, pp. 196–208.

Siminoff, Laura A./Chillag, Kata (1999): "The Fallacy of the 'Gift of Life'." In: The Hastings Center Report 29/6, pp. 34–41.

Simmel, Georg (1996): "Faithfulness and Gratitude." In: Aafke E. Komter (ed.), The Gift: An Interdisciplinary Perspective, Amsterdam: Amsterdam University Press, pp. 39–48.

Sothern, Matthew/Dickinson, Jen (2011): "Repaying the Gift of Life: Self-Help, Organ Transfer and the Debt of Care." In: Social & Cultural Geography 12/8, pp. 889–903.

Sque, Magi/Long, Tracy/Payne, Sheila/Allardyce, Diana (2007): "Why Relatives Do Not Donate Organs For Transplants: 'Sacrifice' or 'Gift of Life'?" In: Journal of Advanced Nursing 61/2, pp. 134–144.

Svenaeus, Fredrik (2012): "The Phenomenology of Organ Transplantation: How Does the Malfunction and Change of Organs Have Effects on Personal Identity." In: Martin Gunnarson/Fredrik Svenaeus (eds), The Body as Gift, Resource, and Commodity: Exchanging Organs, Tissues, and Cells in the 21st Century, Huddinge, Stockholm: Södertörns Studies in Practical Knowledge, pp. 58–79.

Te Puni Kokiri (1999): Hauora O Te Tinana Me Ona Tikanga: A Guide for the Removal, Retention, Return and Disposal of Māori Body Parts, Organ Donation and Post-mortem: Māori and Their Whānau. Wellington.

Titmuss, Richard M. (1997 [1970]): The Gift Relationship: From Human Blood to Social Policy, New York: The New Press.

Tutton, Richard (2002) "Gift Relationships in Genetics Research." In: Science as Culture, 11/4, pp. 523–542.

Waldby, Catherine/Mitchell, Robert (2006): Tissue Economies: Blood, Organs and Cell Lines in Late Capitalism, Durham: Duke University Press.

Webb, Robert/Shaw, Rhonda (2011): "Whānau, Whakapapa and Identity in Experiences of Organ Donation and Transplantation." In: Sites 8/1, pp. 40–58.

15. Transplanting the Uterus
A Reproductive Justice Perspective

Sayani Mitra

1. Introduction

On April 2015, a headline on *The Guardian* (a UK based popular English Daily) read "Baby born from grandmother's donated womb" (Guardian 2015). The article reported the birth of yet another baby boy from the pioneering procedure of uterus transplantation (UT) at Gothenburg in Sweden. The transplanted uterus as stated came from the grandmother of the child born. A very similar headline from India appeared in 2017, which read 'Mom donates womb to daughter in India's first uterus transplant'. Later in 2017, it was reported that the first child born through uterus transplant in the US was conceived using a uterus donated by a registered nurse. It seemed like this new technological advancement had just opened up yet another avenue of gendered responsibility – the moral duty to enable another woman get pregnant by donating a functioning uterus. It provided not just a reproductive alternative for women (including transwomen) to reverse their infertility but also raised questions about the ethics of access, the moral obligations to embrace a risky surgical procedure and the rights to do the same. Although UT is a transplant procedure, the reason for performing and undergoing a UT procedure is reproductive. Hence, I find it extremely crucial to approach the ethics of performing UT through a reproductive justice lens.

UT is a novel experimental procedure designed to provide a clinical remedy for absolute uterine factor infertility that affects 1 in 500 women of reproductive age (Johannesson et al. 2014). This can be caused by hysterectomy for a malignant uterine tumor, benign diseases such as leiomyoma and adenomyosis, postpartum hemorrhage, or a congenital defect such as Mayer-Rokitansky-Keuster Hauser (MRKH) syndrome (Kisu et al. 2018). The process requires transplantation of the uterus from donor to recipient to reinstate the latter's childbearing capacity. The first successful UT procedure was carried out by the same transplant team in Sweden and the first successful childbirth through UT occurred in Sweden during early 2017. Trials in various other countries are now underway (Petrini/Morresi 2017).

Although UT can be performed from both deceased and live donors, all successful UT in Sweden, USA and India have, to date with the exception of Brazil and Ohio (Cleveland, USA), came from live rather than deceased donors (Brännström et al. 2015; Pritchard 2016; Banerjee 2017; Lang 2019). Thus, it can be expected that live uterine transplants would be the dominant form and would give rise to yet another routinized form of clinical labor. If clinically introduced, both deceased and living UT is likely to garner popularity, given the current global demand for surrogacy. This is likely to give rise to new forms of biointimacies that are uniquely regenerative and raise ethical and legal dilemmas, which cannot be neatly resolved by reference to existing protocols on other forms of bodily donation such as kidney or liver. Although scholars have started identifying the possible ethical challenges and risks underlying the use of UT in respective countries (Arora/Blake 2014; Hammond-Browning 2016), it remains to be seen how UT will be made available as a fertility option around the world.

The rates of clinical trial successes has established UT as a 'hope technology' (see Franklin 1997) like most other reproductive and transplant technologies. With each successful trial, the surgical procedure is continuously evolving and has led to the pioneering of a range of efficient surgery techniques from open to robotic to laparoscopic (Sánchez-Margallo et al. 2019). With the recent success in a robotic assisted uterine procurement and follow-up, doctors have brought down the time of the procedure by almost half, claiming to have devised a technique that completes surgery for donors in 7:50 hours and that of the recipient in 6:50 hours as opposed to the previous duration of 11:50 hours as recorded by the Swedish team (Wei et al. 2017). A team at Baylor in the US has further brought down the surgery time to five hours for the donor and recipients each. There has been a quick uptake for UT research in countries around the world. So far, twelve countries have already performed successful transplants, 42 women worldwide have received transplanted wombs, over 20 babies have been born until early 2019 in Sweden, USA, Serbia, India, Brazil and Germany (Hammond-Browning 2019; Williams 2018; Scott/Wilkinson 2018; Fabian 2019; Lan 2019) and more trials are on its way. Thus, it only seems reasonable to expect a swift clinical uptake of this procedure in the coming years (see table 1).

With various lines of trials lined up and an overwhelming number of women enquiring about the trial, the ethicists and transplant teams are already contemplating about the ways in which UT could be made available in particular countries. However, unlike other organ transplantation procedures, UT selectively targets women's bodies to achieve biological reproduction. This makes it a gendered procedure. Ethical discussion around UT thus needs to overtly account for the gendered aim and nature of this transplant procedure. Therefore, approaching the medical and social implication of the procedure from the social, political and economic positioning of the women involved in it as donors and recipients is likely to provide a gender sensitive frame for understanding UT. This chapter thus opens up a discussion on the ethics of UT using a reproductive justice approach to offer an ethical analysis from the vantage point of women's (re)productive roles in society.

Year of First Trial	Country and Research team	First successful live birth	Donor and recipient details	Source
2013	Sweden, University of Gothenburg	2014	Live donor (family friend). recipient number five in the original Swedish trial	Radio Sweden 2014
2015	China, Xijing Hospital in Xian,	2019	Live donor mother of the recipient, recipient was a 22-year-old without a uterus or vagina	Pinghui 2015
2016	USA, Cleveland Clinic	2019	Deceased donor, recipient was in mid-30s with uterine factor infertility[1]	Scottie and Saeed 2019
2016	USA, Baylor University Medical Centre at Dallas	2017	Live donor 36-years-old registered nurse, recipient with absolute uterine factor infertility	Sifferlin 2017
2016	Germany, University hospital of Tübingen	2019	Live donors, two recipients both born with labia but without a vagina and uterus	Schmidt 2019
2017	India, Galaxy hospital Pune	2018	Live donor who was the mother of the recipient, recipient was 28-year-old with non-functional uterus after abortion and a miscarriage	Thompson 2018
2016	Czech Republic, Prague Motol hospital	2019	Deceased donor, recipient was 27-year-old	Willoughby 2019
2016	Brazil, University of Sao Paulo	2017	Deceased donor, 45-year-old mother of three who died from a rare type of stroke; recipient was a 32-year-old woman born without a uterus	Weintraub 2018
2017	Serbia, University Children's Hospital in Belgrade with Swedish Team	2020 (IVF procedure and the birth took place in Sant'Orsola Hospital in Bologna, Italy)	Live donor the identical twin of the recipient, recipient was a 38-year-old Serbian woman, was born without a uterus due to a congenital malformation	Uterus Unique 2018
2018	Lebanon, Bellevue Medical Centre in Mansourieh			Hovsepian 2018

Table 1: A Timeline of the Ongoing Uterus Transplant Trial Successes around the World

1   https://edition.cnn.com/2019/07/09/us/first-us-baby-transplanted-uterus-of-dead-donor-trnd/index.html (accessed June 29, 2020)

The concept of reproductive justice was developed by the SisterSong organisation in the US. This approach combines concepts of reproductive rights, social justice and human rights to argue that reproductive justice can only be achieved when women have suitable life conditions in place to make their reproductive health decisions (ACRJ 2006). Hence, it upholds that reproductive polices need to focus on the societal needs and group sentiments to understand the rationale behind women's reproductive decision-makings. The underlying assumptions defining the ethics of UT from a reproductive justice standpoint is likely to account for the larger societal factors that impacts women's understanding and engagement with this reproductive option of UT. While this concept overlaps with the concept of ethics of justice, keeping reproductive justice at the center of the discussion on ethics of UT helps specifically account for the tensions shaping women's reproductive roles in society and their relationships with technological interventions.

Therefore, this chapter aims to discuss how a feminized need for fertility, responsibility to donate and the decision to undergo UT deserves a separate ethical and legal framework. Methodologically this chapter is offering an ethical analysis using a normative critique of the UT debate from a feminist standpoint. The analysis is carried out at the backdrop of the ongoing ethical and legal debates from around the world on UT and by narrowing down on issues that specifically requires a gender sensitive explanation. The ethical assumptions steering the discussions in the chapter is enhanced by a reproductive justice approach. In the following section, I will start by outlining the recent debates and ethical issues flagged out by different scholars. This will be followed by a discussion on the key ethical dilemmas that deserves further exploration.

2.   Ongoing Ethical-Legal Debates on UT

UT is both an organ transplant procedure as well as a fertility option. Hence, debates on UT are divided on the lines of *transplant ethics* and *reproductive ethics*.

2.1   Transplant Ethics of UT

2.1.1   Allocation

From the perspective of transplant ethics, there has been concerns regarding the grounds for allocation of uterus, preferences between deceased and living UT and the risks associated with the transplant procedure. The donor registry coordinators in the UK have estimated the availability of only five cadaveric uteri per year (Jonston 2015). Although the introduction of presumed consent might improve the number, it is unlikely to meet the demand for 15.000 women with uterine factor infertility in the UK and 50.000 in the USA, who suffer from urine-factor-infertility (UFI) annually (Zaami et al. 2019). Moreover, unlike other organ transplantation procedure, the principle of the sickest or best prognosis or the longest in the waiting list cannot apply for UT because every woman eligible for UT will have the same chances of success (Persad et al. 2009; Bruno/Arora 2018). A process of fair allocation of uteruses therefore becomes a concern for UT. In addition to medical criteria for donor-recipient matching, some have argued for a ranking system for organ allocation prioritizing those who have difficulties in finding an appropriate donor or are towards the end of their reproductive years (Bayefsky/Berkman 2016). Similarly, low priority has been proposed for those who have gestated and have given birth (Bruno/Arora 2018). Proposals for ranking criteria for uterus recipients based on age, motivation, child-rearing capacity, a minimum financial stability, criminal record check and amount of infertility treatment required has also been in circulation (ibid.). Additional proposed criteria for ranking include a comprehensive evaluation by social worker or psychologist about one's ability to rear a child (ibid.). However, proving recipient's childrearing capacity through comprehensive assessment is seen by others as regressive, who have suggested keeping the requirements limited to adoption screening criteria (Bayefsky/Berkman 2018). Again the criteria concerning the number of children of the recipient has been deemed as unfair since women may desire for additional children as strongly as those without children (Wall/Testa 2018).

Since at present, childbirth after uterus transplantation take place through in-vitro-fertilisation (IVF), it is argued that one's ability to procure embryos be considered as a criteria for inclusion in the donor registry (Bruno/Arora 2018). This clause has been rejected by others since procuring embryo just for being listed would imply women having to undergo IVF without knowing if they will be listed high enough to actually receive an uterus or whether the procured embryo has the actual potential of creating a successful pregnancy conception (Bayefsky/Berkman 2018). Moreover, in future if UT surgeons are able to connect the new uteruses to the fallopian tubes, some recipients might not require the embryos at all (ibid.).

Testa et al. (2018) however argue that for the purpose of uterus allocation, listing and prioritization needs to be dealt separately. The principle of utility and justice for organ allocation as per the Organ Procurement and Transplantation Network (2017) would not hold true for uterus because the utility of a donated uterus can only be defined by the birth of a child and hence all women in need of UT will have the same likelihood of a childbirth. If all potential recipients have the same level of infertility, then waiting time would become the proposed determining factor for organ allocation based on the principle of justice (Testa et al. 2018). However, the ground of defining the waiting time still remains to be decided.

2.1.2 Preference of Deceased versus Living UT

Uterus allocation through deceased donation has been considered to be insufficient because a substantial number of potential deceased uterus donors might have already undergone hysterectomy (Shapiro/Ward 2018). Since deceased donors cannot provide sufficient number of uterus for donation, living donation is likely to be the norm. Although the principle of autonomy has been placed as the ground for respecting living uterus donation, concerns are being raised about UT becoming a coercive practice because till date, donors in UT trials have been mothers or grandmothers of the recipient (Brannenstorm et al. 2014; Shapiro/Ward 2018). Given the harm associated with living donation, along with the possibility of regret and potential threats to donor autonomy and consent; deceased donation has been proposed by some as the preferred model for uterine transplants (Williams 2016). There has been debates on the time of uterus retrieval with ethicists arguing for uterus removal be done after the procurement of other vital organ due to its no-vital role. However, others have suggested its retrieval before cross-clamp and hence before the procurement of other vital organs in order to ensure substantial improvement of uterus quality (Testa et al. 2018). Yet there remains a small risk in terms of viability of other organs. Moreover, if the loss of organs can be avoided with the help of an experienced team and an optimized protocol, supplementary tests would need to be performed on the deceased donor to determine if she qualifies as a uterus donor and seek consent. This may delay the removal and transplantation of vital organs (Mertes/van Assche 2018). Others hope that progress in regenerative medicine and 3D printing could meet the shortage of organs and foreclose the need for living uterine donations (Corin et al. 2018; see also chapter 17 in this book).

Further, other experts have have pointed out the benefits of living donor hysterectomy over deceased donation as the former can provide comprehensive medical history, offer the recipient to be physically and emotionally ready and can be timed in a way to minimize the time between donor hysterectomy and implantation (Wall/Testa 2018). In case of deceased donation, concerns have also been raised about the consent to donate uterus. Blanket consent for posthumous donation in the UK under the National Health Service (NHS) that was given several years ago when certain tissues and organs were not a part of the registry is often treated the same way as blanket consent today (Williams 2018). Therefore, questions have been raised whether it's justified to retrieve tissues without knowing if potential donors are aware of uterus donation as an option and are willing to donate to an experimental procedure (Williams 2018). While some have argued for the surrogate consent to be inappropriate unless one has expressed the desire to donate while being alive (Bruno/Arora 2018), others have argued that the surrogate consent is not just mere reporting but is rather a substituted judgement using knowledge about the donor's personality and interest (Williams 2018).

2.1.3 Risks

Like all other transplant procedures, concerns have been raised about the risk of an experimental transplant procedure that has long operative time and is non-vital (Bruno/Arora 2018). However, the risks of donor hysterectomies are well known and recent robotic and laparoscopic procedures have only brought down the risks by implementing a safer technique using utero-ovarian veins as the sole outflow of the graft (Testa et al. 2018). Moreover, the uterus is seen to have exhausted its function and hence the risks to donors are limited to the transplantation process itself and not beyond (Wall/Testa 2018).

Again while ethicists have highlighted the potential psychological risks for living uterus donors, others have argued that the potential psychological benefits of being able to help cannot be ignored (ibid.). Yet the health risks of undergoing a hysterectomy and narcosis by the donors cannot be underestimated. The risks and harms of living UT are similar to that of a total abdominal hysterectomy. Although the risks are expected to lower with advances in clinical trials, so far living donors have experienced complications requiring surgical, endoscopic or radiological intervention under anesthetic and have experienced infections, urinary hypotonia, leg and buttock pain, and depression (Donovan et al. 2019). Further, it is pointed out that health risks to the recipients and the future child is often neglected in order to respect the informed consent of the former to undergo the procedure and undertake those risks (Robertson 2016). The recipients need to undergo three invasive surgeries – transplantation, caesarean section and removal of uterus that carry sufficient risk. Further, MRKH is usually accompanied by renal problem that can contribute to pregnancy complications.

Moreover, studies have shown that young women who have been on the same immunosuppressant as that of UT, experience prematurity, hypertension and preeclampsia (Armenti 2008; Shapiro/Ward 2018).

Moreover, the donor surgery is argued to be more exhaustive than routine hysterectomies, as it takes 10 times the duration and is associated with a higher rate of ureteral injury (Shapiro/Ward 2018). The impact of immunosuppression, even if for a temporary period of few years cannot be considered as trivial to the health of a woman (ibid.). This makes childbirth risky when the goal should be safe childbirth (Mertes/Assche 2018).

3.   Reproductive Ethics of UT

From the perspective of reproductive ethics, several key concerns have been raised regarding the implications for clinical introduction of UT as a reproductive option for those in need. There have been four main concerns regarding: *the value and meaning of gestational ties*, the *existing guidelines on parental rights, foreclosing of other reproductive alternatives, and transgender reproductive rights.*

3.1   Value and Meaning of Gestational Ties

While UT offers women with the chance of having their own pregnancies (Catsanos/Rogers/Lotz 2013), ethicists are concerned about the questions regarding *the value and meaning of gestational ties*. It has been pointed out that UT raise questions about the social embeddedness of value attached to gestation and its comparison to the value attached to genetic and social parenthood (Williams et al. 2018). Shapiro and Ward are of the view that "It is difficult to conceive how the experience of gestation, especially without parturition, can be sufficiently important to justify the risk to all parties involved in UTx [UT]" (2018: 36). Concerns have been raised about overt valorization of gestation in attempts to justify the significance of UT as it risks portraying life without gestation to be bad, even when gestation is desired (McTernan 2018). Since UT involves both a transplant and assisted reproductive technology (ART) procedure (at this moment), it imposes higher costs and risks on the donor and recipient and questions the permissible amount of risks for both donor and recipient on the pretext of enhancing quality of life (Williams et al. 2018). While some women with UFI may still opt for surrogacy and adoption, argument has been made that the desires of women who choose to use UT to attain motherhood through pregnancy cannot be denied (Testa/Johannesson 2017).

3.2   The Existing Guidelines on Parental Rights

Concerns raised by ethicists on parental rights matches the *existing guidelines on parental rights* during surrogacy and gamete donation. Once donated, the uterus is considered as the "property" of the recipient and thus the transplant team is asked to ensure that the donor and /or their family members understand that they will have no parental right over the future child born using the donated uterus (Bruno/Arora 2018). Further, it is proposed that until the child reaches 18, all contact between the child and the deceased donor's family or living donor should be done through the parents out of respect for the parents' right to choose a birth story (ibid.).

Ethicist have also argued at length about the funding of UT by a public health care system or its coverage under insurance without which it is likely to further widen the inequality of access to reproductive options. Concerns have been raised over funding of a non-life saving procedure by insurance or public funds. Blake (2018) says UT in a private health care system like the US cannot be covered unless health care in general becomes more widely equitable. Since many groups in the country have historically suffered inequality in access to infertility services and childbirth, UT cannot be prioritized. Sandman (2018) looks at the Swedish health care system that is publicly funded to argue that whether UT could be seen as a treatment for absolute uterine infertility (AUIF) should depend upon the relative severity of AUIF as compared to other health care needs and on the effectiveness and cost of UT in comparison to other reproductive alternatives like adoption and surrogacy. Others like Wilkinson and Williams (2015) argue that the case for not funding UT through a public health system like that of the NHS in the UK is rather weak. They are of the opinion that infertility can be viewed as a disorder due to the clear biological causes and effects. So the absence of sufficiently good alternative that could replace UT makes it a case for being funded. However, in order to be funded, UT needs to be established as a safe and cost-effective option and if surrogacy laws get reformed, the rationale for funding UT could get weak (ibid.).

3.3   Foreclosing of Other Reproductive Alternatives

Offering UT as a reproductive alternative is also seen as creating *potential harm* to the position of adoptable children (Lotz 2018). Thus an unintended consequence of offering UT would be to keep people from considering adoption as an option (Shapiro/Ward 2018). Moreover, it is argued that the introduction of UT frames the right to bear a child as not just liberty but claim and hence reinforces a life without birthing a child as a lesser life (Mertes/van Assche 2018). Since UT is often presented as an ethically less problematic alternative to surrogacy, Guntram and Williams (2018) studied the 2016 Swedish government white papers, which considered amending Sweden's existing policy on surrogacy to permit altruistic surrogacy. They showed how the arguments held against surrogacy can also be used against UT. They argued that nations banning surrogacy on moral grounds need to maintain consistency and ban UT as well. But then again, ethicists have argued against offering a simplistic ethical mapping of UT by suggesting a ban. Instead, restrictive measures through regulation by ensuring delay in access to treatment and strict counselling sessions has been recommended as ethical alternatives (McTernan 2018).

3.4   Transgender Reproductive Rights

A debate on UT is incomplete without addressing the possibilities that it creates for *transgender and potentially male reproductive rights and justice*. UT could be a path for transgender pregnancy and in future developed for male pregnancy (Alghrani 2018). However, ethicists remain concerned about the social feasibility of making UT available to transwomen in practice. Given the heteronormative reproductive practices that dominate social mindsets, it is apprehended that while a prospective donor might be willing to donate uterus to a woman with congenital defect, they might not be willing to do the same for a transwoman. Thus, a strategy of organ allocation that includes even transwoman is yet to be established and their disadvantaged position needs to be taken into consideration during framing policies (Spillman/Sade 2018). Moreover, policies directing towards cis-women for uterus allocation by placing clauses like bring your own egg and others might keep transwomen from attaining their goal of becoming a "woman in full" (Spillman/Sade 2018: 33).

4.   Ethical Discussions around UT through a Reproductive Justice Lens

Based on the above discussed transplant and reproductive ethical concerns raised by ethicist regarding the introduction and acceptance of UT as a transplant and fertility alternative in near future, three issues emerge that requires further discussion. The first ethical issue revolves around the designation of UT as a 'non-vital' transplant procedure that simply improves the quality of life and the impact of this categorization on uterus retrieval procedures. The second issue concerns the strategy of uterus allocation and listing and the gendered position of the donor in the process. The third issue revolves around the questions as to whether UT needs to be regulated as another transplant procedure like the other Vascularized Composite Allograft organs (VCAs) or needs to be recognized as an ART. In the following section, I will take up each of these three ethical issues one by one and demonstrate the benefits of approaching the ethics of UT through a reproductive justice approach.

4.1   UT as Improving Quality of Life, Non-Vital Organ

The first ethical issue revolves around the designation of UT as a 'non-vital' transplant procedure that is not life-saving but simply improves the quality of life (Caplan et al. 2007). UT however, is also seen as strengthening reproductive desires to achieve fertility through a risky procedure that could have been avoided in its absence. But once a reproductive technology is clinically introduced and the risks are deemed ethically acceptable by experts, its life changing potentials are tough to deny. While ethicists have discussed the importance of enhancement of quality of life for women who need UT and their moral right for the same, UT still continues to be categorized as non-vital due to its non-life saving role. Bruno and Arora (2018) argued that all lifesaving organs should be removed from the body first before the removal of the uterus. However, others are of the opinion that UT's potential for improving quality of life could be more than other lifesaving transplants like heart or kidney.

Although, UT requires women to undergo a round of risky surgical procedures that includes oocyte extraction, organ transplantation, embryo transfer and hysterectomy, the procedure is demonstrated as 'safe' through the recent successful childbirths. The procedure is also likely to advance further in future to minimize risks and errors. Thus, there remains little rationale behind denying women their rights to access UT once its clinically available. In order to decide on the circumstances under which UT needs to be made available and whether uterus as an organ requires more credit than just being categorized as non-vital, one needs to understand the changing meaning of the uterus made possible through its novel transplantation. The previously 'dormant', 'vacant' uterus or the ones that would become wasteful through hysterectomy now holds a vital future.

Kalindi Vora (2015) outlines that vital organs can be understood as an essential part of one's body and life and can be freed only after being constructed as 'extra' or not needed in its current site by the biomedical discourse. Uteruses like other 'vital' organs (e.g. kidneys) are suddenly seen as surplus once medical technologies are able to utilize and transfer its vitality to another human's body that lacks the same. In the context of organ and tissue donation, it is argued that a fantasy for a regenerative body brings out bioeconomic value from the bodies of others and creates a demand for new sites of surplus (Waldby/Mitchell 2006). Fertility is known to be an innate desire even if socially constructed and validated but is still a powerful desire. Thus, by offering the hope to regenerate the fertile capacities of the recipient, the novel technique of UT creates new sites of surplus, which when extracted and accumulated can prove to be vital for its recipients. The novel transplant technology and social desires of gestating and birthing a child becomes sites of (re)production of the vital capacity of the uteruses. Biology and biological substances are made to matter through the imagination of biotech practitioners and social analysts (Helmreich 2008). Technological possibilities and social desires thus create the avenue of birthing through UT and its mere possibility is likely to turn its desirability as a quintessence for its recipients. A first glimpse of that is already seen in the turnout of women who have registered their interests in the various UT clinical trials all over the world.

In the context of IVF, we know that people do not feel they have tried enough until they have exhausted all their options because even failures can grant the satisfaction of trying (Franklin 2010). UT has thus turned uteruses into a biocapital for the uterine transplant industry by making the procedure available as a reproductive option. Biocapital is discussed by Franklin and Lock (2003) as a form of extraction that involves isolating and mobilizing the primary reproductive agency of specific body parts. Therefore, once the vitality of uterus becomes an extractable commodity, the process of transplantation turns it into a biocapital for the transplant and fertility industry converting it into a vital asset for those who lack it. The vitality of the uterus thus becomes an indispensable reproductive asset for the recipient for whom UT becomes the ultimate means of gestating and birthing a child through their bodies. Although ethicists are of the opinion that undergoing such a risky procedure just for the experience of gestation might not be ethically justifiable when childbirth through the same is tentative, it is the hope for a successful gestation and the social construction of attaining motherhood by experiencing gestation and birthing that makes yet another 'hope technology' like UT highly desirable.

Now that UT is a possible birthing option, the inability to access the same unless one consciously chooses to dismiss this option, is likely to lead to gendered suffering for those women 'in need' (including transwomen). Hence, even if non-life saving, UT is likely to become a vital procedure for many due to what it makes possible. Also unlike other non-life saving transplants like face and hand grafts, UT is temporary and do not hold the same risks of undergoing life-long immunosuppression. While, other non-vital transplants pose similar ethical and moral challenges, unlike face transplant or hand transplant, UT is temporary and involves transfer of reproductive capacity and not a permanent transfer of a physical image or a visible body part, which has its own ethical complexity to cope with. The visible output of the transfer of reproductive capacity through UT is the birth of a child and concerns have been raised about the relational dynamics between the child born out of a transplanted uterus with their known donors. Yet studies on surrogacy have shown such relationships not necessarily causing complexities but often expanding the definition of kinship and giving rise to new roles. Thus, even if it is non-life saving, UT is likely to become indispensable for cis-gendered women[2], who are now aware of its availability as an option as well as transwomen for whom UT, once it becomes compatible for trans-reproduction can be the sole way of attaining biological motherhood. Under such circumstances, by taking on a reproductive justice perspective, one needs to break beyond the vital and non-vital or lifesaving and life enhancing dichotomy and not rank the uterus below other life-saving organs. The procedure requires recognition on its own right and for the gendered dimension attached with it.

Thus, although procurement of vital organ are often prioritized, the ethical importance of a potential good life offered by UT cannot be dismissed (Vong 2018). It has even been argued that if a transplant donor qualifies all listing criteria and has the possibility of retrieval of either heart or uterus, uterus should be retrieved as it will offer a higher quality of life (ibid). UT recipient is likely to give birth to another life whose average span will be higher than the heart transplant recipient and UT is going to improve the quality of life of two persons. On certain occasions, when vital transplants are not likely to improve quality of life significantly while UT can potentially improve quality of life of the recipient, it is argued that there is a need to move away from the typical procurement priority (ibid.). However, although it is argued that UT can at times offer a better quality of life than other lifesaving organ transplants like heart, I would like to argue that life-saving transplants still ought to deserve priority until technological progress can end the need for such prioritization. According biological reproduction a morally higher place over life-saving procedures could essentialize reproduction and offer oppressive frames for women. Having said that, I would also like to argue that procedures for procurement of uterus from deceased whole-body organ donor should be conducted in a way to ensure safe retrieval of uterus. The right of women and transwomen to access a transplantable uterus, if they are clinically suitable to undergo the procedure, should not be constrained should they have the means to do so (financial/insurance, donor available) due to its significance in their lives. Hence, it will be important to prioritize the advances in transplant medicine that would allow for its safe retrieval after the removal of other solid organs. If the same is not possible, techniques for uterus retrieval consuming minimum time prior the retrieval of other vital organs can be considered by transplant scientists as long as that does not risk safe retrieval of other organs. If the same is not possible at all, living UT is likely to become the preferred mode of uterus retrieval even if there is clinical evidence in future about the same success rate and risks of using both types of donation options. Therefore, it might be important to take into account the urgency and vital role of uterus in the lives of its recipients and work towards devising a way for its efficient retrieval.

Making UT a solution might overshadow the sufferings of unsuccessful recipients of UT for whom UT is inaccessible or those who remain involuntary childless for causes other than uterine infertility (Mertes/van Assche 2018). Thus people who cannot afford or access UT would be put on a loop of suffering. Yet once clinically made available, it

---

2 Cisgender is a term for people whose gender identity matches the sex that they were assigned at birth.

is tough to prevent people from desiring for UT and hence care needs to be taken about their efficient and fair access without passing on the burden to the potential donors.

4.2   Uterus Allocation and Gendering the Gift of the Donor

The second ethical issue concerns the strategy of uterus allocation and listing. Organ registries for UT cannot be maintained in the same way as that of other organs like kidney or liver (see chapter 9 in this book). It is tough to prioritize recipients in the listings since every recipient with birthing potential will have the same utility of the UT unlike other transplants where such prioritizations are done on the basis of its utility for the donor (Williams 2018). This requires a major amendment of organ allotment laws across countries. Moreover, as clear from various reports and articles, live uterus donation is likely to be a norm and given the shortage of live organ donors in various parts of the world the question remains as to whether and how demand for uteruses can be met. While several countries have or are moving towards deemed consent (see chapter 2 in this book), even if deceased UT becomes an option, deemed consent as discussed above, is unlikely to meet the high demand of uteruses required for UT around the world. Hence, there is a need to rethink the ethics of allocation of live uterus donation and its sourcing from known or unknown 'altruistic' donors.

Gifts are never 'free'; they inevitably come with strings, making the recipient beholden in crucial ways (Mauss 1925; see also chapter 10 and 14 in this book). "Pure altruism does not exist, except perhaps toward one's children, and bio-evolutionists have pointed out that parental sacrifice hides a form of (genetic) self-interest" (Scheper-Hughes 2007: 508). While studies have confirmed time and again that the joy of giving becomes a form of reciprocation for donors, and transplant teams are expected to carefully ensure effective procedures of informed consent (Gill/Lowes 2008), one needs to take into consideration the gendered dimension of uterus donation. Understanding the gendered dimension is important as it allows the use of reproductive justice as a moral frame to approach women's participation as UT donors. Researchers studying organ donation have long found that social desirability influences donor's decision-making (Russell/Jacob 1993). Few studies that are available from the US and Japan states that the majority of the public is in favour of UT as a reproductive option (Nakazawa et al. 2019; Hariton et al. 2018). Such attitudes could selectively target bodies of women with dormant and yet fertile uteruses, expecting them to 'help' those in need. The gendered availability of uteruses makes it important to deliberate upon the circumstances under which women (and transmen) donate their uteruses. Uteruses are going to come from women and in future even from transmen during their hysterectomy procedures once the transplant medicine is able to accommodate the same. Since uteruses cannot come from the men or women who might have not completed their own reproductive journeys, those women who have completed their reproductive years and transmen might feel socially obliged to consider donation as their responsibility. The pressure of being socially responsible might influence these potential donor's decision-makings and hence needs to be approached from a reproductive justice point of view.

Unlike other live donations like kidney or liver, uterus is not lifesaving but reproductive. Certain studies show that kidney recipients have not directly asked their family members to donate to avoid feeling beholden (Gill/Lowes 2008). Uteruses unlike kidneys are constructed in the transplant discourse as not just 'spare' organs but 'surplus with no further purpose' for the donor. Uterus recipients thus might feel relatively less pressure to compensate the donor for their loss of an organ since the uterus in question did not have a purpose for the latter. Thus their anticipated obligation towards the donor is unlikely to disappear, but will be of a different nature. Hence, recipients might directly expect their family members to donate their vacant uterus to them as an act of female solidarity. Potential donors on the other hand, might feel an urgency to help their daughters or friends to have a child since they themselves have experienced childbirth, which the latter is longing for. Bruno and Arora thus proposed that donor evaluation team should have private conversation with the donors. Pressures of family members in a pronatalist society should be evaluated (Catsanos et al. 2013) and UT donors should have a right to withdraw their consent at any stage (Bruno/Arora 2018). However, it still remains to be seen how this can be efficiently ensured.

Like the donors in the studies on kidney donation, the UT donors in various clinical trials have expressed the joy of being able to help their daughters, sisters or friends (Mitchell 2019). Yet one cannot deny that known directed uterus donation do come with the risk of both unsaid expectations from women to donate or even the possibility of direct coercion holding women in family obliged to donate. On the other hand, as discussed before, it can be expected that in several societies, living donors might not wish to donate their uteruses to a trans women. Further, transwomen might lack the same social capital and support from friends and family willing to assist a transbirth by donating their uterus like a cis-woman. Hence, if reproductive justice is to be achieved one has to think of ways for uterus allocation that would neither selectively target gendered bodies nor selectively deprive access for some on the basis of their sexuality and gender.

Non-directed unknown live uterus donation to some extent is likely to come from menopausal women and transmen once the UT procedure is able to utilize uteruses harvested through hysterectomy. If in future, UT continues to require uteruses with larger grafts vessels, women of menopausal age and transmen could be unnecessarily subjected to a more complex surgical procedure, even when they might give their informed consent to undergo the same.

Based on the lessons from kidney donation, we know that women all over the world are frequently chosen or expected by their family members to be a kidney donor for being the most non-productive member of the family (Scheper-Hughes 2007). Studies on surrogacy have also shown that several altruistic surrogates during the early days of surrogacy have been the mothers or a close friend. Hence, one cannot but be vary of the possibility of women within one's families especially mothers either feeling obliged to help by donating their 'dormant, vacant' uterus to their daughters or a close friend or sister feeling the moral responsibility to 'help'.

Discussing the German Organ donation scenario, Schweda and Schicktanz characterized the laws of living organ donation that is directed towards family and relatives as "mutual family responsibility" (2012: 247), which often take a gendered role. Through empirical research, they have shown that a sense of individual responsibility towards donating organs like kidney or liver often arise out of traditional gendered roles in society expecting women to provide as a carer. Women is their study declared their willingness to 'sacrifice' their heart or both kidney for their children if need be. On many instances, individual responsibility can turn into self-responsibility when people start considering the act of organ donation as indicative of being a good person (Schweda/Schicktanz 2012).

However, the phenomenon of donor regret (Scheper-Hughes 2007) is also common among live kidney and liver donors especially when the transplant fails. For every uterus rejection or failed attempt at childbirth after UT, the donor and in this case women would become selectively vulnerable to feelings of regret. Again the onus of organ gifting can lead to a creditor-debtor relationship between the organ donor and recipient that has been noticed in cases of kidney transplant on the organ watch files (Scheper-Hughes 2007) and which Fox and Swazey describe as "tyranny of gift" (1978: 386).

Although the debt of receiving the uterus as a gift from one's family member could be avoided by some by purchasing organs from the 'poor' and hence outsourcing the labor of donation to deprived parts of the world; the issue of sacrifice, moral obligation or coercion to donate could very well be the reason for uterus selling just like that of kidney donation (see Scheper-Hughes 2007).

Since transnational kidney markets and transnational surrogacy markets are a well known phenomenon, the uterus shortage could soon be met by through cross-border uterine donation through the underground organ markets emerging in Asia, Africa and Middle East (Scheper Hughes 2002; Cohen 2013; see also chapter 11 in this book). Or it could take the form of transnational surrogacy markets like India, Nepal, Mexico, Russia etc. A first glimpse of the same is is visible in the advertisements of medical tourism platforms like Medmonks who have already started promoting low cost cross-border UT opportunities in Pune, India.[3] It suggests that UT is likely to generate cross-border markets and pose distinct sets of ethical, moral, and legal challenges.

Thus, clear ethical frames for live uterine donation needs to be thought through by taking into consideration the local socio-cultural context and developing mechanisms through uterus donation campaigns or awareness drives that frees women and transmen of being responsible by default to donate their uteruses. Live uterus listing and allocation be it directed or non-directed should take into consideration this additional gendered responsibilities associated with the process of uterine extraction that suddenly deems women as hosts with surplus, who might either see it as an opportunity to help their loved ones or an overt or covert obligation. While transplant teams have been offering counselling to potential donors, UT counselling requires an additional perspective on childbirth and parental relationships, which might demand the expertise of counsellors working with egg donors and surrogates.

4.3   The In-Betweeness of UT as a Transplant and Fertility Procedure

The third ethical issue that has been circulating in the ethical debates on UT and yet not been directly voiced is the concern regarding whether UT needs to be regulated as another transplant procedure like the other VCAs or needs to be recognized as an ART. Although UT is a transplant procedure and an output of the advancement in transplant medicine, the purpose of carrying out this transplant is reproductive. Hence, it

---

3 Website of Medmonks: https://medium.com/@medmonks/process-uterus-transplant-india-cost-med-monks-95dec366ef06 (accessed on September 4, 2018)

is bound to raise ethical questions that fall within the domain of reproductive ethics and law, as much as transplant ethics and law.

For the purpose of uterus allocation, parental fitness has been considered by ethicists as a screening criteria. Some have argued that uterine allocation model should replicate the organ allocation model and not adoption policies. Hence parental fitness should not be a criteria for UT allocation since the criteria established by United Network for Organ Sharing (UNOS) for medical fitness cannot be extended to parental fitness (Rogers 2018). Thus psychosocial criteria for assessment could be discriminatory as per the present guidelines and transplant teams are not qualified enough to make these decisions (ibid.). However, the issue of parental fitness is often discussed under the domain of assisted reproductive technologies (ARTs). Bodies like the *American Society for Reproductive Medicine* (ASRM) urge fertility clinics to not provide services that would threaten the future of the child, there is no mandatory regulatory policy in countries like US to determine whom fertility clinics are actually offering their services (ibid.). In contrast, in the UK, the *Human Fertilisation and Embryology Authority* (HFEA) mandates the clinics to conduct child welfare assessment (ibid.). Thus, to be able to accept or contest the significance of reproductive issues like parental rights during UT, laws of uterine allocation would need to take into account the ART regulations or guidelines for fertility clinics in respective countries and merge it with organ transplantation guidelines like the UNOS guidelines.

ART could be available as a fertility option offered by fertility clinics in collaboration with transplant surgeons. The possibility of women feeling morally obliged or being coerced into uterus donation as has happened in the case of egg donation and even kidney donation can also be addressed if UT donors are offered similar psychological and legal support as the egg donors and surrogates by the fertility clinics. Thus, UT ethics needs to draw from the national and international ethical guidelines already in place to safeguard the interests of women participating in similar technology aided reproductive procedures like egg donation and surrogacy. Under such circumstances, regulation would need to safeguard not just the choice of using living or deceased donor or ways of uterus allocation and listings. It needs to also focus on envisioning competent counselling procedures for the donors and ways of ensuring adherence to a set recipient selection process. Private ART clinics offer ART services to anyone medically suitable – irrespective of whether the donors and surrogates work altruistically or commercially. Since UFI is a diagnosis that is likely to come from the domain of fertility medicine and for some through the ART clinics, the extent to which those clinics will be able to freely allocate uteruses to their patients is a question that needs to be reflected upon. Moreover, it is known that the IVF recipients in countries like the UK often travel to Spain or Cyprus to jump the long waiting list of egg donation due to its time consuming and restrictive ART guidelines under the HFEA. A similar pattern is known to be exiting for cross-border kidney exchanges. Clinic might begin to promote the same for UT in future unless the transnational flow of patients is tracked and regulated by prospective source and recipient countries in unison. Hence, for practical regulatory purposes, one cannot lose sight of the precedents set by other ART and transplant practices that UT is likely to replicate.

Like every other fertility option, UT is also likely to raise issues related to cost, availability and most importantly uniformity of access. UT is expensive. It incurs costs for a prolonged period in order to monitor and administer immunosuppressants.

Since until now UT are performed using IVF (the uterus is not being connected to the native fallopian tube) there are additional costs and procedures involved that might not be legally compatible with the existing ART laws in various countries. The procedure could involve cost of maintaining frozen embryos, its plight if the transplant fails, frozen eggs or ovarian tissues (if the recipient have been battling cancer), preimplantation genetic diagnosis (PGD), non-medical sex selection to state a few. In state sponsored programs, it remains to be decided whether the same couples or individuals who have been sponsored for previous surrogacy attempts are covered for UT. Hence, like other ARTs, UT could potentially stratify reproduction further by creating inequalities amongst women across class, country, race and ethnicity. Since incongruent access is likely to leave some women deprived despite their clinical suitability to undergo UT, the issue of access and allocation needs to be approached though the lens of reproductive justice and not through the traditional political economic argument on fair allocation. Moreover, UT is likely to be the only option for transwomen to attain biological reproduction. In future, once UT for transwomen become possible, additional ethical concerns like transwomen's access to egg and embryo donation, uterine donors and non-discriminatory ways of access to UT is likely to be of importance. Such ethical and legal concerns overseeing UT are gendered and is of moral significance. Each of these issues unless dealt carefully threaten to coerce reproductive rights of women and transmen and create new structures of inequalities and reproductive injustice.

Since UT is set to become a reproductive alternative for many in need, compatibility between UT laws and existing ART laws would be key to ensure that the reproductive rights of the donors and recipients of UT receive the same leverage as that of those using other forms of reproductive assistance. Thus, in order to remove all structural constrains from women's and transmen's access to UT, the procedure needs to be categorized as both a transplant procedure and a fertility procedure. This should especially be the case since IVF is the only way through which recipients of transplanted uteruses are birthing children. Through progress in the field of transplant medicine, it might soon be possible for some women to 'naturally' conceive once their fallopian tubes are connected to their ovaries. However, such pregnancies are still likely to be closely monitored by obstetrics and gynecology surgeons. Moreover, IVF would always be an option for some women and transwomen who might not still be in a position to 'naturally' conceive.

Moreover, if the regulation and planning for its systematic allocation fails to balance and merge the transplant and the fertility dimensions of UT, it would be giving higher importance to the biomedical process of uterus retrieval and successful transplantation. Assigning UT the status of quasi transplant and fertility procedure would bring the actual purpose of the transplant to the forefront, would make the response of the bodies to transplanted organs and immunosuppressant visible. It would highlight the often invisible reproductive journeys of women, which otherwise risk getting overshadowed by the biomedicalized transplant narratives of success and failures. Unlike other organ transplants involving kidney or liver, UT is a temporary transplant with a definite goal of childbirth. Attempts to achieve the same starts only in the post-transplantation period. Thus, the post-transplant period does not only become a time of recovery and survival within one's body with a foreign organ but also the period of attaining one's fertility by attempting to conceive, gestate and birth. The politics and ethics of this post-transplant period could only be understood and regulated if UT is approached as both a transplant as well as a fertility procedure. This is crucial in order to understand whether the arrangements fall short of ensuring reproductive justice for the recipients.

5.   Conclusion

In this chapter, I have identified and discussed three key ethical issues at the backdrop of the ongoing debates on UT from around the world. The first ethical issue revolves around the designation of UT as a 'non-vital' transplant procedure that simply improves the quality of life and the impact of this designation on uterus retrieval procedures. I argued that uterus as an organ during a transplantation procedure deserves more credit than simply being categorized as 'non-vital' due to the role it plays in the recipient's lives. Once technology is able to utilize and transfer the vitality of a uterus to the body of another woman who lacks it, its vital capacity becomes extremely desirable and can seem quintessential to cisgender and transgender women to attain fertility. Hence, I argue for breaking out of the 'vital' and 'non-vital' rationale behind organ retrieval and allotment and state that uterus retrieval deserves as much attention as other lifesaving organs, though not more than it. As a possible birthing option, it can cause gendered suffering amongst women who desire to utilize UT to reverse their infertility. Hence, given the vital role of a transplanted uterus in the life of the recipient, transplant scientist must devise a way for safe retrieval of uteruses before or after retrieval of other vital organs as risking the opportunity to utilize a potentially viable uterus might bring increased sufferings.

The second issue that I discussed concerns the strategy of uterus allocation and listing and the gendered position of the donor in the process. I argued that since gifts are never free, there is a need to rethink the ethics of allocation of live uterus donation and it's sourcing from known or unknown live altruistic donors. Since, UT selectively target bodies of women, the gendered availability of uteruses need to be taken into consideration in order to understand the nature of responsibility that UT might bring for women and how that might influence their decision-making. Like the donors in studies on kidney donation, the UT donors from the ongoing clinical trials have expressed their joy at being able to help their loved ones. Yet that cannot dismiss the possibility of holding women and transmen morally obliged to gift their uteruses during their hysterectomies in order to prevent it from going to medical waste. Moreover, the phenomenon of donor regret could further make potential UT donors vulnerable to experiencing failures on instances when UT would fail to cause a successful childbirth. While some recipients might avoid making their family or friends feel obliged to help them by sourcing uteruses from transnational organ markets, even a price for uterus selling as is known, cannot ensure a non-coercive decision-making for donors. Thus, I argue for the need to have clear ethical frames for live uterine donation that takes into consideration the local socio-cultural context and legal scenario. It would also be important to develop mechanisms through uterus donation campaigns or awareness drives for freeing women and transmen of their presumed moral responsibility to donate their uteruses.

The third ethical issue that I discussed revolves around the question as to whether UT needs to be regulated as another transplant procedure like the other VCAs or needs to be recognized as an ART. ART could be available as a fertility option offered by fertility clinics in collaboration with transplant surgeons. Hence, for practical regulatory purposes, one cannot lose sight of the precedents set by other ART practices that UT is likely to follow suit, which are available to anyone deemed medically eligible and often transnationally. Like every other fertility option, UT is also likely to raise issues related to cost, availability and most importantly uniformity of access. UT is expensive and its costs could lead to non-uniformity of access and inefficiency of the national waiting lists. Such ethical and legal concerns can only be addressed if the existing ART laws of the respective countries are taken into consideration alongside its transplantation laws while drafting the guidelines and regulations for making UT clinically available. Therefore, I argued that UT needs to be categorized as both a transplant procedure and a fertility procedure, especially because IVF is the only way through which recipients of transplanted uteruses at present are birthing children. Moreover, if the regulation and planning for its systematic allocation fails to balance and merge the transplant and the fertility dimensions of UT, it would be giving higher importance to the biomedical process of uterus retrieval and successful transplantation while overshadowing the motivations and embodied experiences of women undergoing the transplants.

Therefore, in this chapter, I have stated that UT is likely to alter reproductive norms for women, selectively target bodies of healthy women as sites of extraction and create a new relational dynamics between the donor, recipient and the child-to-be. Hence, I would like to point out that there is a need for a gender sensitive ethical framework in order to understand the nature of risks, hopes and responsibilities that are intertwined with the clinical use of UT. Although UT is a transplant procedure and an output of the advancement in transplant medicine, the purpose of carrying out this transplant is reproductive and is hence bound to raise ethical questions that falls within the domain of reproductive ethics and law, as much as transplant ethics and law.

References

Alghrani, Amel (2018): "Uterus Transplantation in and beyond Cisgender Women: Revisiting Procreative Liberty in Light of Emerging Reproductive Technologies." In: Journal of Law and the Biosciences 5/2, pp. 301–328.

Andrew, Scottie/Ahmed, Saeed (2019): "A Woman Delivered the First Baby in the US Born from the Transplanted Uterus of a Dead Donor." CNN. Availabe at: https://edition.cnn.com/2019/07/09/us/first-us-baby-transplanted-uterus-of-dead-donor-trnd/index.html (accessed April 24, 2020)

Armenti, Vincent T./Constantinescu, Serban/Moritz, Micheal J./Davison, John M. (2008): "Pregnancy after Transplantation." In: Transplantation Reviews 22/4, pp. 223–240.

Arora, Kavita Shah/Blake, Valarie (2014): "Uterus Transplantation: Ethical and Regulatory Challenges." In: Journal of Medical Ethics 40/6, pp. 396–400.

Banerjee, Shoumojit (2017): "India's First Uterine Transplant Performed." The Hindu. Available at: https://www.thehindu.com/news/national/other-states/indias-first-uterine-transplant-performed/article18491542 (accessed September 5, 2018)

Bayefsky, Michelle J./Benjamin E. Berkman (2016): "The Ethics of Allocating Uterine Transplants." In: Cambridge Quarterly of Healthcare Ethics 25/3 pp. 350–365.

Bayefsky, Michelle J./Benjamin E. Berkman (2018): "Toward the Ethical Allocation of Uterine Transplants." In: The American Journal of Bioethics 18/7, pp. 16–17.

Blake, Valarie K. (2018): "Financing Uterus Transplants: The United States Context." In: Bioethics 32/8, pp. 527–533.

Brännström, Mats/Johannesson, Liza/Bokström, Hans/Kvarnström, Niclas/Mölne, Johan/Dahm-Kähler, Pernilla/Enskog, Anders (2014): "First Clinical Uterus Transplantation Trial: A Six-Month Report." In: Fertility and Sterility 101/5, pp. 1228–1236.

Brännström, Mats/Johannesson, Liza/Bokström, Hans/Kvarnström, Niclas/Mölne, Johan/Dahm-Kähler, Pernilla/Enskog, Anders (2015): "Livebirth after Uterus Transplantation." In: The Lancet 385/9968, pp. 607–616.

Bethany, Bruno/Kavita Shah, Arora (2018): "Uterus Transplantation: The Ethics of Using Deceased Versus Living Donors." In: The American Journal of Bioethics 18/7, pp. 6–15.

Caplan, Arthur L./Perry, Constance/Plante, Lauren A./Saloma Joseph/Batzer, Frances R. (2007): "Moving the Womb." In: Hastings Center Report 37/3, pp. 18–20.

Corin, Zoe/Roee, Furman/Shira, Lifshitz/Ophir, Samuelov/Greenbaum, Dov (2018): "How Do You Donate Life When People Are Not Dying: Transplants in the Age of Autonomous Vehicles." In: The American Journal of Bioethics 18/7, pp: 27–29.

Catsanos, Ruby/Rogers, Wendy/Lotz, Mianna (2013): "The Ethics of Uterus Transplantation." In: Bioethics 27/2, pp. 65–73.

Eduardo, Hariton/Bortoletto, Pietro/Goldman, Randi H./Farland, Leslie V./Ginsburg, Elizabeth S./Gargiulo, Antonio R. (2018): "A Survey of Public Opinion in the United States regarding Uterine Transplantation." In: Journal of Minimally Invasive Gynecology 25/6, pp. 980–985.

Fox, Renee C./Swazey, Judith P. (1978): The Courage to Fail: Organ Transplantation and Hemodialysis, Chicago: University of Chicago Press.

Franklin, Sarah (2002): Embodied Progress: A Cultural Account of Assisted Conception, London: Routledge.

Franklin, Sarah (2010): "Transbiology: A Feminist Cultural Account of Being After IVF." In: Scholar and Feminist Online 9/1–2, pp. 1–8.

Franklin, Sarah/Lock, Margaret (2003): "Animation and Cessation: The Remaking of Life and Death (Editor's Introduction)." In: Sarah Franklin/Margaret Lock (eds.), Remaking Life and Death: Toward an Anthropology of the Biosciences, Santa Fe: School of American Research Press, pp. 3–21.

Glenn, Cohen I. (2013): "Transplant Tourism: The Ethics and Regulation of International Markets for Organs." In: The Journal of Law, Medicine & Ethics 41/1, pp. 269–285.

Gill, Paul/Lowes, Lesley (2008): "Gift Exchange and Organ Donation: Donor and Recipient Experiences of Live Related Kidney Transplantation." In: International journal of nursing studies 45/11, pp: 1607–1617.

Guntram, Lisa/Williams, Nicola Jane (2018): "Positioning Uterus Transplantation as a 'More Ethical' Alternative to Surrogacy: Exploring Symmetries between Uterus Transplantation and Surrogacy through Analysis of a Swedish Government White Paper." In: Bioethics 32/8, pp. 509–518.

Hammond-Browning, Natasha (2016): "Womb Transplants-are they Worth the Risk?" In: Bionews, 847.

Helmreich, Stefan (2008): "Species of Biocapital." In: Science as Culture 17/4, pp. 463–478.

Hovsepian, Grace (2018): "First Successful Uterus Transplant in the MENA Region was Completed in Lebanon!" The 961. Available at: https://www.the961.com/uterus-transplant-in-lebanon/ (accessed April 24, 2020)

Johnston, Chris (2015): "Womb Transplants: First 10 British Women Given Go-Ahead." The Guardian. Available at: https://www.theguardian.com/lifeandstyle/2015/sep/29/10-women-receive-go-ahead-for-first-ever-womb-transplants-in-uk (accessed February 13, 2019)

Kisu, I./Kato, Y./Hideaki, Obara/Kentaro, Matsubara/Matoba, Y./Kouji, Banno/Daisuke, Aoki (2018): "Emerging Problems in Uterus Transplantation." In: BJOG: An International Journal of Obstetrics & Gynaecology 125/11, pp. 1352–1356.

Lang, Fabianne (2019): "First Baby Born in the U.S. from Transplanted Womb of Deceased Donor. Interesting Engineering." Available at: https://interestingengineering.com/first-baby-born-in-the-us-from-transplanted-womb-of-deceased-donor (accessed August 21, 2019)

Lotz, Mianna (2018): "Uterus Transplantation as Radical Reproduction: Taking the Adoption Alternative More Seriously." In: Bioethics 32/8, pp. 499–508.

Mauss, Marcel (1925 [1990]): The Gift: The Form and Reason for Exchange in Archaic Societies, London: Routledge.

McTernan, Emily (2018): "Uterus Transplants and the Insufficient Value of Gestation." In: Bioethics 32/8, pp. 481–488.

Mertes, Heidi/Van Assche, Kristof (2018): "UTx with Deceased Donors also Places Risks and Burdens on Third Parties." In: The American Journal of Bioethics 18/7, pp. 22–24.

Mitchell, Natasha (2019): "A Uterus Transplant Made this Woman's Dream Come True, but the Procedure Sparks Ethical Controversy." ABC Science. ABC News. Available at: https://www.abc.net.au/news/science/2019-03-10/future-uterus-transplants-ethical-dilemmas-science-friction/10879024 (accessed August 21, 2019)

Nakazawa, Akari/Hirata, Tetsuya/Arakawa, Tomoko/Nagashima, Natsuki/Fukuda, Shinya/ Neriishi, Kazuaki/Harada, Miyuki (2019): "A Survey of Public Attitudes toward Uterus Transplantation, Surrogacy, and Adoption in Japan." In: PloS one 14/10, pp. e0223571. DOI: 10.1371/journal.pone.0223571

Persad, Govind/Wertheimer, Alan/Emanuel, Ezekiel J. (2009): "Principles for Allocation of Scarce Medical Interventions." In: The Lancet 373/9661, pp: 423-431.

Petrini, Carlo/Morresi, Assuntina (2017): "Uterus Transplants and their Ethical Implications." In: Annali dell' Istituto Superiore di Sanita 53/1, pp. 25–29.

Pinghui, Zhuang (2015): "Woman in China Undergoes Country's First Successful Womb Transplant after Mother Donates Organ." In: South China Post. Available at: https://www.scmp.com/news/china/society/article/1883501/woman-china-undergoes-countrys-first-successful-womb-transplant (accessed April 24, 2020)

Pritchard, Sarah (2016): "First Uterus Transplants from Living Donors Carried Out in the US." BioNews. Available at: https://www.bionews.org.uk/page_136325 (accessed April 24, 2020)

Radio Sweden (2014): "First Baby Born after Womb Transplant. Radio Sweden." Available at: https://sverigesradio.se/sida/artikel.aspx?programid=2054&artikel=5982635 (acessed April 24, 2020).

Robertson, John A. (2016): "Impact of Uterus Transplant on Fetuses and Resulting Children: A Response to Daar and Klipstein." In: Journal of Law and the Biosciences 3/3, p. 710–717.

Russell, Sue/Jacob, Rolf G. (1993): "Living-Related Organ Donation: The Donor's Dilemma." In: Patient Education and Counseling 21/12, pp. 89–99.

Sánchez-Margallo, Francisco M./Moreno-Naranjo, Belén/Del Mar Pérez-López, María/ Abellán, Elena/ Domínguez-Arroyo, José A./Mijares, José/Álvarez, Ignacio S. (2019): "Laparoscopic Uterine Graft Procurement and Surgical Autotransplantation in Ovine Model." In: Scientific Reports 9/1, pp. 1–12.

Sandman, Lars (2018): "The Importance of Being Pregnant: On the Healthcare Need for Uterus Transplantation." In: Bioethics 32/8, pp. 519–526.

Scheper-Hughes, Nancy (2002): "The Global Traffic in Human Organs." In: The Anthropology of Globalization: A Reader 4/2, pp. 270–308.

Scheper-Hughes, Nancy (2007): "The Tyranny of the Gift: Sacrificial Violence in Living Donor Transplants." In: American Journal of Transplantation 7/3, pp. 507–511.

Schmidt, Fabian (2019): "Two Children Born in Germany for the First Time after Uterus Transplant. Deutsche Welle." Available at: https://www.dw.com/en/two-children-born-in-germany-for-the-first-time-after-uterus-transplant/a-48850203 (accessed August 21, 2019)

Schweda, Mark/Schicktanz, Silke (2012): "Shifting Responsibilities of Giving and Taking Organs? Ethical Considerations of the Public Discourse on Organ Donation and Organ Trade." In: Gunnarson Martin/Fredrik Svenaeus (eds.), The Body as Gift, Resource and Commodity: Exchanging Organs, Tissues and Cells in the 21st Century, Stockholm: Södertörn Högskola, pp. 235–266.

Shapiro, Michael E./Frances, Rieth W. (2018): "Uterus transplantation: A Step Too Far." In: The American Journal of Bioethics 18/7, pp. 36–37.

Sifferlin, Alexandra (2017): "Exclusive: First U.S. Baby Born After a Uterus Transplant." TIME. Available at: https://time.com/5044565/exclusive-first-u-s-baby-born-after-a-uterus-transplant/ (accessed April 24, 2020)

Spillman, Monique A./Sade, Robert M. (2018): "A Woman in Full." In: The American Journal of Bioethics 18/7, pp. 32–34.

Testa, Giuliano/Johannesson, Liza (2017): "The Ethical Challenges of Uterus Transplantation." In: Current Opinion in Organ Transplantation 22/6, pp. 593–597.

Testa, G./McKenna, G. J./Gunby, R. T./Anthony, T./Koon, E. C./Warren, A. M./Putman, J. M./ Zhang, L./DePrisco, G./Mitchell, J. M./Wallis, K. (2018): "First Live Birth after Uterus Transplantation in the United States." In: American Journal of Transplantation 18/5, pp. 1270–1274.

Thompson, Alexandra (2018): "Indian Woman who had Three Abortions and a Miscarriage Gives Birth after her Mother Donated her Womb." Mail Online. Available at: https://www.dailymail.co.uk/health/article-6393029/Indian-woman-gives-birth-Asias-uterus-transplanted-baby.html (accessed April 24, 2020)

Uterus Unique (2018): "Not a day too soon. Uterus Unique [Blog]." Available at: https:// uterusunique.se/en/not-a-day-too-soon/ (accessed April 24, 2020)

Vong, Gerard (2018): "The Purported Procurement Priority of Lifesaving Organs over Non-Lifesaving Organs: Uterus Transplants and the Ethical Importance of Potential Lives." In: American Journal of Bioethics 18/7, pp. 25–26.

Vora, Kalindi (2015): Life Support: Biocapital and the New History of Outsourced Labor, Minneapolis: University of Minnesota Press.

Waldby, Catherine/Mitchell, Robert (2006): Tissue Economies: Blood, Organs, And Cell Lines in Late Capitalism, Durham/London: Duke University Press.

Wall, Anji/Testa, Giuliano (2018): "Living Donation, Listing, And Prioritization in Uterus Transplantation." In: The American Journal of Bioethics 18/7, pp: 20–22.

Wei, Li/Xue, Tao/Tao, Kai-Shan/Zhang, Geng/Zhao, Guang-Yue/Yu, Shi-Qiang/Cheng, Liang (2017): "Modified Human Uterus Transplantation using Ovarian Veins for Venous Drainage: The First Report of Surgically Successful Robotic-Assisted Uterus Procurement and Follow-Up for 12 Months." In: Fertility and Sterility 108/2, pp. 346–356.

Weintraub, Karen (2018): "First Successful Uterus Transplant from Deceased Donor Leads to Healthy Baby." Scientific American. Available at: https://www.scientificamerican.com/article/first-successful-uterus-transplant-from-deceased-donor-leads-to-healthy-baby/ (accessed April 24, 2020)

Wilkinson, Stephen/Williams, Nicola Jane (2016): "Should Uterus Transplants be Publicly Funded?" In: Journal of Medical Ethics 42/9, pp. 559–565.

Williams, Nicola (2016): "Should Deceased Donation be Morally Preferred in Uterine Transplantation Trials?" In: Bioethics 30/6, pp. 415–424.

Williams, Nicola Jane (2018): "Deceased Donation in Uterus Transplantation Trials: Novelty, Consent, and Surrogate Decision Making." In: The American Journal of Bioethics 18/7, pp. 18–20.

Williams, Nicola Jane/Scott, Rosamund/Wilkinson, Stephen (2018): "The Ethics of Uterus Transplantation." In: Bioethics 32, pp. 478–480.

Willoughby, Ian (2019): "Woman with Transplanted Womb Gives Birth in Czech Republic for First Time. Radio Prague International." Available at: https://www.radio.cz/en/section/news/woman-with-transplanted-womb-gives-birth-in-czech-republic-for-first-time (accessed April 24, 2020)

Zaami, S./Di, Luca A./Marinelli, E. (2019): "Advancements in Uterus Transplant: New Scenarios and Future Implications." In: European Review for Medical and Pharmacological Sciences 23/2, pp. 892–902.

V. ALTERNATIVES

16. Researching Xenotransplantation
Moral Rights of Animals

Tatjana Višak

1. Introduction

"*Ein Herz für uns*" ("A heart for us"): this is the title of a recent article on xenotransplantation in *Die Zeit*, one of Germany's major newspapers (Steeger 2019). The article describes experimental research taking place in Munich, Germany, in which researchers have cloned and genetically modified pigs. Their aim is that humans, such as the several hundred people currently waiting for a donor heart in Germany, will soon be able to receive the animals' organs. As far back as 1999, a famous Swiss company predicted it would be able to provide 300.000 animal organs for human use by 2010. In 2006, US scientists also expected that the first clinical trials would take place by 2010. At the time of writing it is 2020, and none of these developments have eventuated.

While some people want pigs to have hearts for humans, others feel that we humans should, in a sense, have a heart for pigs and not use them in this way. Is it ethically acceptable to use pigs as resources for spare body parts, and to use non-human primates and other animals as experimental subjects in order to develop the technology? This chapter addresses these and other questions about the ethics of xenotransplantation.

2. Xenotransplantation Research

Deriving from the Greek word *Xénos* ('foreign'), 'Xenotransplantation' refers to the transplantation of *living* organs, tissue, or cells across species boundaries. Tissue transplants from *inactivated* cells, such as the transplantation of heart valves from pigs to humans, do *not* count as xenotransplantation. The same holds for animal-based products that contain only molecules, such as insulin derived from pigs. In case of xenotransplantation of living *organs*, the incoming heart, liver or kidney is connected to the recipient's body and is supposed to perform all normal functions. In case of xenotransplantation of living *tissue*, such as skin, corneas or bones, the recipient's blood vessels are supposed to nourish that tissue, a process called 'vascularization'. Xenotransplantations are 'concordant' when the two involved species have a close phylogenetic, i.e. evolutionary, relationship, such as in ape-to-human transplantation;

otherwise they are 'discordant', as in pig-to-human transplantation (Cooper/Wagner 2012). 'Xenotransplantation' is typically contrasted to 'allotransplantation' (transplantation within a species) as well as to autotransplantation (transplantation within an individual).

Since the end of the 1990s, xenotransplantation research has flourished, mainly in the United States and the United Kingdom, but also in Germany. Accounts of the history of xenotransplantation research typically mention the so-called Baby Fae case, which spurred public debate about the technology and also led to some regulation. In 1984, the surgeon Leonard Bailey replaced the heart of the newborn human, Stephanie Fae Beauclair from Los Angeles, who was born with a severe heart problem, with the heart of a baboon. The baby died 20 days later. The research involving Baby Fae was severely criticized, not least because a surgical procedure that could have cured the baby's heart condition already existed. Moreover, the xenotransplantation couldn't possibly have succeeded, and it was considered foolish to believe it could (Gericke 2014). Dr. Bailey had previously performed at least 160 transplantations between different species, such as sheep, goat and baboon, all of which resulted in the death of both donor and recipient. This was also the outcome of the hundreds of trials by other xenotransplantation researchers undertaken since the early 20th century. For example, Keeth Reemtsman performed 13 chimpanzee-to-human kidney transplantations in 1963–1964, and Thomas Starzl carried out many liver transplants between chimpanzees and human children. Nearly always, the xenotransplantation failed due to hyperacute organ rejection (Gianello 2014). Transplantation medicine in general was in an experimental stage during the 20th century. For example, it was only in 1954 that Joseph Murray first successfully transplanted a kidney between two identical twins.

Nowadays pigs are considered the most likely non-human organ sources for humans. Speaking of 'donor' animals in case of xenotransplantation would be a euphemism, since the animals do not voluntarily *give* their organs. (More appropriate labels might be 'organ sources' or 'transplant victims'.) Pigs are considered suitable due to the size and function of their organs, which are similar to those of humans. Furthermore, the risk of transmitting viruses is smaller for pigs than for species that are more closely related to humans, such as primates. Finally, pigs are relatively cheap and easy to breed. A disadvantage of using pigs, however, is that the human immune system tends to reject pig organs even more rapidly than those of more closely related species (ibid.). Pigs are not only envisioned as a source of solid organs for humans: porcine pancreas and brain cells are being tested for use in the treatment of diabetes and Parkinson's disease, respectively. In the latter case, the brain cells are coated in seaweed, preventing the human immune system from attacking the xenograft while allowing growth factor to move into surrounding brain tissue. Furthermore, pig livers have been used *ex vivo* – i.e. connected to the human body externally – as a temporary support for humans with acute liver failure.

To date, porcine organs have mainly been transplanted into non-human primates as part of efforts to develop the technology. No xenograft recipient, regardless of species, has ever survived for longer than a few months; typically, they die much earlier. It is technically still unclear whether pig hearts, or other living body parts from any non-human species, could ever be modified to function in humans. The major technical problems in xenotransplantation research are (1) the required correspondence of size, structure and function between organs; (2) the hyper-acute rejection of the newly received organ by the recipient's immune system (as well as a rejection on the medium and longer term in cases where hyper-acute rejection was prevented); and (3), the risk of transmitting infectious diseases from non-human animals to humans. Because humans received the HIV and the Ebola viruses, as well as influenza viruses and most recently the Coronavirus, from non-human animals, it is feared that other deadly viruses may cross the species boundary as well. Furthermore, the non-human transplant victims are genetically modified to resemble humans in certain respects, and the human recipients receive drugs to suppress their immune response, potentially paving the way for so-called xenozoonoses: infectious diseases from other species. This concern informs various international laws and regulations regarding xenotransplantation, which range from mandating protective measures for the clinical use of xenotransplantation to temporary bans on its clinical use (Schicktanz 2018). Given these major obstacles, xenotransplantation research is still in an experimental stage.

Nevertheless, some researchers expect new technological developments to bring clinical trials closer. In 2017, US scientists succeeded in removing porcine retroviruses from the genome of pigs by using CRISPR and CAS9 technologies (Niu et al. 2017). Porcine retroviruses are considered particularly dangerous because they have been shown to infect human cells in vitro. If they found their way into humans via transplants, they could not only infect the organ recipients but also spread to other people, and in the worst-case scenario they could cause dangerous new pandemics. Therefore, removing the retroviruses counts as an important achievement. Furthermore, researchers are now able to knock out the pigs' growth hormones, thus allowing them to farm smaller pigs with more human-sized hearts. Furthermore, these pigs are genetically modified to produce a human protein, and to lack a porcine enzyme. Such modifications are meant to prevent the human immune system from destroying the transplanted organ. In addition, the genetically modified pigs in Munich now produce a further protein, which prevents blood clotting in the transplant. These new technological possibilities make clinical trials more likely to happen and have sparked renewed interest in the relevant ethical issues (Wünsch et al. 2014, Mohiuddin et al. 2016, Kemter et al. 2017).

3. Ethics

The ethics of xenotransplantation have been discussed in politics, society and academia for more than a decade (Bartholomew/Auchincloss 1998; Quante/Vieth 2001; Schicktanz 2002; McLean/Williamson 2005). The question at the center of this discussion is whether xenotransplantation research should continue. Some of the arguments put forward in this debate are narrowly anthropocentric (i.e. human-centered), holding that humans should be the sole objects of our moral concern. Accordingly, such arguments typically address the harms and benefits of the technology for humans. In contrast, other arguments are premised on a wider, sentientist perspective, according to which all sentient individuals deserve our moral consideration, and therefore it also matters how the technology affects sentient *non-humans*.

3.1   Harms and Benefits for Humans

Moral theories seek to determine what is morally right or wrong and why this is so. These theories can be divided into consequentialist and non-consequentialist, or 'teleological' and 'deontological', theories. The former evaluate actions *only* on the basis of their consequences, whereas the latter do not, or at least do not *only*, consider consequences. Arguments that evaluate the significance of xenotransplantation for humans typically focus on consequences of the technology. This is not to say that only consequentialists can or do embrace these arguments; even those who hold that other considerations are ethically relevant *in principle* may concede that the potential harms and benefits of this technology should play a major role in its evaluation.

If we are to assess the harms and benefits of xenotransplantation research for humans, we must compare it with alternatives. After all, 'harm' and 'benefit' are comparative notions. By definition, an event benefits me if and only if it leads me to be better off than I would otherwise have been; conversely, an event harms me if and only if it leads me to be worse off than I would otherwise have been. This is the standard, counterfactual account of harm and benefit.

In debates about xenotransplantation it is typically assumed that transplant recipients, and less directly their friends and families, would benefit from the technology. But whether the recipients can be said to benefit depends on how receiving the transplant compares with the counterfactual scenario. If the transplant granted them additional years of life when they would have otherwise died, the transplant benefited them. How great a benefit this was would depend on the quality of the transplants. It also would depend on other factors. For example, transplant recipients might be forced to live with unusual restrictions on their privacy due to being subjected to measures designed to prevent the spread of infectious diseases. They might even have to register their interactions with other people. The restrictiveness of these measures would depend on the remaining risk of zoonoses. The overall benefit to the transplant recipients would also depend on how many people received xenografts. Finally, the extent of the benefit (or harm) would depend on the exact nature of the counterfactual situation. Would people that received a xenograft have otherwise received an allograft? Or would they have died? Since we currently do not know these facts, it is unclear and controversial what the benefits of xenotransplantation would be. (This suggests topics for fur further empirical research, but also for ethical exploration. For example, there isn't much debate in ethics yet about how pig organs should be allocated after the phase of clinical tests.)

One might also wonder to what extent certain pharmaceutical companies or scientists would benefit from advancing xenotransplantation. It is easy to imagine that companies could profit greatly, not least from selling immunosuppressive drugs. And scientists might have a range of motivations for becoming involved in xenotransplantation research. However, these potential benefits do not do much to justify the technology. If the technology could not be independently justified, the fact that some people earned fame or money through it would not make it any more acceptable. On the contrary, it would cast a negative light on those who profited from it.

Promotion campaigns for organ transplantation commonly depict stories of patients whose lives have been prolonged by the technology. These benefits are undeniably relevant. However, such campaigns do not show what benefits might have accrued from spending the same amount of money differently. For example, many diseases could be prevented or cured much more cost-effectively. That is, spending money on transplantation technology has so-called opportunity costs. This gives some indication of the harm caused by the technology: based on the counterfactual account of benefit and harm, the technology is harmful insofar as it consumes resources that could otherwise have provided more benefit to individuals. In times of scarce resources and pressing unmet needs, these opportunity costs are morally significant.

There are other potential harms to consider if xenotransplanations were actually performed on human patients. As already mentioned, viruses could infect transplant recipients and cause new pandemics, although new technological developments are supposed to reduce the likelihood of this scenario. This raises the general question of how to account for risks that have a very low probability but very high stakes. How cautious can we and should we be, and when, if ever, is it acceptable to take such a risk? Should we act according to the precautionary principle, or according to some other principle? A relevant example is how to reduce the risks of zoonoses. For example, it has been argued that trials with humans are unavoidable in the development of xenotransplantation, but that allowing test subjects to interact with other people would be too risky. Therefore, it has been suggested that the bodies of people in a permanent vegetative state could be used for this kind of research, assuming the prior consent of these body-donors (Ravelingen et al. 2004). Others have argued that various safety measures are required before such risks could be taken (Rothblatt 2004). In any case, in medical ethics, the principle of patient autonomy is central, therefore it can be expected that there will be no trials on human subjects without their prior consent. Furthermore, clinical trials are typically performed only on patients who have a real chance of benefiting from the experimental treatment. They receive the experimental treatment in cases in which no other treatment is available that is at least as good as the experimental treatment. This latter condition would not be fulfilled if one used the bodies of body-donors. But arguably this can be justified, given that they consented and that (arguably) no harm can be done to them anymore.

Some authors also conceive of risks related to blurring the boundaries, as it were, between humans and non-humans. The species concept is controversial, as is talk of 'boundaries' in this context. Nevertheless, some authors fear negative effects on the self-conception of organ recipients, and they are also concerned about uncertainty regarding the moral status of the resulting animal-human chimeras, such as the genetically modified pigs that produce human proteins or the humans with porcine organs. The status of these beings is of concern in human-centric approaches, but less so from a sentientist perspective. After all, this perspective holds that sentience, not species membership, determines an individual's moral status.

3.2 Harms and Benefits for Non-Humans

According to the sentientist position, the boundaries of the moral community – those individuals who deserve moral consideration – do not follow species boundaries. Instead, all and only sentient individuals can have interests, such as the interest in not suffering. In other words, all and only sentient beings are subjects of wellbeing. Animal ethicists have argued that discounting the interests (that is the wellbeing) of non-humans just because they belong to another species than we do, is speciesist. Speciesism, according to these authors, is a form of wrongful discrimination, akin to sexism and racism. This is not to say that it is never justified to sacrifice some individuals for the greater good. Whether or not this is ever justified is a perennial debate in ethics. But the fact that we would not be willing to cause the same amount of harm to humans as we do to non-humans has been criticized as being incompatible with the principle of equal consideration of interests (Singer 1975).

In the course of xenotransplantation research, large numbers of non-human animals are harmed due to the way in which they are housed and treated. These animals suffer from inadequate housing conditions that induce behavioral abnormities, anxiety, stress and pain. Furthermore, these animals are ultimately deprived of living full lives, for example when they die due to housing conditions or are killed during experiments. Most must live their brief lives in a laboratory, subjected to invasive and deadly research. For example, experiments undertaken at the University of Munich, Germany, include the following:

1. The hearts of six genetically modified pigs were transplanted into baboons. The baboons received immunosuppressive drugs. A special camera observed the blood vessels in the mucous membrane under their tongue. All the monkeys died between five hours and four days due to organ rejection or heart failure.
2. Two baboons received the hearts of two non-transgene pigs in addition to their own hearts, resulting in a hyper-acute rejection of the new organs. The transplanted hearts swelled up and the animals were killed.
3. In order to study damage caused to transplanted organs, the arms and legs of 19 unconscious monkeys were bound. All blood was removed from their arms and legs and replaced with human blood. The blood vessels in their muscles were observed under microscope. Finally, the monkeys were killed.
4. The hearts of four genetically modified pigs were transplanted into the bellies of baboons. The baboons received immunosuppressive drugs. The transplanted organs swelled to twice their original size and were rejected within two to eight days. The report does not specify whether the monkeys died or were killed (Gericke 2014).

No official numbers exist, but it is estimated that more than a thousand primates have been used for xenotransplantation research of this kind over the past 20 years, particularly in Europe, North America, and Russia (Schicktanz 2018).

Does it make a moral difference whether pigs or primates are used as organ sources? We already saw that there are practical reasons for using pigs. But from an ethical perspective one can ask whether using pigs rather than primates can be justified, and if so, how. If one only considers human interests, the mere fact that humans prefer pigs as organ sources would favor this choice. After all, if only human interests are considered, and if those are better served by using pigs, then this is considered the better option. However, from a sentientist perspective the issue is more complicated. If being used as an organ source harmed non-human primates more than pigs, this could justify the use of pigs according to a sentientist view. It may well be the case that the conditions of breeding, confinement, handling and so on are more harmful for primates than they are for pigs, in the sense that more of the primate's needs would be frustrated under such circumstances. If this were the case, it would count in favor of using pigs above primates. (One could argue that primates would be treated better than pigs, because breeding primates would be more expensive. But I think in both cases ensuring a sufficient quality of the organ is not the same as ensuring a good quality of life for the animal in question.)

Some authors have argued that apes and perhaps also monkeys have a higher moral status than pigs and should therefore not be used. This position is incompatible with sentientism, which grants all sentient animals an *equal moral status*. Here, it is important to distinguish between two claims: that harm to primates matters more than harm to pigs, even if it is the same amount of harm; and that harm to both matters equally, but, due to different interests, an intervention may be more harmful to one species than it is to another. Only the latter consideration is compatible with the principle of equal consideration of interests.

It has been argued that death is more harmful for individuals that have plans for the future. According to such a position, death may be a greater harm for primates, assuming that primates tend to have more plans than pigs (Singer 2011). According to an alternative and more prominent view, though, the harm caused by death is not the frustration of desires but the deprivation of value, i.e. the amount of future welfare that it takes away from the individual (Bradley 2009). According to this view, if the individual would otherwise have had a pleasant future, death is harmful regardless of whether the individual had any plans or desires. Given that a chimpanzee's natural lifespan is about twice that of a pig, if both animals were killed at the same age, the chimp would probably lose more than the pig because he would have otherwise lived longer. According to this deprivation view, even individuals that live entirely in the present – such as human babies, small children, certain mentally disabled humans, and certain non-humans – can be harmed by death. Thus, whether death is a lesser harm for pigs than for primates depends on empirical facts about their capacities, the relevant counterfactuals, and the correct theory about the harm of death.

4.   Moral Rights

When evaluating actions, many ethicists consider not only harms and benefits for individuals but also their moral rights. In general, moral rights function as constraints on what can rightfully be done to someone. For example, people often appeal to the moral right to life in order to argue that it would be wrong to kill a person, even if this allowed us to use her organs to save three lives. Moral rights are often seen as protections of the individual's basic interests. This includes sentient non-human animals, which also have interests. For example, all sentient beings have the interest not to be in pain. We already saw that it would be discriminatory to neglect or discount this interest just because the being in question belongs to a different species. So, non-human animals are considered subjects of rights, and these rights form constraints as to what can justifiably be done to them. The notion of 'animal rights' refers to the rights of sentient non-humans.

Of course, it is not necessarily a rights violation if one suffers due to someone else's actions. But authors who accept moral rights would argue that if someone kicked me in the face simply to hurt me, or killed me in order to harvest my organs, they would be violating my right to bodily integrity. There is no principled reason why sentient non-humans should not have similar rights. And if they have such rights, xenotransplantation and related research is at least prima facie wrong.

In special circumstances, one may have to choose between two unavoidable rights violations. If we had to choose between the death of a pig (for xenotransplantation purposes) and the death of a human (due to organ failure), wouldn't the death of the pig be the lesser evil? If both had a right to life, what would be the right thing to do? Those who appeal to moral rights broadly agree that xenotransplantation is not an example of a so-called lifeboat case. In lifeboat cases, one individual must be thrown overboard to save the other passengers because the boat is too full to carry them all – the question is who this unlucky person should be. But in the case of xenotransplantation, the pig is not in any danger *until we put it there*. Thus, rights views typically hold that xenotransplantation is unacceptable. A right to life, after all, does not entail that others have the duty to save one's life under all circumstances. Rather, it normally entails protection from being killed (Pluhar 1995).

Rights views assume that there is a morally relevant distinction between doing and allowing harm. For example, killing is usually considered a rights violation, including killing another person in order to harvest her organs to save three others. Letting someone die is usually not a rights violation, as in the case of letting a patient die on the waiting list for a transplant. This raises the question of why there should be a right not to be killed but not a right to be saved. One possible explanation is that rights are justified claims on others, and in order for such a claim to be justified, it shouldn't demand too much. It is generally much less demanding for others to refrain from killing than it is for them to save lives. In general, if I require from others that they do not kill me, I leave them free to choose what else to do. If, instead, I require from them to save my life, this may leave them with only one option. According to this view, there is a moral duty to save a life only in exceptional cases in which doing so would not be overly demanding.

Those who accept rights views need to specify the exact rights possessed by a rightsholder. Here, knowledge of the basis of moral rights is helpful. Some authors base rights on interests, i.e. on wellbeing. If rights should protect wellbeing, this already suggests what rights an individual should have: for example, a right to life and to bodily integrity. Other authors ground rights on some form of inherent value. In that view, rights are meant to safeguard an individual's autonomy or even dignity. It has been argued that regarding sentient beings as mere means (or close to mere means) is morally wrong. Along these lines, one can ask whether animal research in general, and genetic modification of animals in particular, entails regarding these animals as mere means (Parfit 2012: 212–233).

It has been argued that for those who accept moral rights, accepting rights for all sentient animals should be a matter of consistency. After all, what could possibly justify accepting moral rights for all humans but not for any non-human? For all plausible grounds for moral rights, it holds that either not *all* humans qualify for rights or that *some* non-humans qualify as well. For example, if only moral agents (i.e. those who can act on the basis of moral principles) possessed moral rights, non-human animals would be excluded, but so too would be human babies, severely mentally disabled humans, and Alzheimer's patients. Thus, those who want to grant special protection to humans but not to non-humans have to face the so-called argument from marginal cases: the relevant capacities are not divided neatly along species boundaries. It is hard to justify that individuals should be treated based on characteristics that are common for members of their group (for example their species) but which they themselves do not possess (Norcross 2004).

Rights views, i.e. moral theories that appeal to moral rights, are typically non-consequentialist. For example, Tom Regan argues that sentient animals (above one year of age) are rights holders because they have a good of their own (Regan 2004). In a similar but more elaborated way, Christine Korsgaard (2016) defends animal rights on what she takes to be a Kantian basis. Those authors, just like others who argue that animals have moral rights, are also passionate defenders of *legal* rights for animals, such as the right not to be killed or injured. Garry Francione (2000) grounds his animal rights theory on the claim that animals have the right not to be property. Those who hold that rights should protect interests are not convinced by Francione's arguments, since they hold that animals do not have an interest in not being property, although they do have an interest in freedom from pain and in continued life. This is because these things promote the animal's welfare, but whether or not an animal is someone's legal property can only *indirectly* influence the animal's wellbeing. Changing its property status is something that could have positive effects on animal welfare, but it is not something that matters to the animals themselves (Cochrane 2012).

A *consequentialist* defender of moral rights, Chris Woodard (2019), recently argued that consequentialists should care not only about determining individual acts that have the best consequences but also about practices that are beneficial if enough people participate in them, such as respecting animal rights. This claim is based on the plausible empirical assumption that respecting animal rights *generally* has positive consequences, even if it may not have the best consequences in every individual case. According to this view, an animal's moral right to life is itself enough reason for someone to refrain from participating in an action that would lead to an animal's death.

Rule consequentialism, a sub-variety of consequentialism, may not accept the a priori existence of moral rights, but it may accept rules that forbid killing innocent individuals, or similar. According to rule consequentialism, an action is right just in case it conforms to the set of rules that, if endorsed by (nearly) everyone, would have the best consequences (Hooker 2002). Such a set of rules could conceivably contain the rule not to perform invasive experiments on non-consenting sentient beings, or the rule not to kill.

Most consequentialists do not accept *moral* rights, but they typically favor *legal* rights for sentient beings. If accepting legal rights has better long-term consequences than not doing so, consequentialism requires that we respect those rights. Thus, it might lead to better overall consequences in the long run not to assess animal experiments on a case-by-case basis but to forbid them across the board in the name of animal rights. Similarly, when classical utilitarians argued against discrimination against women and against slavery, they favored fundamental legal reforms. They did not argue that one should assess on a case-by-case basis whether some instance of slavery did more good than harm. Along these lines, even classical act-consequentialists could argue in favor of legal rights for animals.

Sue Donaldson and Will Kymlicka's (2011) book *Zoopolis* strongly influenced the recent discussion of animal rights in the field of Political Theory. Donaldson and Kymlicka accept that animals have moral rights and, based on this, they spell out which legal rights animals should have. The authors divide sentient animals into three political categories: citizens, denizens, and sovereigns. Legal rights and duties, they argue, should be accorded on this basis, as they are among humans, who all have the same fundamental human rights but also have more specific rights based on membership in one of the three political categories. Thus, just like former slaves, domesticated animals should be accorded citizen status, a move which would be incompatible with using them as a source of organs. A common objection to this argument is that pigs cannot be citizens because it makes no sense to give them the right to vote in elections. However, certain mentally disabled humans count as citizens even though they do not have the right or capacity to vote in elections.

One might object that, given that we routinely kill many pigs and other animals for food, xenotransplantation research cannot be wrong. Nearly no one needs meat, dairy or eggs to survive, or even to stay healthy, yet we routinely harm and kill large numbers of animals for these products. How could it then be wrong to harm and kill a relatively small number of non-humans in order to save human lives? But the mere fact that we harm and kill countless animals for food does not mean that it is morally justified. A sentientist position asks us to reconsider both novel and more traditional forms of animal use.

5.   Conclusion

New technological developments are spurring renewed interest in the ethics of xenotransplantation. But is continued research into xenotransplantation justified? The ethical debate about xenotransplantation features two main lines of argumentation: anthropocentric and sentientist. The former focuses on harms and benefits for humans. The main benefits of continued xenotransplantation research are the potential improvements to the welfare of organ recipients and their loved ones. The extent of this benefit is still unclear, since it depends on the quality of the organs and on the required public safety measures, among other things. The main costs are the opportunity costs: the lost benefits that would have occurred if scarce health care resources had been invested in other, more cost-effective, projects. Other costs include the various risks of the technology for humans, most importantly the risk of zoonoses. By contrast, sentientist arguments consider the interests of all sentient beings on an equal basis. These arguments allow for animal rights, which are meant to protect animal interests and function as constraints against killing and injuring animals for research purposes or as organ sources.

Is xenotransplantation acceptable from a sentientist position? From a sentientist position that grants moral rights to non-human animals, xenotransplantation is clearly unacceptable. A sentientist position that is not based on moral rights would still be likely to accord legal rights to animals, which would also be incompatible with xenotransplantation. At the very least, according to a sentientist position, the welfare of non-human sentient beings would be taken as seriously as that of humans. Whether such a non-speciesist principle of equal consideration would be compatible with xenotransplantation depends on what the consequences of all available options would be for the wellbeing of all concerned individuals.

References

Bartholomew, Amelia/Auchincloss, Hugh (1998): "Xenotransplantaton." In: Peter J. Delves (ed.), Encyclopedia of Immunology, 2nd edition, Amsterdam: Elsevier, pp. 2508–2512.

Bradley, Ben (2009): Well-Being and Death, New York: Oxford University Press.

Cochrane, Alasdair (2012): Animal Rights Without Liberation, New York: Columbia University Press.

Cooper, David K.C./Wagner, Robert (2012): "Xenotransplantation." In: Christian Abee/ Keith Mansfield/Suzette Tardif/Timothy Morris (eds.), Nonhuman Primates in Biomedical Research, 2nd edition, Amsterdam: Elsevier, pp. 391–402.

Donaldson, Sue/Kymlicka, Will (2011): Zoopolis: A Political Theory of Animal Rights, Oxford: Oxford University Press.

Francione, Garry (2000): Introduction to Animal Rights. Your Child or the Dog, Philadelphia: Temple University Press.

Gericke, Corina (2014): "Stellungnahme zu Xenotransplantation." Available at: https:// www.aerzte-gegen   tierversuche.de/de/projekte/stellungnahmen/1151-stellung-nahme-zu-xenotransplantation (accessed January 23, 2020)

Gianello, Pierre (2014): "Xenotransplantation: Past, Present, and Future." In: Giuseppe Orlando/Jan Lerut/Shay Soker/Robert J. Stratta (eds.), Regenerative Medicine Applications in Organ Transplantation, pp. 953–968.

Hooker, Brad (2002): Ideal Code, Real World, New York: Oxford University Press.

Kemter, Elisabeth/Cohrs, Christian M./Schäfer, Matthias/Schuster, Marion/Stein-meyer, Klaus/Wolf-van Buerck, Lelia/Wolf, Andrea/Wuensch, Annegret/Kurome, Mayuko/Kessler, Barbara/Zkhartchenko, Valeri/Loehn, Matthias/Ivashchenko, Yuri/Seissler, Jochen/Schulte, Anke M./Speier, Stephan/Wolf, Eckard (2017): "INS-eGFP Transgenic Pigs: a Novel Reporter System for Studying Maturation, Growth and Vascularization of Neonatal Islet-Like Cell Clusters". In: Diabetologia 60/6, pp. 1152–1156.

Korsgaard, Christine M. (2016): "A Kantian Case for Animal Rights". In: Tatjana Višak/ Robert Garner (eds.), The Ethics of Killing Animals, New York: Oxford University Press.

Mc Lean, Sheila/Williamson, Laura (2005): Xenotransplantation: Law And Ethics, Aldershote: Ashgate.

Mohiuddin, Muhammad M./Singh, Avneesh K./Corcoran, Philip C./Thomas, Marvin L./ Clark, Tannia/Lewis, Billeta G./Hoyt, Robert F./Eckhaus, Michael/Pierson, Richard N./Belli, Aaron J./Wolf, Eckhard/Klymiuk, Nikolai/Phelps, Carol/ Reimann, Keith A./Ayares, David, Horvath, Keith A. (2016): "Chimeric 2C10R4 Anti-CD40 Antibody Therapy is Critical for Long-Term Survival of GTKO.hCD46. hTBM Pig-to-Primate Cardiac Xenograft". In: Nature Communications 5/7, 11138. DOI: 10.1038/ncomms11138

Niu, Dong/Wei, Hong-Jiang/Lin, Lin/George, Haydy/Wang, Tao/Lee, I-Hsiu/Zhao, Hong-Ye/ Wang, Yong/Kan, Yinan/Shrock, Ellen/Lesha, Emal/Wang, Gang/Luo, Yonglun/Qing, Yubo/ Jiao, Deling/Zhao, Heng/Zhou, Xiaoyang/Wang, Shouqi/Wei, Hong/Güell, Marc/Church, George M./Yang, Luhan (2017): "Inactivation of Porcine Endogenous Retrovirus in Pigs Using CRISPR and CAS9." In: Science 357/6357, pp. 1303–1307.

Norcross, Alasdair (2002): "Puppies, Pigs and People: Eating Meat and Marginal Cases". In: Philosophical Perspectives, 18/1, pp. 229–245.

Parfit, Derek (2012): On What Matters, New York: Oxford University Press.

Pluhar, Evelyn (1995): Beyond Prejudice. The Moral Significance of Human and Non-Human Animals, London: Duke University Press.

Quante, Michael/Vieth, Andreas (2001): Xenotransplantation. Ethische und rechtliche Probleme, Paderborn: Mentis.

Ravelingien, An/Mortier, Freddy/Mortier, Eric/Kerremans, Ilse/Braeckman, Johan (2004): "Proceeding with Clinical Trials of Animal to Human Organ Transplantation: a Way out of the Dilemma." In: Journal of Medical Ethics 30, pp. 92–98.

Regan, Tom (2004): The Case for Animal Rights, Berkeley: University of California Press.

Rothblatt, M. (2004): Your Life or Mine: how Geoethics can Resolve the Conflict between Public and Private Interests in Xenotransplantation, Aldershot: Ashgate.

Schicktanz, Silke (2002): Organlieferant Tier? Medizin- und tierethische Probleme der Xenotransplantation, Frankfurt: Campus.

Schicktanz, Silke (2018): "Xenotransplantation." In: Johann Ach/Dagmar Borchers (eds.), Handbuch Tierethik, Stuttgart: Metzler.

Singer, Peter (2011): Practical Ethics, 3rd edition, New York: Cambridge University Press.

Singer, Peter (1975): Animal Liberation, New York: Random House.

Steeger, G. (2019). "Ein Herz für Uns?" In: Die Zeit 25, pp.

Woodard, Christopher (2019): Taking Utilitarianism Seriously, Oxford: Oxford University Press.

Wünsch, Annegret/Baehr, Andrea/ Bongoni, Anjan K./Kemter, Elisabeth/Blutke, Andreas/ Baars, Wiebke/Haertle, Sonja/ Zakhartchenko, Valeri/Kurome, Mayoko/ Kessler, Barbara/ Faber, Claudius/Abicht, Jan-Michael/Reichart, Bruno/Wanke, Ruediger/ Schwinzer, Reinhard/Nagshima, Hiroshi/Rieben, Robert/Ayares, David/Wolf, Eckhard/Klymiuk, Nikolai (2014): "Regulatory Sequences of the Porcine THBD Gene Facilitate Endothelial-Specific Expression of Bioactive Human Thrombomodulin in Single- and Multitransgenic Pigs." In: Transplantation 97/2, pp. 138–147.

17. Envisioning 3D Bioprinting
Scenarios of Organs 'on Demand'

Charlotte Burnham-Stevens & Niki Vermeulen

1. Introduction

The oft-cited game-changing potential of 3D bioprinting in transplantation medicine tends to focus on its promissory power – its capability to 'solve' several key problems associated with traditional organ transplantation and revolutionize modern medicine. Whilst the nascent technology could indeed have some clear benefits, it also brings social and ethical issues regarding its embedding in health care systems, including regulation, ownership and access. Organs become exchangeable alienable objects, subject to the market forces of supply and demand. Thereby, organ bioprinting may risk further commodification of our bodies, increase existing health inequalities, while heightening expectations and desires for 'ideal health'.

In the context of emerging ethical debates on bioprinting, this chapter combines bioethics with insights from Science and Technology Studies (STS) to explore some of these issues further. Building on current ethical and legal scholarship, we are particularly interested in questions regarding ownership of bioprinted organs, e.g. who would be entitled to a bioprinted organ, whether they could be sold, and issues of liability. As real-life examples are not yet available, we use hypothetical narratives as heuristics for thinking through emerging ethical and regulatory issues, in order to provoke questions and stimulate debate. We will argue that the ways bioprinted organs become classified for legal, regulatory and economic purposes has important implications, and must be dealt with as part of the technology's further development and potential use in health care.

2. Bioprinting: Process and Overview

2.1 3D Bioprinting 101

Bioprinting, also referred to as additive manufacturing (Murphy/Atala 2014), or biofabrication (Groll et al. 2016), involves the three-dimensional printing of biological materials: printing living human cells into desired patterns and structures. The field has widely been described as 'coming of age' (Guillemot et al. 2010), incorporating regenerative medicine and tissue engineering (Mironov et al. 2011, 2003). At present, technical capabilities only allow for printing smaller tissues, but there are hopes and expectations that scientists will one day be able to bioprint whole functioning organs. The process involves "layer by layer precise positioning of biological materials, bio-chemicals and living cells" to produce functional 3D structures (Murphy/Atala 2014: 773). An essential component of the bioprinting process is bioink (Gungor-Ozkerim et al. 2018), which contains a mixture of living cells and a form of 'hydrogel' (usually made from natural polymers which can be broken down once inside the body). Research-ers are exploring a number of different approaches for the production of these tissues, and a variety of different printers, bioinks, cell types, and modelling software.

At present, two likely options exist for the types of cells used in bioprinting: dif-ferentiated primary cells (heart cells, lung cells, liver cells), or autologous Induced Pluripotent Stem Cells (IPSCs) (Murphy/Atala 2014).[1] The idea is that cells would come from the patient who is to receive the bioprinted organ. IPSCs are deemed the most promising, because they can be derived from adult cells but are still able to reproduce and develop into almost any type of cell. The bioprinting process as applied in a clinical setting would likely involve the following basic steps:

1. A physician takes a cell sample, likely in the form of a biopsy; or this may be a simple skin-scraping
2. The cells are cultured in a laboratory to produce IPSCs and reproduced and com-bined with other biomaterials to form the bioink
3. 3D images are taken of the organ (MRI, CT scan etc.) and any faults corrected using modelling software
4. The printer is programmed to print the bioink in layers into the organ structure, based on the model provided
5. Possibly, the bioprinted organ is matured for a period of time in a 'bioreactor' before surgical implantation into the patient.

Whilst this process is based on the current discussions of the state of the art, it is a simplified version, still hypothetical, and subject to change. It cannot be emphasized enough that significant technical barriers remain: keeping the cells alive post-printing, vascularization of the organ, timing the scaffold degradation, and scalability of the printing process and the materials – to name but a few (Murphy/Atala 2014). These technical barriers must be overcome before 'on demand' organ printing can be realized, if indeed it ever will be.

2.2   Framing Ethical Issues

Because the potential development of bioprinted organs is not only a technical issue, it is important to think proactively about the social and ethical aspects of this technology, including the embedding of bioprinting in health care practices. The expectations of 3D

---

1   This chapter focusses specifically on IPSCs and not hiPSCs (heterologous induced pluripotent stem cells – taken from cell banks or donors), as their use would not remove the risk of rejection (which is one of the leading causes of transplant failure). However, we acknowledge that there are a number of ethical issues associated with using hiPSCs in bioprinting.

bioprinting are high, and among the numerous benefits cited are its potential to revolutionize the medical industry by removing the need for organ donation (Lewis 2017;
Williams 2014; Savage 2017). 3D bioprinting, it is claimed, will eliminate a number of
ethical issues around difficulties in sourcing (youth) organs, black-market organ sales,
and the many issues associated with xenotransplantation and animal testing. However, the science and research being conducted in 3D bioprinting is still very speculative, and as Gilbert et al. (2017) have highlighted, the overly positive and promissory
media narratives of the technology create ethical implications of their own, especially
for patients who need organ replacement. Against this background, we explore some
of the ethical issues and potential risks of bioprinting, not aiming to be exhaustive or
complete but rather to stimulate discussion.

In an earlier article, Vermeulen and colleagues (2017) provide a horizon scan of
ethical issues, including expectations, safety, social stratification, and ownership.
Because the technological capabilities for bioprinting are still relatively novel, scientists are unable to provide realistic development timeframes, which means that public
and patients' expectations need to be managed. With regards to safety, the significant
risks and likely irreversibility of transplanting living IPSCs into humans are still insufficiently tested, and no significant long-term studies exist to date. The issue of social
stratification (see also Kass 2012; Squier/Waldby 2005) is becoming increasingly prevalent because increasing reliance on complex and expensive health solutions means
that they are often only available to a privileged few.

Bioprinting presents new legal challenges regarding the ownership of biological
materials, and how we categorize them may have a significant impact on future users/
patients. Other issues, such as those relating to intellectual property (Li 2014; Li et al.
2017), are also paramount because they are associated with different stages of the bioprinting process. Intellectual property issues extend to the software, hardware and
biomaterials used, as well as access/ownership of the data used in the bioprinting process, and whether aspects of bioprinting could be patented. Finally, it is possible that
the technology could be used for human enhancement, not just repair. The potential
for humans to bioprint body parts with greater abilities raises a whole other raft of
ethical issues (Boucher 2018).

Consequently, the idea of organ printing 'on demand' presents risks because
organs are seen as 'spare parts' rather than essential components of peoples' bodies; they become exchangeable alienable objects, subject to the market forces of supply and demand. Thus framed, biotechnological knowledge and innovation coincide
with the creation of a paradigm in which every human health problem can be fixed or
influenced. Grunwald (2007) calls this shift an increased contingency in the 'conditio
humana', which highlights the need to rethink the rules and regulations by which we
currently govern our health care practices. Bioprinting risks further commodifying
our bodies and heightens the desire for 'ideal health'. Other qualms include the deval-
uation of the human body and undermining the developing health paradigms of bodily
self-care and disease prevention; what incentive is there to take care of the body you
have if you can just print a new one?

The current uncertain and ambiguous status of the bioprinted organ, epistemologically, physically and legally, creates further issues and exacerbates some of the risks
and ethical considerations mentioned above. A fundamental question that must first
be asked is – what *is* a bioprinted organ? A bioprinted organ would be simultaneously

alive, not alive and capable of giving life; it would be natural *and* artificial, separate *and* embodied, human *and* thing. It is a "boundary crawler" which disrupts the "conventional boundaries and identities of biological forms and categories [...] sitting ambiguously in between those entities that we tend to conceptualize as human subjects and as non-human objects" (Metzler/Webster 2011: 649). It is therefore not clear what form of categorization we are using when we talk about bioprinted organs.

A bioprinted organ could be understood through the lens of 'bio-objects' (Vermeulen et al. 2012; Tamminen/Vermeulen 2019). The common theme in the bio-objectification process involves transforming biological material to produce data or materials that are intentionally different or ideologically separated from the original thing. This lens assists epistemologically and shows how the problem of classifying bioprinted organs makes it difficult to fit them into current regulatory frameworks. Determining how a bioprinted organ is classified will determine its regulation, its legal status and, to an extent, the ethical issues it raises. This becomes particularly clear in discussions of the ownership of bioprinted organs – e.g. how to deal with testing and liability – and of data protection and counterfeiting.

Whilst from an ethical perspective our theoretical approach may be viewed as an account of justice – and much of our analysis could be understood through a justice lens – we do not write as bioethicists but as social scientists. Our methods simply aim to open up questions for debate, using hypothetical scenarios as a way to initiate discussions.

2.3   Using Hypothetical Scenarios

Many traditional science and technology studies (STS) methods and frameworks prove rather difficult to apply to future technologies that are still under development, such as bioprinting. STS often focuses on the here and now: studying laboratories, workshops, companies and publics, with scientists, engineers and users. When discussing emergent technologies, we need conceptual tools that allow us to conceptualize what is to come (Stilgoe et al. 2013). Consequently, we have chosen to combine methods from bioethics and innovation studies to create hypothetical scenarios, which we will then use as a starting point for focused discussion of the regulation of bioprinted organs in health care practices.

Foresight practices are tools that are increasingly used in business and policy-making (see Popper 2008). Two main foresight tools are horizon scanning and scenario planning, which are best used in conjunction to obtain both breadth and depth (Rowe et al. 2017). Horizon scanning presents a brief account of a broad range of issues, using creative processes designed to alert relevant parties (Amanatidou et al. 2012; Van Rij 2010). In contrast, scenario planning tends to focus on one issue and examine it in great depth (Wilkinson 2009). A related practice that is often relied on in bioethics are 'thought experiments' and 'what if' scenarios (Hedgecoe 2004; Swierstra et al. 2009). A well-known example of this was Thomson's (1971) thought experiment regarding a famous violinist being plugged into a woman's body to use her organs, as a means of illustrating and exploring notions of bodily rights. However, principlist bioethical arguments have been criticized by bioethicists and social scientists for their over-reliance on abstraction; the arguments are based on moral principles that do not necessarily reflect the social and medical realities of everyday practice (Hedgecoe 2004;

Petersen 2013; Keulartz et al. 2004; Smits 2006). However, that is not to say that these thought experiments cannot still be extremely useful, as is also shown in the STOA report presenting bioprinting to European policymakers (Boucher 2018).

Our study draws upon a more pragmatist version of scenarios, presenting short narratives that are grounded in the social realities of our existing world and within the context of a particular setting, focusing predominantly on UK and US perspectives. We have devised three narratives/scenarios which can be used as heuristics for stimulating thinking, analysis and debate about the issues associated with bioprinting. We find that the use of stories can be particularly helpful in situations like this, where real-life examples are not yet possible. The 'hypothetical' signifies this speculative character, while we use scenarios that are especially designed to raise questions, provoke discussion, and engage readers and audiences.

3.   Exploring the Legal Landscape

During the preparation stages for your heart transplant, the hospital bioprints two hearts from your tissue – a contingency should there be surgical complications (damage or error to the first replacement heart). This is common practice because widespread use of 3D bioprinted hearts for transplantation is reasonably new. The operation goes smoothly; you now have a bioprinted heart in place of your old one. What happens to the spare bioprinted heart? Do you have rights over it? If the hospital were to damage or lose it, would you have recourse to get it back?

Investing property rights in human beings is one of the most contentious issues amongst bioethicists and legal scholars, because of its close alignment with commodification of the human body. This debate is inherently bound up with how 3D bioprinted organs will be treated from both regulatory and commercial perspectives – as (parts of) a human, or as something else? Understanding the nature of bioprinted organs can be both useful and necessary to figure out how to classify them. Until they are classified, it would be extremely difficult to determine how to regulate, and what rights to attach to, bioprinted organs. The above scenario provides us with a means to explore notions of ownership over human biomaterials. What must be determined here is who owns the actual organ – not the printer or the rights to the software, but the tangible, material *thing*.

Bioethicist Leon Kass points out that we can, do and should "distinguish among that which is *me*, that which is *mine*, and that which is mine as *my property*" (2002: 190). Although this distinction may seem obvious, it is in fact not so clear-cut as a result of emerging biotechnologies. My bioprinted heart is 'me' in the sense that it is literally made from my own cells; but, whilst the bioprinted heart that resides inside my body is undoubtedly "mine", can it (and the spare heart) be understood as "my property"? Quigley (2014: 692) asserts that one of the distinctive characteristics of property is that the owner has a right to exclude it from others, or in other words 'if I own a particular item, you (and everyone else) are under a *prima facie* duty not to interfere with my use of it'. This distinction is fairly self-evident for the bioprinted heart that has been transplanted, as most would agree that everyone is under a duty not to physically interfere with my use of my heart. But what about the spare?

In the UK context, the *Human Tissue Act* 2004 governs the use, retrieval, storage and disposal of human biomaterials. The Act also prohibits any commercial dealings for transplant purposes; however, biomaterials such as cells and tissues that are not removed for the purposes of transplant are not governed by this prohibition (ibid.: 679). This means that third parties, usually researchers or biotechnology companies, are legally permitted to sell tissues and cells, although "the individuals who are the source of those biomaterials cannot" (ibid). This double standard has already been pointed out (Kass 2004; Rostill 2014) because it appears that we *do* allow commercial ownership and trading of human tissues by third parties, we just deny those rights to the original owner. Legal possession of body parts, even by third parties, can be understood as a type of "transient guardianship" (Lucassen/Wheeler 2010: 190) because it can only be owned and sold by medical professionals and researchers in specific ways and for specific purposes. Nevertheless, we are yet again confronted with a problem of categorization: Is the bioprinted organ to be treated as a natural organ, which therefore could not be sold? Or should it be classed as a mass of tissues and cells, and thus open to commercial dealings?

3.1   The "Landmark" Legal Cases

A useful starting point on the ownership of human biomaterials is the US Ruling of Moore vs. Regents of the University of California. The case involved a cell line, derived from the spleen of John Moore. After years of treatment for Leukemia, which involved taking his spleen and subsequent tissue samples, Moore's Doctor and hospital researchers patented and commercialized Moore's cell lines – which proved highly lucrative – without his knowledge or consent (Harbaugh 2015). Moore sued the hospital for a share in the profits, but the Court ruled against him on the basis that allowing patients to dictate future uses of their biomaterials would produce potentially "chilling" effects on medical research (ibid: 175). This ruling is often interpreted as in line with the "Lockean labor" (ibid) theory: the scientists and medics involved would have "labored" (ibid) to assemble the materials – in the case of bioprinting to make the organ – which would therefore give them ownership rights. However, Quigley (2014) notes that this US case cannot necessarily have a direct influence in the UK or elsewhere but can merely indicate how claims about commercial property rights in organs may be treated.

In the realm of reproductive tissues, the legal scene appears very different. In the US case of Davis vs. Davis, which aimed at determining what should be done with cryopreserved embryos, the courts determined that "the embryos 'potential for human life' entitled the genetic parents to 'decision-making authority'" over them (Harbaugh 2015: 177). In this case, the argument for personal autonomy triumphed. In the UK, a similar case came before the courts, in which Natallie Evans requested the right to implant embryos that she had made with her previous partner (Dyer/McVeigh 2007). Both UK and EU courts sided with the rationale of personal autonomy, ruling against her and granting her partner the right to refuse the use of his materials. Many legal battles regarding the ownership rights of fertilized embryos result in the would-be parents being declared legal owners of the embryo. They therefore have the ultimate right to decide its uses (destruction, research or donation), even though clinicians have 'labored' to create them. Some legal scholars suggest that even though the cases of Moore and Davis are apparently contradictory, they can be reconciled on the basis that embryos have a different status to spleens, due to their "potential for human life" (Harbaugh 2015: 187). This raises the question of the status of a bioprinted organ. Although the similarities between an embryo and a bioprinted organ are fairly clear – they are both new things made from patients' cells – both must be manipulated by doctors to achieve existence, both are made using advanced technologies, and both are imbued with a great deal of promissory value. The key difference is that, because it can grow into a human, the embryo has the potential for personhood rights, whereas a bioprinted organ does not. Despite difficulties in categorizing bioprinted organs, we doubt anyone would attempt to argue that it had the potential to be a 'person'. The bioprinted organ could therefore be seen as not 'life-generating' but merely *life-sustaining*, and so would be unlikely to be granted special status. That is not to say, however, that it *should* not be granted special status.

Our last foray into legal scholarship takes us to a 'landmark' UK court case with regards to ownership of human biomaterials (Rostill 2014; Quigley 2014; Hoppe 2009). The Yearworth case involved a number of men who had stored their sperm with an NHS trust prior to undergoing chemotherapy, which can cause infertility. However, the facility stored the sperm incorrectly and the sperm perished. The donors subsequently sued the NHS trust for negligence, arguing their case on the basis of property rights, and the courts ruled in their favor. This marks the first time that a tissue donor has been recognized as having property rights over their biomaterials (ibid). Hoppe (2009) argues that this ruling can be understood as the UK courts paving the way for property rights to be recognized in any tissue removed from the body. However, a number of other legal scholars refute this (Harmon 2010; Rostill 2014), arguing that the case in question is not quite the bellwether of change that it is often purported to be. The specificity of the case and its context would not necessarily extend to other biomaterials, such as bioprinted organs.

3.2   Managing Body Ownership: How Would it Work?

Having ascertained the uncertainty of the legal landscape with regards to property rights in human biomaterials that have been separated from the body, the next question is whether one *should* have such property rights. If yes, then under what circumstances? Quigley (2014: 692) suggests that philosophical conceptions of property have "use" and "control" as their key features, two features which would allow people to derive income from these uses. As we have already established, the people from whom the biomaterials originated rarely have this right, even though third parties *are* permitted to do this under the *Human Tissue Act*. Fears of commodification and undue restrictions on medical research are the key drivers of this policy, although it has been noted that granting powers of control over uses does not mean that commodification would be rife. It would not be inconceivable to devise a system in which donors would be able to own and control the uses of their biomaterials without having the right to sell them. Under the current system, property rights are not "unfettered" (ibid), even when dealing with traditional objects of property. For example, prescription drugs provided to you by your general practitioner (GP) are technically yours, but they are not yours to do with what you want as it is illegal to gift or sell them to others. Thus, just because you own something does not mean that you are necessarily allowed to derive income from it, or use it in whichever way you please.

Having delved into some of the legal arguments about where we stand with ownership of biomaterials, the purpose of this exercise is to ascertain what, if any, control one might have over a bioprinted organ. Although a bioprinted organ will have been made from *your* cells, they will have undergone a significant amount of transformation in order to be printed into a functioning organ. Would this give your doctor the right to determine uses, as with the 'Lockean labor' theory used to underpin the Moore case? Would ownership rights only extend insofar as the hospital had a duty of care over your organ, as seen in Yearworth? Or would the fact that it was made from *you* mean that you could circumscribe its uses, as with the autonomy arguments put forward in reproductive tissue cases? In the latter case, one might also pose the question, what (if any) restrictions will there be on what you can do with the organ? These questions point to significant gaps in our current understandings about what control we have over our tissues, and how these gaps might be exacerbated in a hypothetical world in which we could bioprint spare body parts from a tissue sample. The substantial grey areas and uncertainties would suggest that the rights of each party in the bioprinting process must be established a priori.

4.   Regulation, Safety and Liability

Imagine you are a year along from the bioprinted heart transplant you received previously. All is well, and your bioprinted heart appears to be functioning much the same as your previous one. But then you start experiencing problems. A fault is subsequently detected that may prove fatal if not addressed; your heart specialist concludes that it must be replaced. It is currently unclear what has caused the fault, but the medical professionals believe that a replacement bioprinted heart would be the best course of treatment, and that they may be able to understand the reason for the fault post-surgery. You agree, and a new heart is bioprinted prior to the second surgery, which is implanted without issue. You have now undergone two surgeries, which both involve significant recovery time. When something goes wrong, and a bioprinted organ fails, whose fault is it? Is there someone to blame? Can it be prevented from happening again?

The legal definition and treatment of a bioprinted organ is still unclear. Should it be treated as we would currently treat a donor organ? As Gilbert et al. (2018) have pointed out, this would be inappropriate because a donor organ has already been proven to work in its previous owner's body. Under the current regulatory regime, the bioprinted organ must therefore be treated as either a product or a device. However, no scholars, as yet, have provided any serious suggestions as to how 3D bioprinted organs might be regulated. Some authors have examined the current system and raised serious questions about the ability of our existing regulations to deal with 3D bioprinting (Wolf/Fresco 2016; Li/Faulkner 2017; Gilbert et al. 2018). Similar concerns have been raised about personalized and/or regenerative medicine products (Faulkner 2016; Faulkner/Poort 2017).

Gilbert and colleagues (2018), have focused on the ethics of testing this type of technology. Pointing at an acknowledged lack of available regulatory directives, they argue that the treatment can be understood as "part medical device, part biological" (ibid.: 85). It does not fit neatly into any category because it is an inherently personalized treatment that would need to be scaled up on an industrial level to meet the needs of a variety of different patients (ibid). It is also problematic because a bioprinted organ is not intended to treat any specific disease; a recipient's problems may arise from an assortment of different diseases, genetic problems, and environmental factors. Furthermore, the safety and efficacy requirements that have come to be expected in contemporary medical care would be extremely difficult to meet through our existing frameworks. As Wolf and Fresco (2016) point out, the output of a 3D bioprinter contains information and materials from multiple different sources. The bioink, the cells, the programming software, the scan/image on which the organ will be based, and the bioprinter all come from different people and places.

4.1   Current Regulatory Landscape

Under the EU regulatory system, the European Medicines Agency (EMA) controls and provides directives on the regulation of various types of product. At present, the regulation of Advanced Therapy Medicinal Products (ATMP) would likely be the most relevant to bioprinting. The ATMP regulation was originally introduced as a result of the increasingly diverse forms of product that do not fall into the drug or device category. Brevignon-Dodin (2010: 121) highlights that it was designed to be "tailored yet flexible enough to keep pace with scientific progress", although some have questioned whether this has been successful (see also Faulkner/Poort 2016). The EU provides the overarching regulation and individual countries may have their own authorities which have further requirements. In the UK context for instance, the two relevant authorities are the Human Tissue Authority (HTA) and the Medicines and Healthcare Regulatory Agency (MHRA). Thus, in order to get market approval in the UK, a bioprinted organ would need to comply with requirements of EU regulation for ATMPs, along with those set out by the HTA and MHRA.

Examining the existing regulatory regime, a number of scholars highlight its complexity and variability. According to Faulkner and Poort (2017), the ATMP regulations were supposed to be radically different from existing directives, namely in its flexibility for including a variety of different products. However, as a result of a combination of factors and the instrumental role of "pharmaceutical industry lobbying" (ibid.: 215), the resulting ATMP regulation is remarkably commensurate with the existing requirements for pharmaceuticals, such as the requirements for placebo-controlled clinical trials. The imposition of a pharmaceutical frame on ATMP regulation effectively encourages the regenerative medicine industry to produce products that fit a "'medicines' rather than a 'devices' paradigm" (ibid.: 226). Faulkner's analysis of the marketing of regenerative medicine in the UK shows that there is a tendency for developers to choose "non-mainstream gateways to market in preference to central pathways" (2016: 322). These include the 'hospital exemption' and the 'specials' routes, which are two separate but similar pathways for bypassing EU regulation, so that unlicensed products may still be delivered in a clinical setting, provided they are 'non-routine' (Mittra et al. 2014). Significantly, the fact that several ATMPs must go through 'exemption' routes would suggest that the ATMP regulation is not quite as flexible as it is purported to be.

Li et al. (2017: 4) assert that a bioprinted product has "the characteristics of an ATMP and some similarity to an ATMP-device combination". However, according to the flowchart provided by the UK government (2015) to help developers understand if their product would fall under ATMP regulation, a 3D bioprinted organ would be considered 'outside the scope'. But what about regulating bioprinted organs as devices? Faulkner (2016) suggests that an increasing number of tissue-engineered products are being designated as medical devices by developers, because the regulatory pathway is seen as less stringent than the ATMP/pharmaceutical route. However, the medical device route would not be without complications either, as Morrison et al. (2015) note that the customized nature presents further challenges. Still others, such as Gilbert et al., suggest that because 3D bioprinted organs are "individualized, custom-made devices" (2018: 85) (because each organ would be personalized for each patient), under current rules they would technically be exempt from regulation. Therefore, we are in a position where all commentators on 3D bioprinting disagree on how it would be regulated, and whilst most point to the inadequacy of our current system for dealing with these technologies, it appears that few alternative ideas are forthcoming.

4.2   Problems of Testing and Standardization

Whilst some scholars have speculated about how 3D bioprinting will be regulated under the current system, one of the key concerns remains how it would be possible to meet our existing requirements for clinical testing. The existing gold standard for testing safety and efficacy is the randomized controlled trial (RCT), in which one group is provided with a placebo treatment (or the current best treatment) in order to comparatively determine a treatment's efficacy. Because this is the existing practice for regulatory approval, it raises questions as to how appropriate this paradigm is for testing emerging biotechnologies (Gilbert et al. 2018). One of the reasons 3D bioprinting seems so promising is the fact that it can be personalized, which means that this testing model would be highly inappropriate. Furthermore, as Gilbert et al. point out, "how could it be morally acceptable, given the severe risk of major harms, to test the safety of an organ which has been specifically made for me with my own stem cells on someone else?" (ibid.: 82). This question certainly merits further attention from bioethicists, policymakers, and clinicians alike. The unique nature of each bioprinted organ, and its function in different individuals, is not necessarily something that can be standardized to the extent that we currently demand.

The requirement for animal testing in the preclinical phase of any trials would need to be met before any further testing could be carried out. In their analysis of the regulation of cultured red blood cells, Mittra et al. (2014: 186) have noted that there were significant issues with the animal testing phase. Similarly, the use of animal cells combined with bioink in animal models would not constitute the same product as using human cells. Whilst it would theoretically be similar, there may be doubts as to the extent that we can compare them effectively for safety and efficacy purposes. Alternatively, testing human cells that have been bioprinted into organs in animals would trigger an immune response in the receiving animals which would likely not occur in humans, so the findings would be flawed in those circumstances too. As Mittra et al. (2014) assert, this problem has been noted with other regenerative medicine products and is one that the European regulatory system has yet to resolve. Whilst the bioinks and the composite materials that are combined with the cells to make the organ could be tested and likely standardized, the personalized nature of the individual organ and

the physical characteristics would make any type of product standardization very difficult. This means that the safety of the product/organ cannot be assured because there
can be no standard by which it is measured.

However, it has been noted that even if the actual product faces standardization
issues, the *process* in which a 3D bioprinted organ is produced may adhere to a standard process – in terms of the software, the use of the bioprinters, and the creation of
the bioinks and their infusion with cells (Gilbert et al. 2018). Nevertheless, when and
if researchers reach the point of human testing, the ethical considerations of testing
the transplantation of bioprinted organs on healthy volunteers seem positively absurd.
How could one possibly justify replacing a healthy organ with a bioprinted one to
ascertain the safety of the process in other individuals? Should the first 3D bioprinted
organs then be tested on those who are already sick? And how could we use a placebo
group or next best treatment? Gilbert et al. (2018) point out that existing gene therapies, where biologically engineered cells are injected into the body, have similar issues
of efficacy and safety that have been described above. However, unlike gene therapies, 3D bioprinted tissues would have to replace an existing organ, which could not
be adequately preserved, thus making the process irreversible. Therefore, Gilbert and
colleagues note that participation in an experimental trial of a 3D bioprinted organ, if
unsuccessful, may preclude patients from accessing further existing treatments, thus
further disadvantaging them. In addition, it may also prove difficult to undertake longitudinal studies of the safety and efficacy of bioprinted organs. The likely use of IPSCs
as the building blocks for the bioprinted organ may mean that we cannot truly understand its safety until longitudinal studies are completed. Take, for example, the case of
a woman who had stem cells injected into her face as a cosmetic treatment, and, some
time later discovered fragments of bone growing in her eyelids (Jabr 2012). Or another
case, which involved a quadriplegic woman who underwent stem cell therapy in her
back, as part of an approved clinical trial, and 8 years later discovered a 'nose' (which
was in fact a growth of nasal tissue secreting mucus) growing on her spine (Wilson
2014). The issue with IPSCs is that they have the ability to grow into numerous different types of tissue. It is worth noting that in the same clinical trial mentioned above,
the majority of other participants saw improvements, and recovered some movement
and sensation, thus highlighting the individual variability of stem cell therapies and
our limited understanding of them. We also acknowledge that there is a significant
ethical difference between stem cell therapies for cosmetic reasons and those carried
out for life-saving treatment, but the examples above are merely intended to demonstrate the current lack of knowledge about the long-term effects in this area.

The consequences of a nose growing on one's back, or a bone at the surface of one's
skin, whilst not ideal, have not yet proven fatal. However, what if a fragment of bone
was to grow inside a vital organ? This scenario raises the need to address our current
problems with emerging biotechnologies and how we test and manage them. We need
to develop new regulatory regimes for the testing of bioprinted organs, which pays
attention not only to the actual thing at the moment of creation/medical intervention,
but also to sustainability.

4.3   A Look at Liability

Alongside issues of regulation and testing, is necessary to determine responsibility and liability when things go wrong. As Wolf and Fresco (2016) highlight, prior to implanting a bioprinted organ into a patient, who would have the final say as to its viability? And should anything go wrong post-implantation, will it be possible to establish what or who is at fault? If you receive a heart transplant from a donor and the heart malfunctions (i.e. you get an infection or there is physiological damage), you do not have recourse for litigation against the donor. However, if you have a pacemaker or another similar medical device in the UK and a malfunction is proven to be the result of manufacturer error, under the Consumer Protection Act 1987 you would have the right to take the manufacturers to court with a product liability claim. Furthermore, in the US, an increasing number of medical device manufacturers are beginning to provide guarantees on their heart devices in order to entice hospitals to use their products (Kelly 2015). If this trend continues, warranties for medical devices and products might become more commonplace. This further increases the regulatory complexities of bioprinted organs because their classification may have ramifications for any liability claims. Because they are artificially made, the reason for any malfunction may exist independently of the patient; nevertheless, it is unclear whether a bioprinted organ would be considered a 'product' for the purposes of law. Li and Faulkner (2017) highlight the difficulties of fitting bioprinting into existing regulatory regimes, and our analysis of bioprinted organs underlines those difficulties.

Faulkner and Poort have asserted that there are two types of regulatory adaptation; "commensuration"; which involves "the stretching and maintenance of a pre-existing legal framework"; and "replacement", which requires the "breaking of existing classifications and establishment of a novel regime" (2017: 209). In their analysis of the ATMP regulation, they conclude that although the stretching and flexibility of existing regulation may seem the most pragmatic, it may produce further confusion and complications. Having a flexible regulatory framework risks a lack of clarity of the rules and standards. However, as Faulkner and Poort state, considering the rate at which new developments are made, we must certainly doubt whether "old rules" are capable of addressing the "new risks" (ibid.) that come with new forms of biotechnology. Bearing in mind that the usual starting point for legislators is to investigate whether new technologies can fit into the existing regulatory framework, our discussion suggests that it is likely 3D bioprinted organs will not.

5.   The Dark Side: From Black Markets to Counterfeits?

Imagine a world where bioprinters are available to purchase at a reasonable sum and can be used in a do-it-yourself (DIY) context to print organs on demand. Although in some countries, organ bioprinting would perhaps be available through national health services, there are many countries worldwide where the cost of treatment is not provided by the state. With the right skills, expertise and equipment, the less lawfully inclined can open up an illicit organ bioprinting workshop, where the uninsured, undocumented and vulnerable are able to purchase custom bioprinted organs much cheaper than from legitimate sources. In these workshops, there are no regulatory requirements, tests, guarantees or responsibility regarding the safety or build quality of these organs. Just as some doctors and hospitals worldwide still implant stolen organs, will this also be the case for 'counterfeit' bioprinted ones? Will the black market in organs ever really disappear, or will it simply transform, reshape and adapt to exploit the vulnerable in new ways?

One of the problematic, but widely cited, benefits of 3D bioprinting technology is that it promises to solve the problem of illegal trade in human organs (Li 2014; Li/Faulkner 2017; Gilbert et al. 2018). The logic behind this is that if we can bioprint new organs, the current issues of supply and demand will disappear, eliminating organ trafficking altogether. However, whilst aspects of the current market may become less prevalent, the assertion that the black market or illegal trade of organs will disappear may be somewhat premature. We suggest that it is more likely that the advent of 3D bioprinting may simply contribute to changing this trade's format, altering its processes, but nevertheless still hurting those amongst us with least access to resources.

Beyond notions of *supply and demand*, common themes amongst scholars regarding the black market in human organs (Cohen 2013; Scheper-Hughes 2000) are *inequality* and *exploitation*. Just because we may have the power to solve one specific problem does not mean that inequality and exploitation will disappear. As suggested above, there are other ways that this inequality might manifest in a world where we can bioprint body parts. The cost of equipment may turn out to be cheap, but the product may be very expensive – because the cost of production and the cost of sale do not always have a direct correlation, and also vary per country. For example, according to Cohen (2013: 282) the average yearly cost of an immunosuppressant regimen for someone who has received a kidney transplant in the US is approximately $20,000 per year. However, according to an NHS England (2013) report, the cost of providing the same service in the UK is £5,000 per year. Considering the disparity in health care costs of drugs, and the complexity of bioprinting and variety of expertise required, it would not be inconceivable that the cost of a bioprinted organ may be so high in some countries that it would lead to medical tourism. This also depends on whether a bioprinted organ is available from national health care services, private insurance companies, neither, or both.

This scenario also raises questions about who should receive a bioprinted organ, and with what priority. For example, what about patients who have already received donated organs? Should they be entitled to have their 'second-hand' organs replaced with 'self-grown' organs? And existing living donors? For people who have altruistically donated a kidney, should they be entitled to have a new spare bioprinted one in the space where their donated one was? Whilst we are not suggesting that the answer should be 'no' to any of the above questions, these factors would nevertheless pose extra strain on an already strained health care system, and the advent of a new technology will not magically make these issues disappear. 'Transplant tourism' (Cohen 2013; Scheper-Hughes 2005) may well still persist, but in a different format – perhaps more aptly transformed into 'implant tourism' where people in need of new organs shop around and travel to where the wait time for implanting a bioprinted organ is lower and the price is cheaper.

Linked to this problem is a fundamental question: should bioprinted organs be considered a profitable technology or part of standard medical care? As appears to be the common theme, how a bioprinted organ is classified will have a significant impact on its use, and the associated issues. If it goes the 'pharmaceutical route' and is considered patentable and profitable (Li 2014; Harbaugh 2015), then counterfeiting may become a genuine issue. There is already a booming trade in 'knock-off' prescription drugs, and these pharmaceutical counterfeits are one of the most lucrative areas in the global economy of counterfeit goods (Behner et al. 2017). It has even been suggested that "more than half the counterfeit pharmaceuticals sold today are fraudulent versions of treatments for such life-threatening conditions as malaria, tuberculosis, HIV/ AIDS, and even cancer" (ibid: 5). Considering the prevalence of this problem, it may seem somewhat surprising that the majority of reflections on the ethics or social consequences of 3D bioprinting appear to dismiss the possibility of counterfeiting as a problem. In fact, Li and colleagues (2017) appear to be the only scholars thus far that have taken counterfeiting seriously. We would contend that the risk of counterfeiting would be linked to bioprinting's treatment with regards to intellectual property, including whether the technology can (or indeed should) be patented.

6.   Conclusion

The uncertainty surrounding the classification of bioprinted organs that has been outlined here becomes inherently entangled with problems of regulation and intellectual property, which are in turn bound up with the legal definition of bioprinted organs. New ways of thinking about bioprinted organs, either as bio-objects, or using another theoretical lens, may be required to determine what new regulations or legal rights, if any, need to be introduced. Being not fully human, nor fully artificial, but biological material inherently connected to a person, the bioprinted organ and its treatment fall outside our current categorization boundaries.

By means of a legal scenario, we have highlighted that the ownership of a bioprinted organ is not clear-cut due to its ambiguous status, and legal scholars have yet to determine how it should be treated or if changes must be made. Looking at regulation, we have suggested that rather than follow a 'commensuration' model, new purpose-made regulation may be required to govern bioprinted organs. Just as new laws and regulations were introduced with the advent of organ transplantation, the same may be needed for bioprinted organs. Looking at testing, the RCT model of clinical trial appears inappropriate for the testing of bioprinted organs because both the ethical and practical considerations would make it extremely difficult. And considering the vast potential for harm caused by errors, the software (i.e. the modelling programs used by bioprinters) should meet stringent standards to prevent any glitches or security concerns. How this technology is controlled and made available also creates further risks; if it is only made available at a high cost, it may not solve the organ shortage as easily as it is claimed. The way that this technology is treated for legal, regulatory and economic purposes will have important social and ethical implications and must be dealt with as part of the technology's further development and potential use in health care.

References

Amanatidou, Effie/Butter, Maurits Carabias, Vicente/Könnölä, Totti/Leis, Miriam/Saritas, Ozcan/Schaper-Rinkel, Petra/van Rij, Victor (2012): "On Concepts and Methods in Horizon Scanning: Lessons from Initiating Policy Dialogues on Emerging Issues". In: Science and Public Policy 39/2, pp. 208–221.

Behner, Peter/Hecht, Marie-Lyn/Wahl, Fabian (2017): "Fighting Counterfeit Pharmaceuticals: New Defenses for an Underestimated – and Growing – Menace." In: Strategy & Insights (PwC Industry report), pp. 1–24.

Boucher, Philip (2018): "3D Bio-Printing for Medical and Enhancement Purposes." In: European Parliamentary Research Service, Scientific Foresight Unit (STOA): Brussels, pp. 1–19.

Brevignon-Dodin, Laure (2010): "Regulatory Enablers and Regulatory Challenges for the Development of Tissue-Engineered Products in the EU." In: Bio-Medical Materials and Engineering 20/3, pp. 121–126.

Cohen, I. Glenn (2013): "Transplant Tourism: The Ethics and Regulation of International Markets for Organs." In: The Journal of Law, Medicine & Ethics 41/1, pp. 269–285.

Dyer, Clare/McVeigh, Karen (2007): "Woman Loses Battle to Use Frozen Embryos Created with Her Ex-Fiance." In: The Guardian, April 11.

Faulkner, Alex (2016): "Opening the Gateways to Market and Adoption of Regenerative Medicine? The UK Case in Context." In: Regenerative Medicine 11/3, pp. 321–330.

Faulkner, Alex/Poort, Lonneke (2017): "Stretching and Challenging the Boundaries of Law: Varieties of Knowledge in Biotechnologies Regulation" In: Minerva 55/2, pp. 209–228.

Gilbert, Frederic/O'Connell, Cathal D./Mladenovska, Tajanka/Dodds, Susan (2018): "Print Me an Organ? Ethical and Regulatory Issues Emerging from 3D Bioprinting in Medicine." In: Science and Engineering Ethics 24/1, pp. 73–91.

Gilbert, Frederic/Viaña, John Noel M./O'Connell, Cathal D./Dodds, Susan (2017): "Enthusiastic Portrayal of 3D Bioprinting in the Media: Ethical Side Effects." In: Bioethics 32/2, pp. 94–102.

Groll, Jürgen/Boland, Thomas/Blunk, Torsten/Burdick, Jason A./Cho, Dong-Woo/Dalton, Paul D./Derby, Brian/Forgacs, Gabor/Li, Qing/Mironov, Vladimir A./Moroni, Lorenzo/ Nakamura, Makoto/Shu, Wenmiao/Takeuchi, Shoji/Vozzi, Giovanni/ Woodfield, Tim B. F./Xu, Tao/Yoo, James J./Malda, Jos (2016): "Biofabrication: Reappraising the Definition of an Evolving Field." In: Biofabrication, 8/1, pp. 1–5.

Grunwald, Armin (2007): "Converging Technologies: Visions, Increased Contingencies of the Conditio Humana, and Search for Orientation." In: Futures 39/4, pp. 380–392.

Guillemot, Fabien/Mironov, Vladimir/Nakamura, Makoto (2010): "Bioprinting is Coming of Age: Report from the International Conference on Bioprinting and Biofabrication in Bordeaux (3B'09)." In: Biofabrication 2/1, pp. 1–7.

Gungor-Ozkerim, P. Selcan/Inci, Ingas/Zhang, Yu Shrike/Khademhosseini, Ali/Dokmeci, Mehmet Remzi (2018): "Bioinks for 3D bioprinting: an Overview." In: Biomaterials Science 6/5, pp. 915–946.

Harbaugh, Jeremy T. (2015): "Do you Own your 3D Bioprinted Body? Analyzing Property Issues at the Intersection of Digital Information and Biology." In: The American Journal of Law and Medicine 41/1, pp. 167–89.

Harmon, Shawn H.E. (2010): "Yearworth vs. North Bristol NHS Trust: A Property/ Medical Case of Uncertain Significance." In: Medicine, Health Care & Philosophy 13/4, pp. 343–350.

Hedgecoe, Adam M. (2004): "Critical Bioethics: Beyond the Social Science Critique of Applied Ethics." In: Bioethics 18/2, pp. 120–143.

Hoppe, Nils (2009): Bioequity – Property and the Human Body, Farnham: Ashgate.

Jabr, Ferris (2012): "In the Flesh: The Embedded Dangers of Untested Stem Cell Cosmetics" In: Scientific American, December 17.

Kass, Leon R. (2004): Life, Liberty, and the Defense of Dignity: The Challenge for Bioethics, San Francisco: Encounter Books.

Kelly, Susan (2015): "Medical Device Makers Beef up Product Guarantees to Woo US hospitals" In: Reuters, July 8.

Keulartz, Josef/Schermer, Maartje/Korthals, Michiel/Swierstra, Tsjalling (2004): "Ethics in Technological Culture: A Programmatic Proposal for a Pragmatist Approach." In: Science, Technology & Human Values 29/1, pp. 3–29.

Lewis, Tim (2017): "Could 3D Printing Solve the Organ Transplant Shortage?" In: The Guardian, July 30.

Li, Phoebe (2014): "3D Bioprinting Technologies: Patents, Innovation and Access." In: Law, Innovation & Technology 6/2, pp. 282–304.

Li, Phoebe/Faulkner, Alex/Griffin, James/Medcalf, Nick (2017): "Mass Customisation Governance: Regulation, Liability, and Intellectual Property of Re-Distributed Manufacturing in 3D Bioprinting." Project Report IfM: Cambridge.

Li, Phoebe/Faulkner, Alex (2017): "3D Bioprinting Regulations: a UK/EU Perspective." In: European Journal of Risk Regulation 8/2, pp. 441–447.

Lucassen, Anneke/Wheeler, Robert (2010): "Legal Implications of Tissue." In: Annals of the Royal College of Surgeons of England 92/3, pp. 189–192.

Metzler, Ingrid/Webster, Andrew (2011): "Bioobjects and their Boundaries: Governing Matters at the Intersection of Society, Politics and Science." In: Croatian Medical Journal 52/5, pp. 648–650.

Mironov, Vladimir/Kasyanov, Vladimir/Markwald, Roger R. (2011): "Organ Printing: from Bioprinter to Organ Biofabrication Line." In: Current Opinion in Biotechnology 22/5, pp. 667–673.

Mittra, James/Tait, Joyce/Mastroeni, Michele/Turner, Marc L./Mountford, Joanne C./ Bruce, Kevin (2014): "Identifying Viable Regulatory and Innovation Pathways for Regenerative Medicine: A Case Study of Cultured Red Blood Cells." In: New Biotechnology 32/1, pp. 180–190.

Morrison, Robert J./Kashlan, Khaled N./Flanangan, Colleen L./Wright, Jeanne K./ Green, Glenn E./Hollister, Scott J./Weatherwax, Kevin J. (2015): "Regulatory Considerations in the Design and Manufacturing of Implantable 3D Printed Medical Devices." In: Clinical and Translational Science 8/5, pp. 594–600.

Murphy, Sean V./Atala, Anthony (2014): "3D Bioprinting of Tissues and Organs." In: Nature Biotechnology 32/8, pp. 773–785.

NHS England (2013): NHS Standard Contract for Adult Kidney Transplant Service. Schedule 2 – Service Specifications. Available at: https://www.england.nhs.uk/ wp-content/uploads/2014/04/a07-renal-transpl-ad-0414.pdf (accessed June 30, 2020)

NHS England (2019) Statistics about Organ Donation. Available at: https://www.
organdonation.nhs.uk/supporting-my-decision/statistics-about-organ-donation/
(accessed June 30, 2020)

Petersen, Alan (2013): "From Bioethics to a Sociology of Bio-Knowledge." In: Social Science & Medicine 98, pp. 264–270.

Popper, Rafael (2008): "How are Foresight Methods Selected?" In: Foresight 10/6, pp.
62–89.

Quigley, Muireann (2014): "Propertisation and Commercialisation: On Controlling the
Uses of Human Biomaterials." In: The Modern Law Review 77/5, pp. 677–702.

Rostill, Luke David (2014): "The Ownership that Wasn't Meant to Be: Yearworth and
Property Rights in Human Tissue." In: Journal of Medical Ethics 40/1, pp. 14–18.

Rowe, Emily/Wright, George/Derbyshire, James (2017): "Enhancing Horizon Scanning
by Utilizing Pre-Developed Scenarios: Analysis of Current Practice and Specification of a Process Improvement to Aid the Identification of Important 'Weak Signals'." In: Technological Forecasting & Social Change 125, pp. 224–235.

Savage, Maddy (2017): "The Firm that Can 3D Print Human Body Parts" BBC news,
November 15.

Scheper-Hughes, Nancy (2000): "The Global Traffic in Human Organs." In: Current
Anthropology 41/2, pp. 191–224.

Scheper-Hughes, Nancy (2005): "The Last Commodity: Post-Human Ethics and the
Global Traffic in 'Fresh' Organs." In: Aihwa Ong/Stephen J. Collier (eds.), Global
Assemblages: Technology, Politics, and Ethics as Anthropological Problems, Mal-
den, MA: Blackwell Publishing, pp. 145–167.

Shapiro, Robyn (1998): "Who Owns Your Frozen Embryo? Promises and Pitfalls of
Emerging Reproductive Options." In: Human Rights 25/2, pp. 12–13.

Smits, Martijntje (2006): "Taming Monsters: the Cultural Domestication of New Technology." In: Technology and Society 28/4, pp. 489–504.

Squier, Susan/Waldby, Catherine (2005): "Our Posthuman Future: Discussing the
Consequences of Biotechnological Advances." In: The Hastings Center Report 35/6,
pp. 4–7.

Stilgoe, Jack/Owen, Richard/Macnaghten, Phil (2013): "Developing a Framework for
Responsible Innovation." In: Research Policy 42/9, pp. 1568–1580.

Swierstra, Tsjalling/van Est, Rinie/Boenink, Marianne (2009): "Taking Care of the
Symbolic Order. How Converging Technologies Challenge our Concepts." In:
Nanoethics 3/3, pp. 269–280.

Swierstra, Tsjalling/Boenink, Marianne/Walhout, Bart/van Est, Rinie (2009): "Converging Technologies, Shifting Boundaries." In: Nanoethics 3/3, pp. 213–216.

Tamminen, Sakari/Vermeulen, Niki (2019): "Bio-objects: New Conjugations of the Living." In: Sociologias 21/50, pp. 156–179.

Thomson, Judith (1971) "A Defense of Abortion." In: Philosophy & Public Affairs 1/1, pp.
47–66.

UK Government (2015): "ATMP Flowchart for Determining the Regulatory Status of
Tissue and Cell-Based Products." Available at: https://assets.publishing.service.
gov.uk/government/uploads/system/uploads/attachment_data/file/397735/Copy_
of_ATMP_flowchart_4a_finalised.pdf (accessed June 30, 2020)

Van Rij, Victor (2010): "Joint Horizon Scanning: Identifying Common Strategic Choices
and Questions for Knowledge." In: Science and Public Policy 37/1, pp. 7–18.

Vermeulen Niki/Tamminen, Sakari/Webster, Andrew (2012) (eds.): Bio-Objects: Life in the 21st Century, Aldershot: Ashgate.

Vermeulen, Niki/Haddow, Gillian/Seymour, Tirion/Faulkner-Jones, Alan/Shu, Wenmiao (2017): "3D Bioprint Me: a Socioethical View of Bioprinting Human Organs and Tissues." In: Journal of Medical Ethics 43/9, pp. 1–7.

Wilkinson, Angela (2009): "Scenarios Practices: In Search of Theory." In: Journal of Futures Studies 13/3, pp. 107–114.

Williams, Rhiannon (2014): "The Next Step: 3D Printing the Human Body." In: The Telegraph, February 11.

Wilson, Clare (2014): "Stem Cell Treatment Causes Nasal Growth in Woman's Back." In: New Scientist, July 8.

Wolf, Marty J./Fresco, Nir (2016): "My Liver is Broken, Can you Print Me a New One?" In: Müller, Vincent C. (ed.), Computing and Philosophy: Selected Papers from IACAP 2014, Cham: Springer, pp. 259–269.

18. Considering the Role of Public Health
Organ Shortage, Global Justice, and the Paradox of Prevention

Hagai Boas, Nadav Davidovitch & Michael Yudell

1. Introduction

What are the chances that a 13-year-old child with end stage renal disease (ESRD) will undergo a kidney transplant, or at least be treated with dialysis? Sadly, the answer is not only clinical but also sociological in nature, deeply rooted in economic, political, and social structures. If, for example, this child lives in a lower- or middle-income country, her chances of being diagnosed in time to receive such care are low (Muralidharan/White 2015; Muller 2016). However, if this child was born in a Scandinavian country, she would have a good chance of receiving a transplant that would lengthen her life by many years.

The gap between organ demand and available supply, even in countries where it has been reduced slightly in recent years, is abysmally large. Patients across the globe die every day awaiting a needed organ. In the United States, for example, a significant disparity between organ supply and demand remains, even as a record number of transplants have been performed. Data from early 2020 provided by The United Network for Organ Sharing indicates that 112.605 Americans are in need of an organ transplant. But in 2019 there were only 39.718 successful organ transplantations (from both living and dead donors). Supply is not meeting, nor will meet, demand (UNOS 2020).

We all know that health disparities exist. In transplant medicine, however, disparities and equity are generally discussed by bioethicists in terms of access to transplantation for ESRD and other chronic health conditions that lead to transplant. In this paper, we show why transplant bioethics alone cannot solve many of the problems facing transplant medicine, and we turn instead to public health for answers. In general, public health employs policies of prevention to address conditions *before* they develop into chronic or fatal diseases. We believe there is an unmet need to discuss prevention in the context of organ transplantation and to explain how public health ethics approaches could both contribute to reducing the organ shortage and provide moral guideposts for such an approach. As public health practitioners, we also believe our moral obligation is to assist those with inherited, chronic, and acute conditions *before* transplants become necessary. Thus, in this paper we argue that the field of transplant medicine will be better able to address its challenges if it incorporates prevention modalities and public health ethics into an overall approach that seeks to reduce the costs and health burden of diseases associated with the need for organ transplant.

2.   Background: Public Health Ethics

Public health emerged as an organized discipline during the 19th century with the goal of improving the health of the nation (Porter 1999; Berridge/Gorsky/Mold 2011). While its initial interests focused on infectious diseases, sanitation, and hygiene, over time, its scope has grown to include health promotion and address the rise of chronic diseases and health inequalities. Yet, emerging and re-emerging infectious diseases – from HIV to SARS to SARS-CoV-2 – constantly remind us that the battle against contagious diseases is far from over. In many parts of the world, the 'double burden' of both infectious and chronic diseases imposes a growing burden especially upon low- and middle-income countries, which have limited resources and struggle to meet the challenges of long-existing problems associated with infectious diseases and the rapid rise in cardiovascular diseases, diabetes, cancers and obesity-related conditions (Bygbjerg 2012).

Furthermore, low- and middle-income countries are also burdened by the interaction of poverty, scarce health-related resources, and a high burden of chronic disease. For example, according to estimates from the Global Burden of Disease study in 2015, globally more than 2 million people died in 2010 because they had no access to dialysis, mostly among the poor (Crews/Bello/Saadi 2019). Such statistics point to a major crisis of chronic kidney diseases (CKD) globally, including the uneven distribution of CKD among poor people. A public health approach can broaden the discussion to include a focus on prevention efforts, which are a less costly and more sustainable approach to the transplantation crisis.

It should go without saying that this is not a solution for many patients currently in need of and waiting for organs. It is, however, about the need to include a public health perspective to improve investment in programs that seek to reduce the burden of disease in conditions ranging from diabetes to cirrhosis to hypertension – in order to alleviate the downstream need for transplantation itself. A public health approach is beneficial because it adds to quality of life, it is easier and less costly to accomplish than cure, and it reduces health inequalities. Take the example of diabetes: it can lead to CKD, and primary prevention campaigns targeting populations at-risk for diabetes may have the beneficial impact of preventing diabetes itself and thereby reducing the further downstream need for organ transplantation. We would rather approach populations this way, instead of treating those with high rates of chronic kidney diseases (which are significantly more prevalent in low socioeconomic groups) and can lead to end stage renal failure and alter organ transplant (especially in low-socioeconomic populations) (Nicholas et al. 2015).

The ethical challenges of organ donation have become more pressing as transplantation has become more efficient (Jonsen 2012; Veatch 2000). But despite the efforts of academic bioethicists and policy makers to assuage the public's fears about being a donor, organ donations around the world remain low. This is due to several factors, including fears about risks from the procedure (Sanner 1994) and widespread concerns about how to measure brain death prior to organ harvesting (Belkin 2014). These concerns are compounded by imperfect policies for both increasing donorship and fairly selecting the individuals to receive a donor organ (Chattergee et al. 2013).

Answers to these challenges may lay outside of traditional bioethics and clinical discourse. Here, we turn to public health ethics and practice for guidance on novel strategies to address organ shortages and global disparities in transplant. Viewing organ transplantation through a public health ethics, rather than a clinical ethics lens, helps brings to the fore very different ethical concerns, and calls into question why most organ transplant-related resources go to costly medical solutions instead of upstream prevention efforts.

There is very little literature examining how prevention efforts related to kidney, liver, and heart disease, as part of wider public health efforts, could help reduce demand for organs. Leading journals on organ transplantation rarely publish on this topic. Existing literature on organ transplantation and prevention yields mainly articles discussing prevention of post-transplant complications, showing that even prevention-focused discussions are almost exclusively focused on clinical aspects.

Current discussions have not adequately served the public's health, nor has the public health ethics and prevention discourse. We believe that this has severely constrained popular and policy discussions about transplantation. The bottom line is this: prevention is necessary in order to reduce organ shortage and the inequalities that often accompany the scarcity of resources; we can address the fundamental problem of scarce resources by preventing the need for transplant itself. As we describe below, such a shift has implications not only for academic debate, but for how policy makers and the general public understand and prioritize the challenges currently facing transplantation and organ procurement.

2.1   Normative Framework of Public Health Ethics

Public health is a function of the complex relationship between the social actions of the state, institutions, and groups of citizens, and is best conceptualized by understanding the socio-philosophical basis of the relationship between the individual and the state. The liberal approach to public health focuses on the right of an individual to defend his/her freedom in the face of coercive state actions, even when these actions are carried out in the interest of the greater good (Bayer/Fairchild 2004; Kass 2001). On the other hand, a communitarian approach views public health care as part of community welfare (cf. Walzer 1983). The authority of the state in public health is broad, permitting extensive interventions in the private sphere. Hence, critics view public health care as open to exploitation by the state, which can engage in coercive practices, trampling on individual rights. Traditional issues of contention have included measures such as vaccination, quarantine, medical examination of immigrants, forced sterilization, and other eugenic measures. (Alberstein/ Davidovitch 2011). Mutual trust between the public and health systems has long been recognized as integral to the long-term success of policy initiatives. Yet, trust cannot be assumed, and trust building should be a fundamental part in planning and program implementation (see also chapter 4 in this book). The view of health systems as socio-political entities, or even tools to achieve social justice, underscores the importance of trust in obtaining equality and equity in health promotion (Ezezika 2015).

The allocation of resources is one of the central aspects of public health ethics, with values such as equity and cost-effectiveness playing key roles, and different potential public health programs competing for limited public resources. How can we balance efficiency with equity and individual rights with the public good, and what institutions are the most appropriate to carry out the public health agenda? The distribution of organs for transplantations faces these very ethical challenges, including understanding organ shortage as not just an individual problem but a societal one, and addressing overall organ supply and demand through a prevention-driven approach that reduces the need for transplant by improving the public's health. Framing organ shortage this way forces us to also consider the fundamental causes of chronic diseases, their uneven distribution within and between societies, and the greater burden this uneven distribution (or health disparity) places on poor people and low- and middle-income countries.

While prevention provides a novel approach to thinking about how to improve care for patients and populations, we must also turn to public health ethics for theoretical justifications as to why we should take such an approach. As we have already stated and is widely described in the literature, bioethics tends to privilege the individual, insuring, for example, the protection of those enrolled in research studies, of patients in clinical settings, and of the fair distribution of organs for transplant. By contrast, public health ethics provides a moral foundation to protect the health of populations. For example, a public health ethics approach can help institutional review boards weigh potential harms to populations in research that may be associated with outcomes that fuel stigma and discrimination. Public health ethics can also give practitioners and policy makers alike a way to consider how to balance individual rights with the need for collective sacrifices in cases such as quarantine or mandatory public health laws, including requirements for vaccination, use of motorcycle helmets, and automobile seatbelts.

The ethical principle of justice – which, according to Gostin and Powers, emphasizes "the fair disbursement of common advantages and the sharing of common burdens" (2006: 1053) – is central to a public health ethics approach to reducing the burden of disease, especially if that disease or condition disproportionately impacts vulnerable communities globally. Focus on such "fair disbursement" (ibid.) creates obligations for public health actors to work towards ameliorating health inequities by addressing determinants of health. Ideally, this would happen in multiple domains, including local, state, and federal government efforts, NGO engagement on these issues, and through communities who fight to redress public health disparities. There are disparities between rich and poor nations in terms of transplant infrastructure; a woman in Pakistan, for instance, has less access to dialysis treatments or to transplantation than a woman at same age with the same medical condition in the West (Ghods 2015). There are also disparities between rich and poor countries in terms of the burden of chronic and infectious disease that can lead to transplant (Sakhuja/Sud 2003). Such disparities are rooted in health determinants, including poverty, health infrastructure, environmental hazards, education, and culture, among others.

Approaching transplant through the lens of prevention raises several important practical and ethical issues that are rooted broadly in public health ethics, specifically in the concept of justice. First, in this context prevention itself must be seen as a public good. If diseases are prevented in the first place and people are thus healthier – for example, a reduction in diabetes and hypertension that can lead to kidney transplant, a reduction in alcohol consumption and/or the prevalence of hepatitis B and C may lead to a decrease in liver failure, and a reduction tobacco use can lead to a decrease in coronary artery disease – then prevention has had the desired effect of both reducing the individual burden of disease and preventing illness in the first place, thus reducing the demand for organs. Because many of the diseases that can lead to organ failure and transplant are not evenly distributed within populations and between societies, the prevention of illnesses that can lead to transplant is satisfying a justice-based approach.

We can also look to more granular aspects of public health ethics, including the role of human rights and social justice theory, in considering how public health ethics can inform our approach to the ethics of transplantation. A human rights approach, for example, offers a universal framework to advance justice in public health, elaborating the freedoms and entitlements necessary to realize dignity for all and create, as Jonathan Mann once wrote, "what are the societal (and particularly governmental) roles and responsibilities to help promote individual and collective well-being" (1996: 924). Indeed, preventing disease that leads to transplant will protect and promote the pre-conditions of human health, as it is focused on social and economic determinants of health.

With international law evolving to address threats to health, a rights-based approach transforms the power dynamic that underlies public health. Moving from human rights to social justice is crucial because social justice is viewed central to the mission of public health. It has been described as the field's core value: "The historic dream of public health [...] is a dream of social justice." (Beauchamp 1999: 105) Two aspects of social justice – promoting health on the population level and fair treatment of the disadvantaged are fundamental aspects of public health. This understanding leads us to consider the multiple causal pathways to numerous dimensions of social inequities. These include poverty, substandard housing, poor education, unhygienic and polluted environments, and social disintegration. Thus, to understand prevention and its implication for transplantation, all these should be taken into consideration.

Global statistics shine a light on the impact of social inequalities on transplant medicine. For example, a major challenge for low-income countries is the complete lack of transplant infrastructure. Only twelve per cent of low-income countries worldwide report, for example, any kidney transplant infrastructure, and all transplants in those countries come from live donors. Furthermore, the global burden of chronic kidney disease – which can have both infectious and non-communicable causes ranging from diarrheal diseases to malaria to pre-term birth – have unequal impacts on populations between low- and middle-income countries and wealthy nations because of the lack of transplant infrastructure (Luyckx et al. 2018)

The Sustainable Development Goals, rooted in a justice approach to public health and adopted by all United Nations member nations, seek to redress persistent disparities multiple domains, including health, education, and the impact of climate change. (United Nations 2020). Sustainable development goal three specifically addresses health – "ensure healthy lives and promote well-being for all at all ages" (ibid.) – and can be applied to the social and environmental determinants of health that lead to both the inequities that produce the unequal burden of infections and non-communicable diseases globally, and the conditions that lead to poor or non-existent organ transplant infrastructure in low- and middle-income countries. Only by developing specific policies that addresses these disparities can we begin to reduce the burden of diseases that lead to a need for organ transplant, thus reducing the demand. This justice-based approach to organ transplant is not a solution to this crisis; however, preventing the need for a significant number of transplants would be a step in the right direction. (Luyckx et al. 2018) Further research is needed to quantify how prevention would both improve the health of populations impact by communicable and non-communicable disease, but also concomitantly how the demand for transplant would change.

2.2   The Paradox of Prevention

Finding the right balance between the more individual-focused, clinically oriented model of health care and public health prevention and community-based approaches, with strong emphasis on social, economic and political determinants of health, remains a global challenge that impacts resource allocation and availability. While many declare that prevention is better than cure (as it adds quality of life, is easier to accomplish, and is often cheaper), in practice prevention is regularly marginalized and deprioritized, and it is generally the first to face cuts during times of fiscal austerity. Harvard's former dean of their School of Public Health, Harvey Feinberg, described this as the 'paradox of prevention' (Feinberg 2013).

As Feinberg points out, the paradox is driven by several challenges, including that prevention's successes are generally invisible, that prevention lacks drama and immediacy, and that it generally requires time-consuming investment with delayed success. Such barriers have, in large part, occluded the application of prevention and public health principle to organ donation. Saving one person's life by transplant will always look more appealing than preventing kidney failure, when apparently nothing 'happened': the transplant is not needed and there is no drama. The current challenge is how to leverage the public's awareness of, and personal connection to, conditions that necessitate transplantation and move both the public and policy makers to develop ethical strategies to subvert the paradox of prevention.

Despite the potential benefits of a population-based prevention approach, it remains the least common strategy and an example of Feinberg's 'paradox of prevention'. The need for prevention-based strategies in transplant medicine are obvious: organ transplants are very expensive. In 2017, Fortune magazine, following the consulting firm Milliman, estimated the cost of kidney transplantations to be 415.000 USD and a heart transplant to be 1.4 million USD (Rapp/Vendermey 2017). In a more recent review, Fu et al. (2020) suggest that associated rise of transplantation costs, certain patient groups may not benefit from transplantation in a cost-effective manner compared with dialysis. Their analysis underscores that transplantation is indeed expensive, but it is cost effective, especially for young people on dialysis. The huge cost of transplants has led to the creation of inequalities related to who has access to transplantation care. It has also led to black markets for organs, both within and between countries (Scheper Hughes 2000). The burden of organ demand on low- and middle-income countries is particularly acute, considering that non-communicable diseases that can lead to organ failure, such as diabetes, are on the rise, especially in poor populations (Crews et al. 2019). Without fundamental structural change, and a change in priorities, the public health and ethical dilemmas related to organ transplant cannot be adequately addressed. The paradox of prevention is more than just a heady concept; it is a barrier to reducing suffering and establishing the best care for patients and populations globally by preventing the need for transplantation.

The principles of public health – distinct from those of clinical medicine, which are more focused on medicalized treatments of individuals in clinical setting – are based on a population approach, an approach to health that aims to improve the health of the entire population and to reduce health inequities among population groups. In order to reach these objectives, this approach looks at and acts upon the broad range of factors and conditions that have a strong influence on our health. Its components include: (1) a focus on primary care prevention and health promotion; (2) targeted studies of the economic, political, and environmental factors that may affect populations and cause diseases; and (3) implementing and translating these studies into policies and ways in which the modification of social and environmental variables may promote public health aims (through active social and political involvement) (Scutchfield/Keck 2009).

3.   The Social Determinants of Supply and Demand in Organ Transplants

Organ shortage is a universal problem, its severity varies across countries, and it is influenced by social, cultural, economic, and political factors between nations. A public health approach to organ shortage maps these differences and seeks ways of limiting the demand in the first place. Above we have described general differences between a bioethics approach and a public health ethics approach. Below we propose how to analyze organ shortage from the perspective of public health ethics, and how this perspective sheds light on two limitations in the current transplant ethics discourse: how the global burden of disease drives up demand in kidney transplantations, and how different socio-cultural approaches to brain death impact the supply side of organ transplantation.

3.1   The Global Burden of Kidney Diseases

The International Society of Nephrology estimates that 850 million people worldwide suffer from CKD. It is hard to assess how many of them will develop ESRD and will need to undergo a transplant or use dialysis machines in order to sustain their life. It is clear, however, that preventing CKD patients from becoming ESRD is a primary mission for public health. Li et al. (2020) define three lines of prevention of CKD. First, intervention before the onset of renal disease; second, diagnosing and prompt treatment before the condition worsens; and third, managing an existing condition to prevent disease progression and complications. Following this categorization of primary, secondary and tertiary lines of prevention, it is possible to focus on different factors of, and tailor a prevention policy for, CKD in each country or global region.

Li et al. evaluate the risk factors for de novo CKD and pre-existing CKD progression as follows: around 50 per cent suffer from diabetes, approx. 25 per cent have hypertension, and ten to 20 per cent are obese. Less than ten per cent have polycystic kidney disorder, a direct heredity condition of CKD that can lead to ESRD. Most of CKD could have benefited from a prevention policy that would create structural changes that encourage them to conduct a healthy way of life (Li et al. 2020).

Studies have shown the low awareness of people with CKD to their condition. This finding was significant in both publicly funded health systems such as in Quebec, Canada (Verhave 2014), as well as in privately funded health systems, including the US health care system. Ene-lordache et al. (2016) found low awareness of CKD symptoms in six different regions of the world. In low-income countries, they found risk factors to be human immunodeficiency virus (HIV) infection, tuberculosis, and exposure to toxins. These factors comprise up to 40 percent of CKD patients, and they are different from the risk factors that Li et al. (2020) found in high-income countries. These differences call for a different line of prevention in different global contexts. Whereas prevention would focus on boosting awareness of the hazards of salt and sugar-rich diets in high-income countries, other preventive measurements are needed in regions the main causes of CKD are from infectious diseases. Yet in both contexts, however, not only are risk factors different, but they tend to be unevenly distributed across low and high socio-economic status.

Prevention of CKD is in large part a matter of raising awareness of risk factors for CKD. It is not clear who bears the responsibility of addressing this awareness and what role health systems, and more broadly the state, have in boosting this awareness and helping populations to make healthy choices. The questions of awareness and responsibility entail a much more detailed and longer discussion than we can develop here. The importance of awareness and prevention, however, is clear: it can save the lives of many on today's lengthening transplantation waiting lists. Identifying risk factors and populations at risk and develop healthy policies to strengthen primary prevention could reduce the burden of waiting lists and the need for transplantation (Li et al. 2020; Ene-Lordache et al. 2016). Prevention strategies should also include secondary prevention (early detection of illnesses) and tertiary prevention for those target populations that are not yet on the waiting lists but are prone to develop conditions that might lead them to end-stage diseases. The paradox of prevention lies in the understanding that prevention is advisable both from clinical, social and economic perspectives, yet prevention is generally less prioritized. It is only when face organ shortage that we start to think of prevention.

3.2 Social Solidarity and Organ Donation

Whereas prevention can help reduce the demand for organ transplantations, public health measures can also help to boost the supply of organ donations. In contrast to many other medical therapies, organ replacement cannot be performed without the cooperation of the public. Advanced and sophisticated as it is, transplant medicine cannot do without a collective willingness to donate organs. This is the point where public health can ease the burden of organ shortage by focusing on how to increase organ donations rates.

These efforts vary from one social context to another; each context poses its own difficulties and challenges. Generally, scholars point to the controversy over brain death (Youngner et al. 2002), bodily conceptions (Schweda/Schicktanz 2009), and lack of information (Rady et al. 2012) as central factors hindering organ donation. Researchers have also identified that these barriers are more evident in specific social groups such as racial and ethnic minorities (Johal et al. 2018; Li et al. 2019; Suliman et al. 2019) and are also impacted by socioeconomic status (Shah et al. 2018). These sociological features pose a challenge to policy-makers to encourage less inclined populations to donate organs. The premise is that if such social and cultural barriers could be removed by educational campaigns, there will be less reluctance to organ donation within these populations. We suggest that a public health approach to problems of organ donation should prioritize fostering social solidarity, thus creating a different context in which organ donations decisions are made, before addressing the specific barriers to donation itself.

Although seemingly self-evident, social solidarity is an ambiguous concept within public health (Dawson/Verweij 2012). Prainsack and Buyx (2011) define it in terms of costs that one pays for the sake of a collective good and point to organ donation as an act that builds social solidarity. Durkheim, on the other hand, defined solidarity as "pre-contractual," (2014 [1893]: 158) that is it precedes rational acts towards the collective good. For both definitions, the link between solidarity and acts on behalf of the collective might be tautological, deserving further analysis. It is not clear whether social solidarity is simply 'out there'; if not, how can it be fostered? Is it an explanation for altruism and voluntary acts, or is it a different separate concept?

Nonetheless, researchers have suggested that social solidarity as a motivation for organ donation must be built on reciprocity (Schweda/Schicktanz 2009). Siegal and Bonnie (2006) have called to replace altruism with social solidarity, which they also base on the concept of reciprocity. For them, solidarity defines one's group belonging, and within this belonging one can expect reciprocal acts. These acts are not oriented toward a complete stranger, as in pure altruism, but rather to someone who shares some social characteristics with the donor.

In more than one sense, such reciprocity already exists in the ethical repertoire of organ donation. Organ donation from family members reflect the same logic: one donates to her kin member only due to their family connections. A public health approach would expand this feeling of a family to the community, thus fostering solidarity. This requires an ethical shift, since such donations will be based on a much closer resemblance between the donor and recipient than in blind altruistic donations.

Such an approach can already be found in organ donation prioritization policies (Lavee/Brock 2012), in donations in return to a future prioritization of a family member in need of an organ (Martin/Danovitch 2017), and in private agencies that match recipients according to the donors' grouping conditions. These initiatives, however, run the risk of being more exclusive than inclusive, turning organ donation to something akin to a club membership.

We believe that a public health approach to social solidarity in organ donation should consider first the public's good in terms of equity and equality. Although the state or any public agency cannot enforce organ donations, just as it cannot authorize organ sale, we do believe that social solidarity, alongside altruism, is a productive concept to work with in organ donation. Social solidarity's benefit lies in a stronger commitment of the group's members towards each other. In a model promoting both solidarity and altruism, where social solidarity leads to donations within the in-group members, and altruistic donations to strangers are allocated according to shorter waiting lists, it is possible to increase the supply of organ donations. Such a model can be multi-level: a communal-oriented approach to encourage donations among community members, where solidarity might be stronger, and a nation state-level approach to encourage altruistic donations towards strangers in need.

4.   Conclusion: Reassessing Organ Transplantation from the Viewpoint of Public Health

This paper began with a claim: that to reduce organ shortage, policy makers must shift from understanding transplant needs as largely clinical in nature to an alternative view rooted in public health approaches. This shift can help draw attention to the relationship between chronic and infectious disease that disproportionately burdens lower- and middle-incoming countries (and people living in poverty more generally), the impact that such diseases have on the need for transplantation, and how we should approach their prevention from a social and economic determinants of health perspectives. A separate but parallel discussion using concepts from public health ethics can also inform the discussion on reducing organ shortage needs by developing alternative models for procuring organs for transplant.

Organ shortage is a product of concrete factors that can be addressed directly by focusing on fundamental causes rooted in the social, environmental, economic and political determinants of health. Framing organ donations and organ shortage within such a context can help us to develop an understanding of why certain questions are being asked instead of others, and to develop mechanisms to build alternative approaches based on public health ethics frameworks. Such an approach has the potential to reduce the burden of suffering, promote primary prevention and other public health-oriented activities, and thus enrich current discussions of organ donation shortage and lead to more deliberate actions.

References

Alberstein, Michal/Davidovitch, Nadav (2011): "Apologies in the Health Care System: From Clinical Medicine to Public Health." In: Law and Contemporary Problems 74, pp. 101–125.

Bayer, Ronald/Faichild, Amy L. (2004): "The Genesis of Public Health Ethics." In: Bioethics 18, pp. 473–492.

Beauchamp, Dan E. (1999): "Public Health as Social Justice." In: Dan E. Beauchamp/ Bonnie Steinbock (eds.), New Ethics for the Public's Health, New York: Oxford University Press, pp. 105–114.

Belkin, Gary (2014): Death before Dying: Medicine, History and Brain Death, Oxford: Oxford University Press.

Berridge, Virginia/Gorsky, Martin/Mold, Alex (2011): Public Health in History, London: Open University Press.

Beauchamp, Dan (1999): "Public Health as Social Justice." In: Dan E. Beauchamp/Bonnie Steinbock (eds), New Ethics for the Public's Health, New York: Oxford University Press, pp. 105–111.

Bygbjerg, Christian I. (2012): "Double Burden of Noncommunicable and Infectious Diseases in Developing Countries". In: Science 337/6101, pp. 1499–1501.

Chattergee, Paula/Atheendar, Venkataramani S./Anitha Vijayan/Wellen, Jason R./
Martin, Erika (2013): "The Effects of State Policies on Organ Donation and Transplantation in the United States." In: JAMA Internal Medicine 175/8, pp. 1323–1329.

Crews, Daidr/Bello, Aminu/Saadi, Gamal (2019): "Burden, Access, and Disparities in
Kidney Disease". In: Kidney International 95/2, pp. 242–248.

Dawson, Angus/Verweij, Marcel (2012): "Solidarity: A Moral Concept in Need of Clarfi-
cation." In: Public Health Ethics 5/1, pp. 1–5.

Ene-Iordache, Bogdan/Perico, Norberto/Bikbov, Boris/Carminati, Sergio/Remuzzi.
Andrea/Perna. Annalisa/Islam, Nazmul/Flores Bravo, Rodolfo/Aleckovic-Halilovic,
Mirna/Zou, Hequn/Zhang, Luxia/Gouda, Zaghloul/Tchokhonelidze, Irma/Abra-
ham, Georgi/Mahdavi-Mazdeh, Mitra/ Gallieni, Maurizio/Codreanu, Igor/Tog-
tokh, Ariunaa/Kumar Sharma, Sanjib/ Koirala, Puru/ Uprety, Samyog/Ulasi, Ife-
oma/Remuzzi, Giuseppe (2016): "Chronic Kidney Disease and Cardiovascular Risk
in Six Regions of the World (ISN-KDDC): a Cross-Sectional Study." In: The Lancet
Global Health 4, pp. e307–e319.

Ezezika, Obidimma C. (2015): "Building Trust: A Critical Component of Global Health."
In: Annual Global Health 81/5, pp. 589–592.

Feinberg, Harvey V. (2013): "The Paradox of Disease Prevention: Celebrated in Principle,
Resisted in Practice." In: JAMA 310/1, pp. 85–90.

Fu, Rui/Sekercioglu, Nigar/Berta, Whitney/Coyte, Peter C. (2020): "Cost Effectiveness
of Deceased Donor Renal Transplant versus Dialysis to Treat end Stage Renal Disease: a Systematic Review." In: Transplantation Directions 6/2, pp. e522.

Ghods, Ahad J. (2015): "Current Status of Organ Transplant in Islamic Countries." In:
Experimental and Clinical Transplantation 13, Suppl 1, pp. 13–17.

Gostin, Laurence O./Powers, Madison (2006): "What Does Social Justice Require
For The Public's Health? Public Health Ethics and Policy Imperatives." In: Health
Affairs 25/4, pp. 1053–1060.

Johal, J./Bains, H./Churchward, D./Brand, S./Malik, S. (2018): "Quantitative Study of
the Beliefs and Attitudes Toward Organ Donation and the Opt-Out System Among
the Sikh Community in the United Kingdom." In: Transplantation Proceedings
50/10, pp. 2939–2945.

Jonsen, Albert R. (2012): "The Ethics of Organ Transplantation: A Short History." In:
AMA Journal of Ethics 14/3, pp. 264–268.

Kass, Nancy E. (2001): "An Ethics Framework for Public Health." In: American Journal
of Public Health 91/11, pp. 1776–1782.

Lavee, Jacob/Brock, Dan W. (2012): "Prioritizing Registered Donors in Organ Allocation: An Ethical Appraisal of the Israeli Organ Transplant Law." In: Current Opinion in Critical Care 18/6, pp. 707–711.

Li, P.K./Garcia-Garcia, G./Lui, S.F./Andreoli, S./Fung, W.W.S./Hradsky, A./ Kumaras-
wami, L./Liakopoulos, V./Rakhimova, Z./Saadi, G./Strani, L./Ulasi, I./ Kalan-
tar-Zadeh, K. (2020): "Kidney Health for Everyone Everywhere – From Prevention
to Detection and Equitable Access to Care. Blood Purifications." In: Blod Purifica-
tion. DOI: 10.1159/000506966

Li, Miah T./Hillyer Grace, C,/Husain Ali, S./Mohan, Sumit (2019): "Cultural Barriers
to Organ Donation among Chinese and Korean Individuals in the United States: a
Systematic Review." In: Transplantation International 32/10, pp. 1001–1018.

Luyckx, Valery A./Tonelli, Marcello/Stanifer, Jhon W. (2018): "The Global Burden of Kidney Disease and the Sustainable Development Goals." In: Bull World Health Organ 96/6, pp. 414–422.

Mann, Jonathan (1996): "Health and Human Rights." In: British Medical Journal 312/7036, pp. 924–925.

Muller, Elmi (2016): "Transplantation in Africa – An Overview". In: Clinical Nephrology, Supplement 1, 86/13, pp. 90–95.

Martin, Dominique E./Danovitch, Gabriel M. (2017): "Banking on Living Kidney Donors – A New Way to Facilitate Donation without Compromising on Ethical Values." In: The Journal of Medicine and Philosophy 42/5, pp. 537–558.

Muralidharan, Aditya/White, Sarah (2015): "The Need for Kidney Transplantation in Low- and Middle-Income Countries in 2012: An Epidemiological Perspective." In: Transplantions 99/3, pp. 476–481.

National Institute of Diabetes and Digestive and Kidney Diseases: "Kidney Disease Statistics for the United States". Available at: https://www.niddk.nih.gov/health-information/health-statistics/kidney-disease (accessed January 25, 2020).

Nicholas, Susan B./Kalantar-Zadeh, Kaymar/Norris, Keith (2015): "Socioeconomic Disparities in Chronic Kidney Disease." In: Advances in Kidney Chronic Disease 22/1, pp. 6–15.

Porter, Dorothy (1999): Health, Civilization, and the State: A History of Public Health From Ancient to Modern Times, New York: Routledge.

Prainsack, Barabara/Buyx, Alena (2011): Solidarity: Reflections on an Emerging Concept in Bioethics, Swindon: Nuffield Council on Bioethics.

Rady, Mohamed Y./McGregor, Joan L./Verheijde, Joseph L. (2012): "Mass Media Campaigns and Organ Donation: Managing Conflicting Messages and Interests." In: Medicine, Healthcare and Philosophy 15/2, pp. 229–241.

Rapp, Nicolas/Vandermey, Anne (2017): "Here's What Every Organ in the Body Would Cost to Transplant. In: Fortune Magazine, Sept. 14. Available at: https://fortune.com/2017/09/14/organ-transplant-cost/ (accessed June 30, 2020)

Sakhuna, Vinay/Sud, Kamal (2003): "End Stage Renal Disease in India and Pakistan: Burden of Disease and Management Issues." In: Kidney International 63/83, pp. S115–S118.

Sanner, Margareta A. (1994): "Attitudes towards Organ Donation and Transplantation: A Model for Understanding Reactions to Medical Procedures after Death." In: Social Science and Medicine 39/1, pp. 1142–1152.

Scheper-Hughes, Nancy (2000): "The Global Traffic in Human Organs." In: Current Anthropology 41/2, pp. 191–224.

Schweda, Mark/Schicktanz, Silke (2009): "The 'Spare Parts Person'? Conceptions of the Human Body and their Implications for Public Attitudes towards Organ Donation and Organ Sale." In: Philosophy, Ethics and Humanities in Medicine 4/4, pp. 1–10.

Scutchfield, Douglas F./Keck, William C. (2009): Principles of Public Health Practice, Boston: Cengage Learning, 3rd edition.

Shah, Malay B./Vilchez, Valery/Goble, Adam/Daily, Michael F./Berger, Jonathan C./Gedaly, Roberto/DuBay, Derek A. (2018): "Socioeconomic Factors as Predictors of Organ Donation." In: Journal of Surgical Research 221, pp. 88–94.

Siegal, Gill/Bonnie, Richard J. (2006): "Closing the Organ Gap: A Reciprocity-based Social Contract Approach." In: The Journal of Law, Medicine and Ethics 34/2, pp. 415–423.

Suliman, Sarah T./Carlson, Jermey/Smotherman, Carmen/ Gautam, Shiva/Heilig, Charles W./Munroe, Charisa/Bridges, Ledetra./Ilic, ljubomir M. (2019): "Effect of Race and Ethnicity on Renal Transplant Referral." In: Clinical Nephrology 92/5, pp. 221–225.

United Nations (2020): Sustainable Development Goals: Knowledge Platform. Available at: https://sustainabledevelopment.un.org/sdgs (accessed January 22, 2020)

United Network for Organ Sharing (2020): Unet data. Available at: https://unos.org/data/transplant-trends/ (accessed January 20, 2020)

Veatch, Robert (2000): Transplantation Ethics, Washington DC: Georgetown University Press.

Verhave Jacobien C./Troyanov, Stephan/Mongeau, Federic/Fradette, Lorraine/ Bouchard, Josee/Awadalla, Phillip/Madore, Francois (2014): "Prevalence, Awareness, and Management of CKD and Cardiovascular Risk Factors in Publicly Funded Health Care." In: Clinical Journal of the American Society of Nephrology 9, pp. 713–719.

Walzer, Michael (1983): Spheres of Justice. A Defense of Pluralism and Equality, New York: Basic Books.

Youngner, Stuart J./Arnold, Robert M./Schapiro, Renie (2002) (eds.): The Definition of Death: Contemporary Controversies, Baltimore/London: Johns Hopkins University Press.

Contributors

Zümrüt Alpınar-Şencan works as a postdoctoral research fellow at the Department of Medical Ethics and History of Medicine in the University Medical Center Göttingen since January 2018. She has a background in philosophy and holds a doctoral degree in biomedical ethics. Her current research focuses on stakeholders' attitudes towards prodromal dementia diagnosis in a cross-cultural comparison. Her previous works focused on dignity in organ markets debate, organ transplantation, justice and rights in health care and methodology in ethics and bioethics.

Katharina Beier is a postdoctoral researcher associated at the Department of Medical Ethics and History of Medicine at the Göttingen University Medical Center, Germany. She studied political science as well as german philology and literature at the Universities of Greifswald (Germany) and Växjö (Sweden). In 2008, she received her PhD in Political Science at Greifswald University. Her research focuses on research ethics, specifically in the fields of biobanks and big data, and on ethical issues of assisted reproduction and the family. Since 2018 she has been the head of the Unversity of Göttingen's Ombuds Office for Good Scientific Practice.

James L. Bernat is Professor of Neurology and Medicine (Active Emeritus) at the Geisel School of Medicine at Dartmouth in Hanover, New Hampshire, USA where he has been a faculty member since 1976. He received his M.D. from Cornell University Medical College in 1973. His scholarly interests are in ethical and philosophical issues in neurology with a focus on brain death, the definition of death, and disorders of consciousness.

Dieter Birnbacher was Professor of Philosophy at the University of Dortmund from 1993 to 1996 and at Heinrich Heine University Düsseldorf from 1996 to 2012. He is vice-president of the Deutsche Gesellschaft für Humanes Sterben, Berlin, vice-president of the Schopenhauer-Gesellschaft, Frankfurt/M. and member of Leopoldina, National Academy of Sciences.

Hagai Boas heads the Science, Technology, and Civilization Cluster at the Van Leer Jerusalem Institute. His research interests are mainly in the field of medical sociology. His work has been published in leading journals such as *Social Science and Medicine*, *American Journal of Transplantation*, *Science, Technology and Human Values*. Dr. Boas was the lead editor of *Bioethics and Biopolitics in Israel*, a collection of essays and research articles on the social, legal, and political aspects of bioethics in Israel. He publishes articles on vaccinations and social solidarity, brain death and religiosity, popular science, and bioethics. Dr. Boas is an adjunct senior lecturer at the Department of Politics and Government at Ben Gurion University of the Negev and a researcher fellow at the Center of Society, Medicine and Humanism at Ben Gurion University of the Negev.

Charlotte Burnham-Stevens is a life sciences consultant and a graduate from the University of Edinburgh. She completed an MA in Social Anthropology followed by an MSc in Science and Technology Studies, both at Edinburgh. Her research focuses on bioethics of emerging biotechnologies, in particular the field of 3D bioprinting.

Anne L Dalle Ave is a bioethicist at the University Hospital of Lausanne in Switzerland since 2014. She received her M.D. from the University of Lausanne in 2002, and specialized in internal medicine and intensive care medicine before pursuing her career in bioethics. Her interests are in the ethical issues in organ donation and intensive care medicine, in the concepts of life and death, and in the foundations of morality.

Nadav Davidovitch, MD, MPH, PhD is an epidemiologist and public health physician. He is a Full Professor and Director, School of Public Health at the Faculty of Health Sciences, Ben-Gurion University of the Negev in Israel. His research interests: health policy, public health, health inequities, one health/ecohealth, comparative health care systems, public health history and ethics, and global health. He authored or co-authored over 150 papers and book chapters, co-edited six volumes and books and published his work in leading medical and health policy journals, such as the *New England Journal of Medicine, Lancet, Clinical Infectious Diseases, Emerging Infectious Diseases, Journal of Pediatrics, Vaccine, Social Science and Medicine*, and *Law & Contemporary Problems*.

Janet Delgado Rodríguez holds a doctor of Philosophy at the University of La Laguna (2018), and is a Registered Nurse in NICU at University Hospital of the Canary Islands. She is a professor of the Master in Bioethics and Biolaw at the University of La Laguna and the University of Las Palmas de Gran Canaria, and has been an associate professor of the degree in Nursing, Faculty of Health Sciences of the University of La Laguna. She is a member of the Ethical, Legal and Psychosocial Aspects of Transplantation (ELPAT), where she participates in the 'Public Issues' research group. She is also a member of the University Institute for Women's Studies at the University of La Laguna.

Heather Draper is Professor of Bioethics at Warwick Medical School, University of Warwick. Her research in transplant ethics uses traditional philosophical and empirical ethics methods. She has worked on projects on directed and conditional deceased donation (funded by the AHRC), split livers (funded by Queen Elizabeth Hospital Birmingham Charity), living liver donation, parent to child kidney donation and the use of social media (funded by ESRC). In addition, she has contributed to projects on unspecified living donation (BOUnD funded by NIHR) and transplant outcomes (ATTOM funded by NIHR). Heather was a member of the Unrelated Living Transplantation Regulatory Authority and the UK Donation Ethics Committee. She is currently a member of NHSBT's Deceased Donor Family Tissue Advisory Group. She has authored or co-authored 26 academic papers on tissue and organ donation and transplantation.

Solveig Lena Hansen is a lecturer for ethics at the University of Bremen, Faculty 11 (Human and Health Sciences). Previously, she was a post-doctoral research associate at the University Medical Center Göttingen. After an MA in Comparative Literature, she received her PhD in Bioethics at the University of Göttingen in 2016. Her ethical research focuses on organ transplantation, stem cells, and obesity; and on public communication on this topics. She also specializes in the field of narrative bioethics, analyzing the negotiation of bioethical issues in literature, and film.

Klaus Hoeyer is Professor of Medical Science and Technology Studies at the Department of Public Health, University of Copenhagen. He has a background in social anthropology and medical ethics and has worked with organizational aspects of a wide range of technologies. He is currently PI for a project funded by the European Research Council about what he terms intensified data sourcing in health care (www.policyaid. ku.dk).

Søren Holm is a Danish doctor and philosopher. He holds degrees in Medicine and in Philosophy and Religious Studies from the University of Copenhagen, a masters degree in Health Care Ethics and Law from the University of Manchester, as well as a PhD and a higher Danish doctorate from the University of Copenhagen. He is currently Professor of Bioethics at the University of Manchester, UK and part-time Professor of Medical Ethics at the University of Oslo, Norway. He has been researching and writing about resource allocation in health care since the early 1990s.

Anja MB Jensen is Associate Professor in Medical Anthropology at the Department of Public Health, University of Copenhagen. She has conducted several field studies of organ donation and transplantation focusing on the experiences of donor families and hospital staffs. Her present research deals with donation refusals, pigs in experimental transplant research, personalized medicine, and the implications of data sourcing in organ donation policy and practice. Currently, she holds a Carlsberg Foundation Monograph Fellowship writing a book on organ donation in Denmark and the US.

Paweł Łuków is Professor of Philosophy and Ethics. He chairs the Department of Ethics at the Institute of Philosophy, University of Warsaw, Poland; he is the director of the MA Program in Bioethics, and the director of the Center for Bioethics and Biolaw, University of Warsaw. He writes on I. Kant's ethics, bioethics, and philosophy of medicine. His current research focuses on the ethical and legal status of the human body in the context of transplant medicine, human dignity and human rights in bioethical regulation, equal access to health care, protection of human dignity and vulnerability in research, and bioethical policy-making in a democratic society.

Douglas MacKay is an Associate Professor in the Department of Public Policy at the University of North Carolina at Chapel Hill. He is also a Core Faculty Member of the UNC Center for Bioethics and the UNC Philosophy, Politics, & Economics Program. He is currently working on projects concerning the ethics of public policy research, the ethics of organ donation and allocation, and the paternalistic dimensions of welfare policy.

Dominique E. Martin is Associate Professor in Health Ethics and Professionalism in the School of Medicine at Deakin University. She studied Medicine and Arts as undergraduate degrees and completed a PhD in Applied Ethics at the University of Melbourne in 2011. Her bioethics research focuses primarily on issues related to procurement, use, and distribution of medical products of human origin such as organs and tissues for transplantation, as well as ethical issues in nephrology and health professionalism.

Sayani Mitra works as a post-doctoral research associate at the Open University, UK. She is a sociologist with interest in reproductive sociology, reproductive technologies, social reproduction, political economy, migration, ethnography and comparative research. She received her PhD from the Faculty of Social Sciences, University of Göttingen, Germany. She has published her research in peer-reviewed journals and has co-edited a book titled *'Cross-Cultural Comparisons on Surrogacy and Egg Donation: Interdisciplinary perspectives from India, Germany and Israel* (Palgrave Macmillan, 2018).

Alberto Molina Pérez is a postdoctoral researcher at the Department of Philosophy of the University of Granada, Spain. He received his PhD in Philosophy of Biology at the Autonomous University of Madrid. He is a member of the Ethical, Legal and Psychosocial Aspects of Transplantation (ELPAT), a division of the European Society for Organ Transplantation (ESOT), where he participates in the 'Public Issues' working group. His research in bioethics focuses on consent systems for deceased organ donation and the role of the family. He also specialises in epistemology of death determination.

Greg Moorlock is a Senior Teaching Fellow, specialising in bioethics, at Warwick Medical School, University of Warwick. His main research interest is in the ethics of organ donation and transplantation. He completed his doctoral thesis (funded by the Arts and Humanities Research Council) on the ethics of conditional and directed organ donation in 2012. Since then he has worked on projects on the ethics of split liver transplantation (funded by Queen Elizabeth Hospital Birmingham Charity) and the ethical issues that arise from transplant patients using social media to find willing living donors (funded by the Economic and Social Research Council). Greg publishes on the ethics of living donation and is a member of the ELPAT working group on Living Donation. He has authored or co-authored 11 papers on the ethics of organ donation and transplantation and has also written 6 articles on the subject for *The Conversation* (UK edition).

David Rodríguez-Arias is a Ramón y Cajal Researcher in Moral Philosophy at the Philosophy I Department of the University of Granada, Spain. He holds a PhD in bioethics from the University of Salamanca and a PhD in Medicine from the Université Paris-Descartes. His research in bioethics has been mainly devoted to brain death determination, organ transplantation ethics, and end-of-life issues.

Katherine Saylor is a postdoctoral fellow in the Department of Medical Ethics and Health Policy in the Perelman School of Medicine at the University of Pennsylvania,

She completed her doctoral work in the Department of Public Policy at the University of North Carolina at Chapel Hill. Her research focuses on the interplay between individual and public interests in human subjects research and health care policy. She was a policy analyst at the U.S. National Institutes of Health, where she worked on data sharing policies and informed consent for genomics research.

Silke Schicktanz is full-professor at the Department of Medical Ethics and History of Medicine at the University Medical Center Goettingen, Germany. Her research focuses on the cultural and ethical study of biomedicine. She has lead many international cooperations and was visiting researcher at UC Berkeley, San Francisco State University, Tel Aviv University, JNU Delhi, Montreal Université and University of Lancaster.

Mark Schweda is Professor for Ethics in Medicine at the Department of Health Services Research of the University of Oldenburg (Germany). His research focuses on philosophical, bioethical, and socio-cultural aspects of aging, the life course, and human temporality. Among his recent publications are the edited volumes '*Aging and Human Nature*' (with Michael Coors and Claudia Bozzaro) and '*Planning Later Life. Bioethics and Public Health in Aging Societies*' (with Larissa Pfaller, Kai Brauer, Frank Adloff and Silke Schicktanz).

David Shaw is Assistant Professor of Health Ethics and Law at Maastricht University, and Senior Researcher at the Institute for Biomedical Ethics of the University of Basel. He has a background in philosophy and medical law and is a Member of the National Institute for Health and Care Excellence (NICE) Shared Decision-Making Guideline Development Committee, and past member of the UK Donation Ethics Committee. His research is in bioethics, with a special focus on the ethics of organ donation, research ethics and scientific integrity. He has supervised several PhD students to summa cum laude degrees and has over 150 publications in leading medicine, ethics and science journals.

Rhonda M. Shaw is Associate Professor of Sociology at Victoria University of Wellington, New Zealand. Her research interests include the sociology of morality and ethics, empirical research on assisted human reproduction and family formation, human milk sharing, and organ donation and transplantation. Rhonda has published widely in these areas, including articles in *Sociology of Health & Illness, Body & Society, Social Science & Medicine, Qualitative Health Research, Health Sociology Review, Feminist Theory, Australian Feminist Studies, Women's Studies International Forum, Health, Sociological Review,* and *Sociology.*

Peter Sýkora is a Professor of Philosophy at University of Sts. Cyril and Methodius (UCM) in Trnava, Slovak Republic. He is a founder and director of the Center for Bioethics at UCM. He has written on evolutionary biology, bioethics, genome editing and transhumanism. He authored and co-authored numerous articles, chapters and books including '*A Tale of Two Countries: Czech and Slovak Stem Cell Biopolicies*' in '*Contested Cells*' (BJ Capps & AV Campbell, eds) Imperial College Press 2010, '*Altruism reconsidered: Exploring new approaches to property in human tissue*' (with M. Steinmann and U. Wiesing, eds), Ashgate 2009, '*Altruism: Reciprocity/Solidarity Approach*', in: Organ

Transplantation (Weimar, M.A. Bos, J.J.V. Busschbach, eds.) Pabst Science Publishers 2011, *'Germline gene therapy is compatible with human dignity'* (with A. Caplan) in *EMBO Reports* (2017) 18, 2086, *'Germline gene therapy in the era of precise genome editing: How far should we go?'* in: *The Ethics of Reproductive Genetics* (M. Soniewicka, ed.) Springer 2018.

Niki Vermeulen is Associate Professor, Science, Technology and Innovation Studies, University of Edinburgh. She specialises in science and innovation policy and the organisation of research, with an emphasis on scientific collaboration in the life sciences. The interdisciplinary field of biofabrication is one of the areas she studies, working with scientists to further explore social and ethical dimensions of their work. Niki has experience as a policy advisor and consultant in science and innovation policy, is a member of the Royal Society of Edinburgh's Young Academy of Scotland (YAS) and founder of 'Curious Edinburgh'.

Tatjana Višak is an ethicist whose work focuses on welfare, animal ethics, and other fields of applied ethics. She is the author of *'Killing Happy Animals, Explorations in Utilitarian Ethics'* (Routledge MacMillan 2013) and editor of *'The Ethics of Killing Animals'* (Oxford University 2016). She is currently a postdoc at Mannheim University, Germany.

Sabine Wöhlke is Professor for Health Science and Ethics at the Hamburg University of Applied Sciences. Her background focuses on anthropological, cultural and ethical applied sciences. Her main interests are ethical and cultural aspects of organ transplantation, digital health literacy and nursing ethics. She has longstanding experience in qualitative social-empirical research in the field of patient-centered communication and shared decision making. She is member of the Clinical Ethics Committee of the University Medical Center Göttingen and a member of the Ethical, Legal and Psychosocial Aspects of Transplantation (ELPAT), a division of the European Society for Organ Transplantation (ESOT), where she participates in the working group on 'Public Issues'.

Michael Yudell, PhD, MPH is a public health historian and ethicist and is Professor and Chair of Department of Community Health and Prevention at the Dornsife School of Public Health, Drexel University. He holds a PhD and MPH in Sociomedical Sciences from the Mailman School of Public Health at Columbia University. Yudell is the author of several books, including *'Race Unmasked: Biology and Race in the 20th Century'* (Columbia University Press, 2014). Along with Dr. Samuel K. Roberts, Yudell edits the Columbia University Press Series 'Race, Inequality, and Health'. Finally, Yudell is currently Chair of the Pennsylvania Secretary of Health's Newborn Screening and Follow-up Technical Advisory Board.

Social Sciences

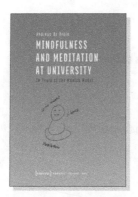

kollektiv orangotango+ (ed.)
This Is Not an Atlas
A Global Collection of Counter-Cartographies

2018, 352 p., hardcover, col. ill.
34,99 € (DE), 978-3-8376-4519-4
E-Book: free available, ISBN 978-3-8394-4519-8

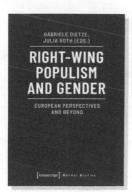

Gabriele Dietze, Julia Roth (eds.)
Right-Wing Populism and Gender
European Perspectives and Beyond

April 2020, 286 p., pb., ill.
35,00 € (DE), 978-3-8376-4980-2
E-Book: 34,99 € (DE), ISBN 978-3-8394-4980-6

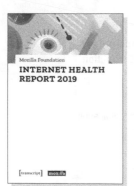

Mozilla Foundation
Internet Health Report 2019

2019, 118 p., pb., ill.
19,99 € (DE), 978-3-8376-4946-8
E-Book: free available, ISBN 978-3-8394-4946-2

**All print, e-book and open access versions of the titles in our list
are available in our online shop www.transcript-publishing.com**

Social Sciences

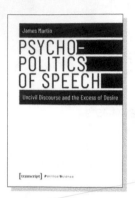

James Martin
Psychopolitics of Speech
Uncivil Discourse and the Excess of Desire

2019, 186 p., hardcover
79,99 € (DE), 978-3-8376-3919-3
E-Book:
PDF: 79,99 € (DE), ISBN 978-3-8394-3919-7

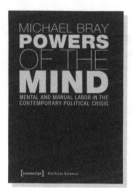

Michael Bray
Powers of the Mind
Mental and Manual Labor
in the Contemporary Political Crisis

2019, 208 p., hardcover
99,99 € (DE), 978-3-8376-4147-9
E-Book:
PDF: 99,99 € (DE), ISBN 978-3-8394-4147-3

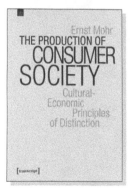

Ernst Mohr
The Production of Consumer Society
Cultural-Economic Principles of Distinction

April 2021, 340 p., pb., ill.
39,00 € (DE), 978-3-8376-5703-6
E-Book: available as free open access publication
PDF: ISBN 978-3-8394-5703-0

**All print, e-book and open access versions of the titles in our list
are available in our online shop www.transcript-publishing.com**